PRACTICING FAMILY THERAPY IN DIVERSE SETTINGS

New Approaches
to the Connections Among
Families, Therapists,
and Treatment Settings

Michael Berger
Gregory J. Jurkovic
and Associates

Foreword by Jay Haley

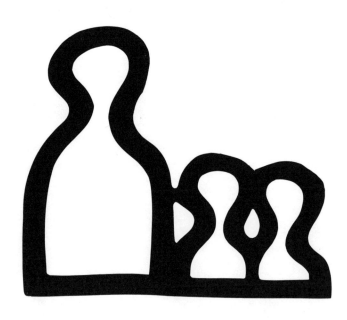

PRACTICING
FAMILY THERAPY
IN DIVERSE SETTINGS

 Jossey-Bass Publishers
San Francisco • Washington • London • 1984

PRACTICING FAMILY THERAPY IN DIVERSE SETTINGS
New Approaches to the Connections Among Families, Therapists, and Treatment Settings
by Michael Berger, Gregory J. Jurkovic, and Associates

Copyright © 1984 by: Jossey-Bass Inc., Publishers
433 California Street
San Francisco, California 94104
&
Jossey-Bass Limited
28 Banner Street
London EC1Y 8QE

Library of Congress Cataloging in Publication Data

Berger, Michael (date)
 Practicing family therapy in diverse settings.

 (The Jossey-Bass social and behavioral science series)
 Bibliography: p. 345
 Includes index.
 1. Family psychotherapy. 2. Problems families—
Services for. I. Jurkovic, Gregory J. II. Title.
III. Series.
RC488.5.B47 1984 616.89'156 83-49256
ISBN 0-87589-591-3 (alk. paper)

Manufactured in the United States of America

The paper in this book meets the guidelines for permanence and durability of the Committee on Production Guidelines for Book Longevity of the Council on Library Resources.

JACKET DESIGN BY WILLI BAUM

FIRST EDITION

Code 8416

The Jossey-Bass
Social and Behavioral Science Series

To our colleague, Carrell Dammann

FOREWORD

This is a lively book exploring a major contemporary issue in the therapy field—what to do about the social systems that impinge on the family-oriented therapist. The various chapters review the influence of hospitals (both medical and psychiatric), court systems, mental health agencies, religious factors, and that vast enterprise known as the educational system (both regular and special). There is even a discussion by a systems-oriented administrator on being in charge of mental health enterprises made up of professionals with opposing ideologies and differing amounts of power. Along with a frank discussion of these systems, the authors offer practical ways for colleagues to work together rather than to oppose each other. The ecological view expressed here has many implications for therapy practice and training as well as for changes in social policy.

Because of the rapid changes today, families seek advice from contemporary experts. A mother wishing to raise her child in the modern way hesitates to turn for advice to her mother because she is old-fashioned and turns instead to a professional in the field of education or therapy. Families also turn to the state, rather than to extended kin, for assistance when their children become unmanageable. As professionals become experts in mothering and managing children, they are also given the power to set parents aside and take over parental functions. The end results are a protective service and juvenile justice system that can remove children from their families and distribute them randomly among the population. While always benevolent, social services can become protective tyrants. They are focused on the child, not the family, and families can become battered and dismembered by professional helpers employed to assist them. A family-oriented therapist called in to deal with a client has a problem not only with the family but with the larger social system. To empower the family to take care of its own, the therapist must first "disempower" colleagues with different views. How to deal with fellow professionals is not taught in universities and must be learned in the day-to-day struggles of the practice of therapy. This book is a valuable guide for the therapist operating in this new jungle.

Just as changes in society affect families, they also affect therapists. When therapy ideology goes through a revolutionary change, clinicians cannot turn to their teachers in the university where they were trained; they are considered too old-fashioned. Instead, therapists go to private training institutes and workshops to hear new teachers offer new approaches. As this process takes place, therapists are not only operating from different ideologies but they are at different stages in the recognition of family involvement in psychological problems. Both client and therapist can be caught among experts who cannot agree on who is part of the problem, far less on what to do about it. In his or her place of work, the therapist finds opposing views, often expressed by older colleagues high in the agency hierarchy. The concern in the past has been with teaching therapists skills and strategies for dealing with clients and their families. Now it is evident that the strategy the therapist chooses must take into account colleagues in the place where the therapy is done. When working in a mental hospital, one must deal with staff members who insist on the rights of the individual to custody and medication, just as when dealing with judges and probation officers in the court system there is opposition to a focus on the family rather than the erring youth. With child abuse problems, people in protective services can be insisting on the separation of child and mother while the therapist is attempting to improve that maternal relationship. Everywhere the individual is still represented, whether child or adult, while the family is not. The educational setting or the mental health clinic restricts therapy operations so that therapists often think longingly about how nice it would be to have a private practice. Yet as this book points out, private practice also has its restrictions. Referral sources have their prejudices, members of families are involved with colleagues, and insurance companies like to decide who is to be considered a patient and for how long.

This book has a variety of contributors, each clarifying, in a refreshingly straightforward way, the social issues involved in a therapy setting. Practical solutions are offered from experience, apparently often painful experience. Exploring the ecology of therapy, the book deals with the next step in the field— once one has learned to develop brilliant strategies for changing families, what is to be done about colleagues whose views affect treatment but differ from those of the therapist?

February 1984   Jay Haley
Codirector, Family Therapy Institute
of Washington, D.C.

PREFACE

This book is about three interrelated ideas that promise to improve the conduct of family therapy. The first idea is that the setting in which treatment occurs (for example, juvenile court, psychiatric hospital, private practice) affects the course of treatment. The second is that many problems involve family members' contact with the very sources that intervene to help the family (for example, school personnel, probation officers). The third is that there are predictable issues that arise when family members deal with particular social agencies and when therapists design and implement systemic interventions within the context of these agencies. Thus, in establishing a workable therapeutic system, the therapist must recognize the interconnectedness of the therapist, the family, and the treatment setting.

These ideas represent a departure from the way we, like almost all clinicians, were trained to do family therapy. We were taught to assume that the unit to treat is the family, that families come to us for therapy, and that our relationship to the family is clearly and explicitly defined. By contrast, we shall be presenting an approach to therapy in which the unit of treatment is idiosyncratically determined for each case and in which the therapist deals with the family members and members of helping systems with whom the family is involved, even though the contract between the therapist and many of these people is not for therapy.

This book is addressed primarily to practitioners working with families in a variety of settings: mental health, child welfare, schools, courts, hospitals, and churches. In an important sense, this is a practical book: The authors have taken the pioneering ideas of Jay Haley, Salvadore Minuchin, and Murray Bowen and have adapted them to the unique demands of these different settings. Hence, the authors' experience and suggestions should enable readers to do more effective family therapy in their own settings.

We think the ideas of this book will also be helpful to persons other than family therapists who either care about the welfare of families or work in settings that affect the lives of families—specifically, parents, teachers, school administrators, school counselors, judges, probation and parole officers, nurses, social workers, hospital administrators, welfare workers, protective service and custody workers, members of the clergy, and business people.

In large measure, the thinking behind this book grew out of the work of the editors and their colleagues at the Atlanta Institute for Family Studies: Douglas Carl, Carrell Dammann, Martha A. Foster, and Michaelin Reamy-Stephenson. Although each of us has worked separately in particular helping systems, our thinking and practice within these systems were guided by our discussions of how to adapt the systemic concepts of Haley, Minuchin, Bowen, Cloé Madanes, and the Mental Research Institute Brief Therapy Group (Palo Alto, California) to the demands of the special contexts in which we each worked. We were delighted to find that this interest was shared by colleagues of ours elsewhere who had worked in and thought about settings with which we were not familiar. Thus, this book represents the thinking of a number of therapists who have worked in a variety of settings and who represent different theoretical orientations (structural, strategic, and Bowenian).

Not only do the authors base their work on different theoretical conceptualizations, but they have participated in the systems they describe at different levels of the hierarchy. Some, for example, worked as administrators; others held staff positions. An additional difference is that several of the authors write from a position within the helping system they describe, while others write from a position outside that system. Because of these differences, although we have asked each of the authors to address a common set of issues (issues set forth in the introductory chapter), we have encouraged them to address these issues as they thought best. The reader will, therefore, note differences in emphasis, tactics, and conceptualization across the chapters. To allow the reader to compare the views of different authors across similar topics, we have, within a particular chapter, included cross-references to other relevant chapters.

The book is divided into five parts. The introductory chapter sets forth the three major ideas of the book. This chapter was read by each of the authors before writing his or her chapter to ensure that each would address these central issues and thus produce a unified book. Part One describes adaptations of systemic therapy in three mental health treatment systems. Chapter Two focuses on the advantages and limitations of family therapy in private practice. Dammann describes the life cycle of the private practitioner and stresses a number of important pragmatic matters, including the effect of economic considerations on the conduct of therapy, relationships with colleagues and the larger professional community, the effects of the different contexts in which private practice occurs (for example, the "lone wolf" versus the "member of the family institute"), and the joys of private practice.

Chapter Three details Reamy-Stephenson's experience in creating an environment supportive of strategic therapy in a private inpatient setting. The author pays particular attention to the importance of viewing all staff members as allies rather than as obstacles, of obtaining the backing of higher administration, and of recognizing and using the analogies between the behavior of patients in their families and with staff and other patients.

In the final chapter of Part One, Carl stresses the necessity for first assessing the structure of the community mental health center and provides a number of suggestions for how and by whom such assessment should be conducted. Viewing the community mental health center as the most appropriate setting for the treatment of chronic patients, Carl discusses various aspects of the mental health center (for example, initial contacts, diagnosis, recordkeeping, and the assignment of staff time) that need to be considered in order to facilitate such treatment.

Part Two focuses on the conduct of systemic therapy in educational settings. Both the authors in this section conclude that therapy in school settings should be organized around educational issues and often should not even be labeled as therapy, since therapy is not a function of the schools. Both authors also pay a good deal of attention to ways in which common school activities such as homework, testing, and staffings can be used to further the goals of therapy. In Chapter Five, Foster discusses the school as a system in great detail, paying particular attention to overlaps in function and jurisdiction between the school and the family and noting a number of ways that therapists can help families and schools collaborate. Berger, in Chapter Six, describes a model program for providing systemic therapy through the framework of a special education program and discusses ways in which special education programs often inadvertently add to the problems of families, as well as discussing predictable issues for therapists who deal with families who have a handicapped child.

Part Three considers the practice of systemic therapy in child welfare and juvenile justice settings. In Chapter Seven, Lewis focuses on the therapist's interactions with protective services, foster care, and adoption services, although special consideration is given to therapeutic work with abused children and their families. She describes various hierarchal imbalances that often develop in transactions among professionals, families, and protective service staff and ways of clarifying or changing structural alignments. How protective service units contribute to the problems of families is also discussed, along with the implications of the potentially lethal nature of child abuse for family therapy; for example, Lewis recommends caution in the use of some strategic maneuvers.

Drawing on his experience in directing a project that provides family therapy to probationers at a juvenile court, Jurkovic in Chapter Eight describes how this setting influences various treatment processes: establishing a therapeutic system, assessment, reformulating the presenting problem, goal setting, and restructuring operations. He points to predictable problems that arise in the therapist/court/family relationship, many of which are traceable to the court's efforts to combine child welfare and legal models. In addition to stressing the importance of working cooperatively with probation officers, Jurkovic considers ways of using juvenile court procedures and practices (hearings, discharge, detention) strategically in the course of family therapy.

Part Four focuses on therapists in medical and clerical settings. In Chapter Nine, Greiner describes the practice of systemic therapy by nonphysician therapists in outpatient and inpatient medical settings, noting how the medical context influences various aspects of treatment. Greiner pays particular attention to triangles between patients and their families, between staff members, and between staff members and patients that are likely to arise. She provides a variety of ways of lowering anxiety in the patient system and the staff system so that issues can be dealt with more directly and productively. Greiner also stresses the advantage to the therapist of being able to intervene with clients without having to label the difficulty as involving a psychiatric condition.

Friedman, in his chapter on the clergy and premarital counseling, makes a similar point, noting that members of the clergy are, by virtue of their ministerial functions, in an ideal position to intervene preventively in the lives of couples. Using premarital counseling as an example of a function through which clerics gain access to families, Friedman details the advantages of a systemic therapy in avoiding or limiting the predictable pitfalls of this type of counseling. He also makes a number of useful suggestions for other ways in which members of the clergy (and nonclerical therapists working in congregational settings) can intervene with families and pays special attention to analogies between the therapist's work with client families, his or her work setting, and his or her own family.

The last section, Part Five, contains two chapters that

provide overviews and integrations of material covered in the book. The first chapter in this section, by Todd, is written from the vantage point of someone who has designed and administered several family-oriented treatment programs in public and private inpatient and outpatient mental health facilities. After reviewing the literature in this area, Todd draws on his personal experiences and observations to discuss aspects of program design, pitfalls, and necessary trade-offs and predictable conflicts with the larger system that need to be considered in implementing family therapy principles in treatment settings. A consistent thread in Todd's chapter is the recognition that systematically oriented programs, like all other programs, have problems, failures, and achievements. His chapter concludes with a helpful list of do's and don't's for the family therapist acting as program designer and administrator.

Jurkovic and Berger conclude with a chapter that elucidates the implications of the ideas presented in the book for practice, training, and social policy. Especially emphasized is the importance of viewing the therapist/client (family)/treatment setting as a basic unit of conceptualization. This chapter will be of particular interest to trainers of family therapy, since it provides a number of specific proposals for training that are consistent with this conceptual framework.

This book is unique in that it tells the practitioner how to operate systemically and effectively in a variety of treatment contexts. The information it contains will increase practitioners' ability to work with family problems that cannot be treated adequately within a traditional office setting. Knowledge of the principles it describes will help therapists deal with a wider range of problems in a larger number of settings. In a similar fashion, this book identifies problems and solutions that will enhance the ability of trainers, supervisors, and consultants to teach trainees how to practice in context.

We wish to note that ours was a truly collaborative effort. Both the order of authorship of the book, therefore, and the order of authorship of our two joint chapters (Chapters One and Twelve) was randomly determined.

Elaine McWilliams, Majella Hardie, and Al Williams diligently, carefully, and cheerfully typed the many drafts of the manuscript. James Kochalka similarly proofread the original draft for us. Duane Rumbaugh, chair of the Department of Psychology of Georgia State University, and Carrell Dammann, director of the Atlanta Institute for Family Studies, provided supportive environments for the writing of this book. Finally, we wish to thank our current families, our families of origin, and our client families for all we have learned from them.

Atlanta, Georgia   Michael Berger
March 1984   Gregory J. Jurkovic

CONTENTS

Part Two: Educational Settings

Part Three: Community Settings

Part Four: Special Settings

Part Five: Broadening the Practice of Family Therapy

THE AUTHORS

Michael Berger is a staff member of the Atlanta Institute for Family Studies and associate professor of psychology at Georgia State University in Atlanta. He is also an approved supervisor of the American Association for Marriage and Family Therapy and a charter member of the American Family Therapy Association. Berger received his B.A. degree (1967) in American studies from Goddard College, his M.A. degree (1969) in history from the University of Rochester, and his M.A. and Ph.D. degrees (1973 and 1974, respectively) in psychology from George Peabody College. He has taught at Wichita State University and, since 1975, at Georgia State University.

Berger has published in a number of areas related to family therapy, family therapy training, and family development. Recent publications include articles in Evan Coopersmith (Ed.), *Family Therapy Collections* (forthcoming), in *The Journal of Strategic and Systemic Therapies* (1983, with Carrell Dammann), in *The Journal of Strategic and Systemic Therapies* (1982, with Debbie Daniels-Mohring), in the *Journal of Marriage and Family Counseling* (1978, with Sally Hughes and Larry Wright), in *Family Process* (1982, with Carrell Dammann), and in *Professional Psychology* (1979, with Luciano L'Abate and others). Berger has a special interest in working with families who have a handicapped child. His publications in that area include articles in Alan Gurman (Ed.), *Questions and Answers in the Practice of Family Therapy* (1982), in *Topics in Early Childhood Special Education* (1981, with Martha Foster and Mary McLean), in *Young Children* (1980, with Mary Ann Fowlkes), and in the *Journal of the Division of Early Childhood* (1979, with Martha Foster).

His current therapeutic and theoretical interests include continuing to extend systemic theory and therapy to include units larger than the family and also to include the inner experience of individuals within a family, the integration of strategic and Bowenian therapies, and family therapy training.

Gregory J. Jurkovic is a staff member of the Atlanta Institute for Family Studies and associate professor and chair of the Clinical Child and Family Psychology area in the Department of Psychology, Georgia State University. He is also an approved supervisor of the American Association for Marriage and Family Therapy. For the past three years he has been directing a privately funded project, the Central Presbyterian-Georgia State Delinquency Project, which provides family therapy to youngsters on probation at an inner-city juvenile court.

Jurkovic received his B.S. degree (1970) in psychology from the University of Iowa and his Ph.D. degree (1975) in clinical psychology from the University of Texas at Austin. He was a predoctoral intern and clinical fellow in psychology in the Department of Psychiatry, Harvard Medical School, Beth Israel Hospital, and later a postdoctoral fellow in clinical child psychology at the Judge Baker Child Guidance Center and Children's Hospital Medical Center, Boston. Before teaching at Georgia State University, he taught at the University of Wyoming.

In addition to his long-standing interest in developmental and family systems approaches to understanding and treating behavior problems in children and adolescents, Jurkovic has become increasingly concerned with the nature of service delivery systems for youngsters and their families, especially juvenile courts and schools. His publications in these areas include articles in the *Journal of Consulting and Clinical Psychology* (1974, with Norman Prentice), in *Psychological Bulletin* (1980), in the *American Journal of Orthopsychiatry* (1982, with Edgar Jessee, Jeffrey Wilkie, and Michael Chiglinsky), and in *Family Process* (1983, with Douglas Carl).

Douglas Carl has been on the staff of the Atlanta Institute for Family Studies since 1979. He served as director of training for the institute from 1981 to 1983. Since 1976 he has developed a special interest in community mental health settings. He served as director of outpatient services in a mental health center in Savannah, Georgia, and in a similar capacity for another such center in Atlanta. Since 1981 he has devoted himself to full-time private practice and training with the institute, and he maintains active consultation roles with public mental health agencies in Georgia and Tennessee. He recently wrote an article (with Gregory J. Jurkovic) to appear in *Family Process* (1983).

Carrell Dammann is founder and director of the Atlanta Institute for Family Studies. Her twenty-year career in the field of family systems therapy began with her exposure to the work of Gregory Bateson during a year Dammann spent as administrative assistant to Margaret Mead. Dammann is particularly interested in strategic family therapy and the integration of the work of Milton Erickson and Jay Haley into a general systems approach. Her publications include articles in Jeffrey Zeig (Ed.), *Ericksonian Approaches to Hypnosis and Psychotherapy* (1982), *Family Process* (1982, with Michael Berger), and the *Journal of Strategic and Systemic Therapies* (1983, with Michael Berger), as well as a bimonthly column on couples therapy for the newsletter of the American Association for Marriage and Family Therapy.

Martha A. Foster is associate professor of psychology at Georgia State University, where she teaches in the clinical child and family psychology areas. She is also a staff member of the Atlanta Institute for Family Studies, involved in practice and training in family therapy. Foster has a long-standing interest in working with families with child problems, particularly families with handicapped or chronically ill children. Her publications include contributions to *Topics in Early Childhood Special Education* (1981, with Michael Berger and Mary McLean), *Journal of the Division of Early Childhood* (1979, with Michael Berger), and *Multivariate Experimental Clinical Research* (1976, with Michael Berger).

Edwin H. Friedman is presently involved in the private practice of family therapy and in postgraduate supervision of family therapists. He is a diplomate of the American Association of Pastoral Counselors and an approved supervisor of the American Association for Marriage and Family Therapy. He has been a consulting supervisor in family therapy at St. Elizabeth's Hospital in Washington, D.C., and a visiting faculty member at the Family Center, Georgetown University Medical School. He is a frequent lecturer and workshop conductor for clergy members and for family therapy professionals. His publications include *Interlocking Triangles: Our Families, Our Congregations and Ourselves* (1984) and chapters in M. McGoldrick, J. Giordane, and J. Pearce (Eds.), *Ethnicity and Family Therapy* (1983), and E. Carter and M. McGoldrick (Eds.), *The Family Life Cycle* (1980).

Doris S. Greiner is an associate professor at the University of Alabama in Birmingham and holds the psychiatric-mental health specialization certification of the American Nurses' Association. In addition to teaching graduate nursing students, she conducts a private family therapy practice. She contributed a chapter to Philip Guerin (Ed.), *Family Therapy* (1976, with Michael Holt).

Helen Coale Lewis is a clinical social worker and marriage and family therapist, in practice in the Atlanta community since 1969 in both family mental health and child welfare settings.

Currently, she is the owner and director of the Atlanta Child Guidance Clinic, where she provides clinical services to families, child custody assessments and expert witness testimony in court, and training for mental health graduate students and postgraduate professionals. She is a nationally recognized speaker on family therapy, child welfare issues, and stepfamilies. She is the author of *All About Families: The Second Time Around* (1980) and of numerous articles on stepfamilies.

Michaelin Reamy-Stephenson is the director of extramural training at the Atlanta Institute for Family Studies. Her professional affiliations include the National Association of Social Workers Clinical Registry; the Academy of Certified Social Workers; the American Association for Marriage and Family Therapy, in which she is an approved supervisor; the Georgia Association for Marriage and Family Therapy, in which she is public relations chairperson; and the allied staff of Brawner Psychiatric Institute. Reamy-Stephenson's experiences living in other cultures in Africa and the Middle East contribute to her interest in the process of reality construction and its applications to clinical practice and the training of strategic systems therapists. In addition to conducting ongoing training in strategic/structural therapy at the Atlanta Institute for Family Studies, she has presented numerous workshops focusing on radical assumptions of strategic therapy and systemic therapy with highly dysfunctional individuals, families, and broader interfacing systems. Her publications include an article on nonobjective reality in the *Journal of Strategic and Systemic Therapies* (June 1983).

Thomas C. Todd is director of the family therapy training program at Bristol Hospital, Bristol, Connecticut, where he has been on the faculty since 1975. He has served as director of psychology training at the Philadelphia Child Guidance Clinic (1970-1975) and as chief psychologist and chief of Putnam Community Services at the Harlem Valley Psychiatric Center in Wingdale, New York (1976-1983). Todd is best known for his work with Duncan Stanton on family therapy for drug abuse, described in *The Family Therapy of Drug Abuse and Addiction* (1982, by M. D. Stanton). While Todd's publications and training workshops have covered a variety of family therapy topics, his main area of expertise is strategic therapy, which is the topic of his forthcoming book, tentatively titled *Paradoxical Prescriptions*.

PRACTICING
FAMILY THERAPY
IN DIVERSE SETTINGS

New Approaches
to the Connections Among
Families, Therapists,
and Treatment Settings

1

Michael Berger
Gregory J. Jurkovic

Introduction: Families, Therapists, and Treatment Settings

From a systemic point of view, the central point about the treatment context is that the unit of treatment always includes the therapist. This point has been insufficiently stressed in works on family therapy and family therapy training. Indeed, even systems-oriented clinicians often describe the therapist as if he or she were a free agent acting unilaterally on the family. This mistake is understandable because the systemic view of the unit of treatment presents the clinician, as Jay Haley (1981, p. 177) has noted, with a disturbing logic: "He must disbelieve the notion that the observer, or therapist, is not part of the system being observed. When he describes a person in terms of a social dilemma, he must logically include himself and his treatment setting in the description of the problem. With this view there is an argument that there is no outside place to stand or take an objective view. The behavior of family members, and their fantasies for that matter, are partly determined by the person examining the family."

As Haley notes, not only does the therapist unavoidably participate in the problem, but his or her efforts to solve the problem are also constrained by the treatment context, the setting in which therapy is conducted. Different settings constrain the therapist in different ways. In some of the settings discussed in this book (schools and churches, for example), the major aims of the setting are not therapeutic. In such settings it may be impractical to conduct therapy explicitly. Rather, the therapist in such settings may achieve better results by framing what he or she does in terms of the overt goals of the setting. For example, in educational settings, the therapist can focus on the problems the child is having in school and meet with school personnel and family members about the child's school problems, using those problems as a lever to make the changes, at school or at home, that are necessary to solve the problem.

By contrast, some treatment settings are set up explicitly for the conduct of psychotherapy (for example, private practice settings, mental health centers, and psychiatric hospitals). Even here, however, the procedures and values of the setting may conflict with the procedures and goals of a systemic family therapy. For example, the family therapist in a traditional inpatient psychiatric facility who works to return patients to their families as quickly as possible may be working at odds not only with other staff members who are oriented to long-term, individual therapy but also with hospital administrators whose job is to fill, not empty, beds.

Other problems stem from administrative procedures that are based on the assumption that the client is always an individual. In some state mental health systems, for example, a therapist who wishes to meet with a family is required to open charts on each family member and, after each session, to write individual progress notes for each family member as if each were an identified patient. Most insurance policies similarly assume that the psychiatric patient is an individual and that individual therapy, therefore, is the appropriate (and hence reimbursable) treatment.

Still other difficulties arise because of clients' involvement with a number of therapists who often hold different views about the case and whose interventions conflict and negate one another. In inpatient settings, for example, a client may easily have an individual therapist, a group therapist, and a therapist who works with the client and his or her family. Or a client may be involved with a number of agencies whose decisions clearly affect treatment. One of the authors once participated in a case management meeting called to coordinate the efforts of the forty-seven helping agencies involved with a particular client.

Other problems concern the amount of support that different settings will give for certain kinds of systemic interventions and the amount of trouble that upset or dissatisfied clients can cause for the therapist. For example, sending a paradoxical letter to family members directing them not to change is often one way of increasing the chances that change will occur. However, although this strategy may be effective in a private practice setting in which all the therapist risks is his or her reputation with the particular family, it can create serious administrative and even legal problems in public settings that must answer to taxpayers, judges, superintendents, and others who might misinterpret such an intervention.

Such settings, however, have advantages. Therapists working in an agency or group setting that offers ample professional resources and backup—for example, the use of consultants sitting behind a one-way mirror during difficult sessions—are free to use more powerful family systems interventions than clinicians working alone in private practice or in a less supportive public practice context. A striking statement of this point is the response of an experienced family therapist who was asked what he would do if he were the therapist to a patient like President Reagan's assassin, John Hinckley, Jr., and Hinckley's family: "It would depend on whether I was seeing the family at the agency where I work or in my private practice. At the agency I'd probably work the way I feel is right. I'd probably not listen too closely to the young man's words since, if I did, I'm sure I'd become inducted and begin to see the young man as being crazy and forget the serious process issues of how this crazy talk functions for everybody in the family. In private practice, on the other hand, I imagine I'd medicate and possibly hospitalize. It's terrible to say, but this Hinckley stuff has gotten to me. Not that it's shaken my theoretical framework so much as it has made me feel less free to use that framework without adequate supports" (quoted in Beroza and Friedman, 1982, p. 15).

This therapist's words highlight the importance of collegial support for interventions that may upset clients or other members of the public; another important factor is how insulated economically the therapist is from the opinions of clients. It should be easier to risk upsetting clients in a public practice, where therapists are paid a salary and client fees go to the agency, not the therapist, than in private practice, where the therapist's income may be quickly and directly affected by clients' negative opinions of his or her work. The treatment given John Hinckley and his family is a good example of these points. The fact that a worker at a public mental health center refused to involuntarily hospitalize Hinckley when he talked about killing people received much less publicity and discussion in the popular and the professional press than the advice allegedly given by Hinckley's private psychiatrist to his parents.

One crucial pragmatic question that must be asked about the therapist and the treatment setting is whether the therapist has control over relevant aspects of the case. Haley (1980) has discussed in detail how therapists working with the families of inpatients often fail because the therapist does not control hospital discharge and readmission. Analogously, a nonmedical therapist who lacks control over the medication given to clients may encounter difficulties. Indeed, when working with families involved with other helping persons and agencies, the therapist often does not control important aspects of the case—whether, for example, a client will receive a jail sentence or be placed in probation by a court, or whether a child will be promoted or transferred to a special education classroom by a school. Our general position is that although it is better for the therapist to have as much control over the case as possible, there is usually sufficient flexibility in a given situation so that a therapeutic solution can be found. Many of the chapters to follow offer useful means of successfully handling situations in which the therapist does not control all aspects of treatment.

Unit of Treatment

From a systemic point of view, any unit of intervention is arbitrarily defined and chosen. Family therapists are well aware that it is arbitrary and acontextual to conceptualize the individual as a discrete unit, divorced from the family and the rest of the intimate environment. It is just as arbitrary to view the family as a real unit in nature rather than as a cut into an ecosystem that contains both smaller units (such as individuals or subsystems within the family such as siblings or the marital dyad) and larger ones (the family social network or the community and its institutions). It is more useful to view the family as part of a complex of interconnected living systems ranging from the biological to the sociocultural (Scheflen, 1980; Spiegel, 1971). The structure of each of these systems is not thought of as causing the behavior of subordinate systems but, rather, as constraining their functioning, limiting their flexibility. Within this perspective, behavior not only is affected by but also influences several levels of systems at once. Thus, behavior that appears dysfunctional at one level (dysfunctional for the family, for example) may be seen as functional at other levels (the extended family or the community). It is therefore important not to confuse levels in assessing the significance of a particular behavioral pattern (Hoffman, 1971).

Haley (1976, p. 4) has stated with characteristic brevity the basic issue for therapists regarding the unit of treatment: "The obligation of the therapist is to define the social unit he can change to solve the presenting problem of a client." It is the argument of this book that, for many problems, the social unit that the therapist will need to change includes the helping systems and persons with which family members are involved. The kinds of experiences that lead to such thinking can be seen in a beautiful clinical example provided some years ago by Hoffman and Long (1969). A family they were working with experienced a number of crises and changes as a result, in large measure, of the actions of agencies with which the family was involved. The family, which consisted of a mother and father, a daughter away at college, and a daughter in high school, came to the au-

thors' attention at the social services department of a neighborhood health center. At that time, the family was involved with
at least the following other agencies: (1) the housing authority,
which was trying to evict the family because their income was
too high for the low-income project, (2) Bellevue Hospital,
where the husband had been taken after he had spells after
drinking and where he had been diagnosed as epileptic, (3) the
social services department of the health center, which had been
contacted by the housing authority agent in the hopes of finding a doctor there who would certify the husband as too ill to
work (if he stopped working, the family would lose his income
but would be able to remain in the housing project), (4) the
physician who had originally seen the husband at the health
center several years before and who, on the basis of notes taken
by the social worker in the husband's social history, had diagnosed the husband as an alcoholic, (5) another physician at the
health center who had been contacted by the housing agent
when the agent felt that the first physician would not cooperate
by certifying the husband as too ill to work, and (6) a lawyer
from an antipoverty program who told the agent that the first
physician's letter would not prevent the family from being
evicted from the housing project. At this point in the story, the
husband quit his job, and in the family's efforts to work out the
changed economics of its life, the family was then involved with
the following agencies: (1) various departments of the health
center, (2) Office of Economic Opportunity legal services, (3)
the housing authority, (4) the husband's union, (5) the Veterans
Administration, (6) workers' compensation, (7) a private loan
company, (8) the family's church, (9) a settlement house, and
(10) the college attended by the older daughter. Given the magnitude and complexity of this family's involvement with various
helping systems, unless the complexity of the family's relationships to helping systems had been grasped, the situation of the
family would have been misunderstood and intervention mis-
directed.

Hoffman and Long enunciate the moral of this story and
the logic of an ecological approach: "In studying paradoxical
systems in human affairs, the usual emphasis has been on the

conflicts between levels of message exchanged by persons in on-going relationships, mainly families. . . . This is too narrow a view when one starts to look at lower-class city families, which, being poor, uneducated, isolated, and often from an alien culture, cannot go through the smallest life crisis without becoming encrusted with parentlike figures who represent the acculturation and controlling systems of the wider society. These systems seldom act collaboratively and are more often than not in conflict with one another. As a result, a person may be caught in a paradoxical situation in a family which is in turn caught in paradoxical situations within the systems designed to help the family or person" (p. 214).

We would amend Hoffman and Long's statement in only one way: It is not only the inner-city poor who are significantly influenced by contact with social agencies and institutional practices in the wider society. Indeed, it is a commonplace notion in sociology and anthropology to see the task of the family as being precisely that of mediating between the needs and demands of its members and of institutions and settings outside the family. Unfortunately for intervention, the logic of a contextual approach has come to be confined almost exclusively to work with populations thought to be underprivileged in some way, such as the poor or families with a schizophrenic or handicapped child, or to special situations, such as crisis intervention. This is so despite the existence of the work of Milton Erickson (as described in Haley, 1973), of Haley (1976, 1980), of the Palo Alto Brief Therapy Group (Watzlawick, Weakland, and Fisch, 1974; Fisch, Weakland, and Segal, 1982) and of Minuchin (1970, 1974), work that clearly demonstrates the usefulness of an ecological approach in the general practice of systemic therapy.

Minuchin (1974) eloquently states the case for attending to other contexts in addition to the family. In order to both maintain a sense of continuity and adapt to change, the family, he argues, is forced to continually transform the relationship of family members to one another so as to accommodate both to the inner pressures for change arising from developmental changes in family members and subsystems and to the outer pressures coming from demands to accommodate to the major social settings that have influence on family members. When stress arises from the contact of a family or a family member with extrafamilial influences, the therapist's task, Minuchin advises, is to assess both the situation and the flexibility of the family structure.

If the family has made adaptive changes to support the stressed member but the problem continues, the therapist's main input may be directed toward the interaction of that member with the stressing agent. If the family has not been able to make adaptive changes, his main input may be directed toward the family.

For example, if a child is having problems in school, the problem may be related basically to the school. If the therapist's assessment indicates that the family is supporting the child adequately, his major interventions will be directed toward the child in the school context. He may act as the child's advocate, arrange a transfer, or arrange for tutoring. But if the child's problems in school seem to be an expression of family problems, the therapist's major interventions will be directed toward the family. Both types of intervention may often be necessary [pp. 62–63].

Although a contextual approach to family intervention is not novel, it has certainly not been widely adopted in the family therapy field. A crucial reason has been the lack of detailed information for interested practitioners that would guide them in working successfully at the interface between families and helping agencies. Aponte (1976a) has described the family/school conference as one method of dealing with issues between family members and school personnel in situations when a child is seen as being in difficulty in school but not at home; Minuchin, Rosman, and Baker (1978) have described an effective method of collaboration between family therapists and pediatricians in the handling of psychosomatic conditions in children; and illuminating case examples are to be found in the work of Erickson, Haley, Minuchin, and the Palo Alto Brief Therapy Group. However, little literature is available describing the predictable issues that arise when family members deal with other helping systems such as the schools, the courts, the medical system, and the clergy or detailing how therapists can work effectively with issues involving family members and helping agencies. A major aim of this book, therefore, is to provide guidance for the systems practitioner who is unwilling to reduce all problems to issues within the family and who is ready to work with a treatment unit that will include the family and the helping agencies with which family members are involved.

Predictable Issues

One structural variable that has consequences for how the therapist will be able to work with the family and helping systems is whether the therapist works for the helping systems involved or is economically independent of them. Although the chapters to follow will explore the nuances of these different arrangements, at least one issue will be touched on here—how does the therapist who is not employed by the helping system enter the system?

Generally, therapists enter the helping system in one of two ways: Either persons within the helping system (referral persons) send the family to the therapist, or the therapist decides that it is necessary as part of treatment to deal with the helping system. In the first case, it is crucial that the therapist understand the relationship of family members to the referral person. Family members will often treat the therapist in particular ways because of their relationship to the referral person and their understanding of the reason they were sent to the therapist. (An excellent discussion of these issues can be found in Palazzoli and others, 1980.) For example, to display loyalty to the referral person, family members may think they need to defeat the therapist and thus prove that she or he could not be more helpful to them than the referral person. Or, as often happens with court referrals, family members may think they must merely attend therapy, with their loyalty to the referral person or agency judged not by whether they change but by whether they attend therapy faithfully. Or the referral person may have an agenda of his or her own for the therapist. For example, one of us treated the family of a client who was on parole. The ostensible aim of the therapy was to have the client's family reorganize so as to return the identified client to work, a condition of his parole. Having failed to return the client to work, the therapist informed the parole officer, who then asked the therapist to certify the client as being psychiatrically unfit to work so that his parole would not have to be revoked. The logic of this request was that, according to the recordkeeping system used by the parole officer's agency, if the client had a "legitimate reason" (such as a psychiatric condition) for violating the conditions of parole, he would be considered a successful case for the parole officer, whereas if the client was returned to prison for violating parole, he would count as a failure for the officer.

However the therapist enters the helping system, it is important that the therapist understand the place of the referral person in the helping system to avoid unwittingly entering into coalitions with the referral person that would impede the progress of therapy. Coalitions in the helping system that cross levels of the hierarchy in that system are as likely to result in pathological behavior in organizations as cross-generational coalitions are in families (Haley, 1980).

Coopersmith (1982) has recently called attention to a number of important questions that therapists must consider when assessing a family's involvement with other agencies, regardless of how the therapist came to deal with these agencies: (1) What is the relationship between the family and the agencies; that is, do the agencies involved define the family's need and the boundaries within which family and agency staff will interact, or is the action more symmetrical, more a negotiation among equals, and if so, are the different parties agreeable or antagonistic? (2) What are the enduring triangles between the family and the various agencies and between the different agencies themselves? (3) Are the agencies overly involved in different aspects of the family's life, thus undercutting family competence and preventing the family from using its own resources? (4) Do the agencies blame the family or individual family members for their problems? (5) What function does the family play for the various agencies? What occurs in the agencies because of the attention paid to this family, and what would happen if the particular family (or a particular kind of family) improved? (6) What are the agencies' agendas for the family? Is the therapist being asked to help the family change or to adjust the family to its place in a dysfunctional system?

Many treatment issues are shared by both therapists who work for the helping system and those who do not. One major difference between working just with a family and working with a family and a helping system is the role of the therapist. The therapist rarely enters the helping system as a therapist to the people in that system. Rather, he or she must define some sort of role that simultaneously puts the therapist into a collaborative relationship with the members of the helping system, does not violate the hierarchy of that system, and still allows the therapist to solve the client's presenting problem.

To do this, the therapist must understand how the helping system is organized (its structure and the hierarchical relationships among the various persons the therapist encounters in the setting) and what its functions are. Understanding the hierarchical relationships among persons in the setting is important so that the therapist will not enter into coalitions that cross levels of that hierarchy. The therapist also needs to take into account the functions of the setting so that he or she will not ask persons in that setting to do something either opposed to the purpose of the setting or irrelevant to it. Different settings have different functions. For example, schools exist to teach students things; special education settings exist to aid students thought to require additional assistance in order to learn; clerical settings exist to help congregation members deal with spiritual issues and correctly carry out the rituals of their religion; and court settings exist to regulate the behavior of felons and, perhaps, to rehabilitate them. Thus, a therapist working in a school setting needs to frame the issues he or she is working on as having something to do with a child's educational performance, while a therapist working in a court setting needs to focus attention on the fact that therapy is helping clients obey the law and the court.

Like family members, different members of a particular

helping system have divergent ideas about how they should function with regard to the therapist's client. This is especially true in settings that have competing or conflicting missions, such as schools, courts, or child welfare settings. It is essential that the therapist understand how the different individuals in the setting view the problem, what they have tried to do to solve it, and how they think the therapist can be helpful. Therapists will be more successful if they pursue these questions in a spirit of "we are all working together to solve this problem" than if they attempt to directly define the individuals in the helping system as part of the problem. To do this, a therapist must join with the various members of the helping system and with the family to create a joint and workable reality in which the client's problem can be solved. For this purpose, the therapist will need the same skills required in joining with family members: the ability to speak the language of different persons and to comprehend their divergent realities; the ability to communicate to all the persons involved that the therapist has their best interest at heart; and the skills to convince people that the therapist can help them solve their problem (Haley, 1976; Minuchin, 1974; Watzlawick, Weakland, and Fisch, 1974).

Aponte (1976a) provides a nice example of how to work with a helping system in a discussion of a family/school conference. The therapist entered the case when a school-aged boy's mother called the mental health clinic saying that the school counselor had indicated the boy needed help. Finding out from the mother that the boy was not perceived as a problem at home, the therapist asked permission to call a family/school conference so that everyone involved could better understand the problem at school. The therapist then phoned the school counselor to indicate that the mother had acted on her suggestion and requested a joint conference, stressing that the therapist needed to understand the problem at school better, that the family was willing to attend (and thus, implicitly, collaborate with the school), and that the therapist viewed school personnel as a resource for solving the problem rather than as part of the problem.

The conference included the principal, the school counselor, the boy's homeroom teacher and another teacher who the counselor had said was very involved with the boy, both parents, and the boy himself. At the conference it became clear that the boy had a bad relationship with his homeroom teacher and that the school counselor (who was protective of the boy) had contacted the mother when the boy racially slurred the teacher. It further became evident that the boy did better, both academically and behaviorally, with his two other teachers, whose classes were smaller. In addition, it became clear that the mother could not get the boy to mind at home but the father could. On the basis of this information, the therapist validated the perceptions of all the participants and asked the principal to consent to a suggestion that the boy be removed from the home room and that he spend the time normally spent in the home room engaged in studying, with his father as his tutor. The principal did so and the suggestion was implemented. The school counselor was to call the father every day to give him the boy's academic assignment, and the therapist met every two weeks with the family and the counselor to review the progress of the new arrangement.

The maneuvering of Aponte and his cotherapist (Lynn Hoffman) here was exemplary. The therapists managed to convey to all the participants that the therapists could be helpful to them; they respected the hierarchy of the school by validating the perceptions of all the school personnel and by requesting the principal's consent to implement a change in the school's procedure; they were respectful of the family's hierarchy as well, validating the role of the father, who, in this particular family, was seen as the head of the household. And they were able to solve the client's presenting problem.

Interestingly, Aponte and Hoffman accomplished all these tasks without explicitly defining their role in the helping system of the school. As will be evident from the chapters that follow, this is a common, though not invariant, procedure that therapists follow when they work with helping systems. Sometimes it is possible to achieve the therapist's aims by clearly defining his or her role, sometimes it is best to avoid an explicit role definition, and sometimes the therapist does well to define

his or her role slightly differently to each of the various participants dealt with.

Another feature of working with helping systems is that
they often have, as part of their own functioning, idiosyncratic
procedures and occurrences that can be utilized for therapeutic
purposes. For example, in working with the courts, it is often
possible to use an oncoming brief incarceration as a lever to demand that the juvenile offender begin to act more independently in the family setting before he or she will have to survive independently in jail (see Carl and Jurkovic, 1983). For another
example, one important and frequent occurrence in the lives of
families who deal with special education settings is the staffing,
a meeting between the family and school personnel in which
educational plans for the child are made and reviewed. One of
us has frequently used these staffings either to intensify issues
crucial to treatment (to highlight, for example, parental disagreements about the nature of the child's condition and the
appropriate treatment) or to solve the presenting problem (Berger, in press; Berger and Fowlkes, 1980; Foster and Berger,
1979). Or, to give an example from yet another setting, Friedman, who is both a rabbi and a Bowenian therapist, writes in
his chapter for this book about the use of a traditional ministerial function, premarital counseling, to further such goals of
therapy as opening up previously cutoff family relationships or
discussing previously toxic (and undiscussed) family issues.

Finally, in keeping with a systemic perspective that assumes a reciprocity of influences between different parts of a
system, we recognize that, no matter what the units with which
the therapist directly deals, systemic interventions may have un-
expected consequences for the helping agency, sometimes posing
dilemmas for the agency. As an example, one of us (Jurkovic)
directs a family intervention project for youngsters on probation at a large inner-city juvenile court. In recent months probation officers have indirectly accused him and his coworkers
of aligning with the parents against them. Apparently, parents
have begun requesting that the officers assume a less active and
intrusive role in supervising their children. They now want to
control their own troublesome offspring. This, of course, direct-

ly challenges the probation officers' responsibilities as defined by the judge, while reflecting positive changes in the parents' executive functioning at home. We are silently pleased with this new development and view it as a by-product of family therapy, although we have not overtly directed parents to question the probation officers' authority. In our opinion, the court would be well advised to reorganize in such a way that probation officers assumed less direct responsibility for their charges. In the meantime, however, we are caught in a conflict between the parents and officers—a triangle that is interfering with treatment.

Although such conflicts vary across settings, we suspect that their formal qualities are similar. Many doubtless take the form of triangles that cut across different levels of the system and thus involve hierarchy violations and boundary disputes. What are these triangles, and how do they interlock in different settings? How does the therapist avoid confusing one level with another while unraveling these structures?

Therapists too, of course, may be a part of such triangles. Indeed, as they work to help family members assume greater responsibility for solving their own problems, agencies that have increasingly permeated the family's boundaries will likely be challenged in various ways to redefine their relationship to those they serve. The agency may make adjustments or perhaps blame the therapist or the family.

By attending more closely to the effects of their interventions on the ecology of the therapeutic system, practitioners will doubtless find themselves in a better position to help families and agencies adapt effectively to each other. Along these lines, we are interested in the changes, however small, that therapists have directly initiated in agency administration, policies, and procedures. To return to an earlier example, as a means of modifying conflictual patterns of interaction among probation officers, therapists, and families, we have now reached an agreement with the officers that they will meet with us and the families early in the treatment process to clarify boundaries and responsibilities. This procedural shift has improved the situation considerably, although it appears to have uncovered another set of concerns pertaining to the role of the probation officers vis-à-vis the judges and the nature of the hierarchy in the court system. More information is needed from an ecosystemic perspective about modifications that might be made in the operations of different agencies and, equally important, about the ripple effects of planned changes that therapists have witnessed in their work in these agencies.

Conclusions

In this introductory chapter we have stressed the importance of viewing families, family therapists, and helping agencies as parts of an interdependent whole. Such a systemic view has implications for the family therapist's understanding of both the context and unit of treatment, as well as for the way he or she practices. In this volume experienced family therapists will describe in depth contextual features of their work in and with different helping systems. Special emphasis will be placed on the kinds of predictable problems and opportunities they have encountered in trying to better arrange the situation for symptomatic individuals and their families. It is our hope that this discussion will improve the practice of family therapy and encourage the construction of more ecologically valid theories of behavior and behavior change.

2 Carrell Dammann

Private
Practice

Family therapists in private practice are in a unique position. On the one hand, they are "free agents"—free to select or refuse to treat clients and to set their own procedures for intake and evaluation. They are unencumbered by the often rigid guidelines of an agency or the requirement to provide services to all comers as described in other chapters of this book. On the other hand, they must deal with the involvement of the full range of social service agencies and institutions, including referring persons, employee assistance programs, and other professionals in private practice. Private practitioners, therefore, must be constantly alert to evaluating, joining, and working with all the systems that may involve themselves in helping an individual or family in difficulty. In this chapter I will consider the pragmatics of a systemic private practice, relationships with colleagues and the larger professional community, and the joys of private practice as a setting for therapists who wish to be useful parts of their community.

Pragmatics of a Systemic Private Practice

The very context of working on a direct fee-for-services basis has significant impact on the treatment process and can encourage both creativity and mediocrity in therapy. The pressures to join with the family to keep them from dropping out of therapy are much different in private practice, where income depends directly on hours of work done, than in an agency where the salary does not vary if a family drops out. The immediacy of financial consequences of many of the private practitioner's decisions can lead to pressure to become inducted into the system of a vocal and reluctant family member who threatens to drop out or change therapists. Likewise, the same pressures may push the creative edge of the therapist to "join a family at their view of reality" rather than label behaviors as resistant and have a family drop out because someone feels disqualified. This situation often comes up with an overinvolved parent, for example, who is insistent that the child, the identified patient, is very disturbed and needs individual treatment and that there is no need for the family to come in. The therapist is faced with accommodating to the parent's demands or having the parent find a therapist who will. The danger here is in either being very rigid and losing the case or totally agreeing to the parent's demands and losing the systemic perspective on the problem. The identified patient will usually accommodate the parent by escalating the symptom at this point. An intermediate strategy is to accommodate to the parent's view of reality that the child is disturbed and needs individual treatment. The therapist can then use a few individual sessions strategically and work at finding a way to show that the parent and other family members are the only logical persons to help the identified patient with a particular piece of the problem.

Concern about financial consequences can also lead a therapist to either compromise or take damaging shortcuts to please or placate a referral source or another therapist who is involved in the family, or such concern may be the inspiration for the family therapist to join and include those parties as a part of a broader system with whom he or she must work. A couple was referred to me by another therapist in town who was seeing the wife individually. It was clear from the referral phone conversation with the wife's therapist that the therapist was strongly allied with the wife in reviewing the husband as the "sick" one who needed to be fixed. As a family therapist, I felt that this uncontrolled alliance would undermine my ability to reframe the problem as a systemic one. I suggested a recess from individual therapy so the couple could put their energy into resolving relationship issues for a short time. The individual therapist did not agree to this, since he felt things were too critical to allow a recess. I then suggested the couple call back at a time when a recess seemed more appropriate. The financial pressures of private practice can often influence a therapist not to stick to her guns on such an issue even when she feels strongly that she is right about a limit or boundary, not only for fear of losing a particular case but for fear of losing a referral source. This issue of working with referral sources and multiple therapists will be discussed in more detail later in the chapter.

Initial Contacts. The financial consequences of private practice also affect a wide range of treatment decisions, such as length of phone contacts, home and school visits, and extent of collaboration with other helping agencies or persons. The proper consideration and use of all these ancillary but necessary therapeutic tasks are much easier when working on salary, where reimbursement for time is automatic. In private practice, when such time-consuming contacts are done on a fee-for-service contract, the decision whether and how to bill for these contacts and the negotiation of such fees with the client are necessary parts of the therapeutic relationship.

One area that is critical and all too easily shortcut is the initial phone contact. Many forms of therapy involve a lengthy assessment process before commencing a therapeutic contract. In family systems therapy, however, particularly if using a problem-focused, strategic approach, assessment and intervention are part of the same process. The very first phone contact initiates both the assessment and the intervention process. For therapists who work and think systemically, the first phone contact is a context in which "one cannot not intervene" (Fisch, Weakland, and Segal, 1982; Haley, 1976; Keeney, 1982). Another factor that differentiates the importance of initial phone contacts in systemic therapy and in other therapies is the issue of membership in the initial session. This is clearly not an issue in individual therapy, and therefore little attention or training has been focused on initial phone contacts. However, in systemic therapy, the omission of a critical member or failure to have clear agreements about expectations during the first contact and initial session can seriously handicap the therapist and be very costly to correct later in the therapeutic process. Often the most crucial battle for structure takes place in the early contacts: "Fortunately, most families do not present us with . . . a crisis in the first interview. But many families do engage in some form of struggle over membership at meetings. So predictable is this challenge that we have given it a name: the battle for structure" (Napier and Whitaker, 1978, p. 10).

For example, a father made an initial phone contact regarding a twenty-three-year-old daughter who had been in and out of psychiatric hospitals for ten years, since her parents had divorced. She was presently out of control, making threats and destroying property. She had been hospitalized for containment, but there was no expectation that this was a solution, since it had been tried so many times in the past. The family had been referred for family therapy. In the initial phone contact, I asked who was involved with the daughter at present, although she was living with friends. She had frequent contact with her mother and younger brother. She would harass her mother at work and at home both by phone calls and by visits. Her father and stepmother would often rescue her or bail her out when she got into trouble. I said I would need agreement that the mother, brother, father, and stepmother would come in along with the identified patient. The father insisted that his present wife and his ex-wife could never be in the same room together because his ex-wife, the girl's mother, would refuse. He had ended their marriage by leaving his wife for a younger woman. His first wife had never met "the younger woman" and was no less angry than she had been the day he left her, years before. I then asked permission to call the girl's mother to discuss this problem, and the father agreed. The mother confirmed the father's story. The only thing more forceful than her anger at her husband was her desperation about her daughter's craziness and unrelenting harassment of her in front of friends and customers. The phone calls gave me a chance to join with each parent in an intensely adversarial system individually before the first session. I got the mother to agree that down the road, if I felt it was necessary, she would agree to attend a session with the husband's new wife. I agreed to meet with the mother, father, brother, and identified patient. I also stated that although it might never be necessary to bring in the new wife, I could not undertake the therapy unless I was assured that they would all come in if needed. With this agreement, therapy was begun. The importance of this agreement was the mother's acknowledgment that her concern about changing her daughter's behavior had priority at this point over holding her old grudge.

Clearly, this kind of careful negotiation with key family members before the first session is critical to establishing a workable therapeutic relationship. The example just given nicely illustrates both the level of assessment and the extent of intervention that takes place before a family ever walk into your waiting room for an initial session. Failure to push for the possible inclusion of the new wife could have obscured the dramatic connection between the mother's old anger and the daughter's symptoms. Therapy could have later become embroiled in a struggle over whether the new wife needed to be included.

Of course, not all initial contacts are this complicated or critical; some, indeed, take only five minutes. However, knowing the value of the initial phone contacts and being committed to use them diagnostically and strategically are necessary skills for the family therapist in private practice. Talking carefully to referring agents or other therapists involved with the case is often also required. The time and financial pressures of a busy private practice can often tempt a therapist to cut this process short, a temptation that should be acknowledged and avoided.

Handling Crises. Because systemic therapists work in a directive fashion with more than one family member, they are more likely to have crises and emergencies that result from the beginnings of change in the system. This, coupled with the fact that many family therapists use hospitalization minimally and prefer to help families use the intensity of the crisis to push for a change, results in a fair number of lengthy phone calls that involve therapeutic consultation. Learning to handle and use these calls is a critical part of strategic therapy.

Recently, I saw a couple with a severely symptomatic wife and a passive-aggressive husband. The couple were in extreme marital crisis, with the husband threatening divorce. Several sessions led to the development of a symptom prescription of their usual sequence. It was fairly clear that this would lead both to a crisis and to some change in the system. Several days later the wife called, saying the husband was threatening to leave. I negotiated for the husband to spend one night in a motel to get away from the very anxious wife, who wanted to talk compulsively all night about their problems. The wife finally agreed he could leave if he would come back the next day, since that was better than having him leave permanently. I then spent several hours that night and the next day on the phone with the wife. This consolidated my relationship with the wife, laying the groundwork for her to follow through on critical interventions later in therapy. In addition, I was able on the phone to coach the wife not to pursue the husband when he returned the next day. She was coached to tell him how glad she was to have him home but under no circumstances to ask why he had left or to talk about their problems. This broke their usual sequence and was a major breakthrough in their therapy.

The issue of charging for such phone calls must be dealt with ahead of time. A written policy statement may be given to all families, to be signed at the initial session, that states fee schedules on charges for phone calls, sessions that run overtime, home or school visits, and conferences with other helping professionals. If payment is being handled by a third party, such as an agency, clearance for such charges needs to be discussed with the agency person making the referral before therapy is begun.

Payment Issues. In general, third-party payments are a major issue in negotiating initial contracts with clients, whether the third party is an agency, a business, or an insurance carrier. The type and extent of services and providers covered often affect the kind of treatment people can afford and thus the kind of treatment they choose. If such concerns are not dealt with carefully at the outset, disagreements about payment can seriously damage the therapy process.

There are also some situations in which the therapist will feel obligated to offer treatment without reimbursement. I was seeing a family with a highly emotional, very scapegoated fifteen-year-old daughter who was seriously suicidal. I was unable to successfully engage the family in treatment, and after eight or nine sessions the family refused to come anymore. The daughter wanted to continue therapy on her own, but the family, being furious with her, refused to pay for it. The daughter agreed to pay $5.00 per hour out of her part-time earnings. I saw her for several years at $5.00 an hour, working to help her change her role in the family. Although the girl did not remain suicidal and used the therapy productively, my evaluation of her suicidal potential had been the impetus for my offering to contract at a reduced fee.

In another case, I worked with a couple with problems of severe wife abuse. The husband was being extremely abusive and terroristic. He dropped out of treatment, forbade his wife to continue, and refused to pay for any services. The wife wanted to continue treatment but was not ready or strong enough to make the decision to leave him. My decision was to continue to work with the wife at no charge until she was in a geographically safe place.

Relationships with Colleagues and the Professional Community

There are two major issues concerning the private practitioners' collegial network and the larger professional community. The first is the effect of working with a group of colleagues who do not share a systemic way of thinking about problems. The second is how to deal with situations in which a couple or family are referred for therapy and one or more members are already in individual therapy with another therapist. Common to these two issues is the financial pressure to stay on the good side of referral sources, or to work in a collegial setting that may produce a strong referral network, or to collaborate with other professionals. This pressure can have subtle but profound influences on treatment decisions and the process of therapy.

These pressures may be particularly acute for the young

or beginning private practitioner, who is usually the most in-secure both financially and in terms of confidence in his or her therapeutic skills. The more seasoned practitioner has often learned from experience many of the pressures and pitfalls of therapeutic decision making. However, the seasoned practi-tioner, dependent on a particular referral base or collegial net-work, may have more chronic problems identifying a repetitive systemic dilemma in his or her network.

Within one's own work group, a colleague's place in the hierarchy will strongly influence the effect of that therapist's opinion on your thinking or decisions. Similarly, differences in status or hierarchy will intensify the effect of any triangles with other professionals in the community. These differences may re-flect different professional affiliations or may involve issues of seniority within a given profession. In an organizational setting, these hierarchal differences are usually an important part of the bureaucracy and cannot be violated without serious conse-quences. It is not unusual for the beginning family therapist to encounter one or more such hierarchal relationships with per-sons with a different epistemology. It is difficult not to be in-timidated or discouraged by input from prestigious figures who, though often supportive of "family therapy," do not share a systemic epistemology.

There are several types of private practice settings in which to do family therapy. Often a fairly predictable developmental sequence occurs as a professional moves into the private arena.

The Lone Wolf. Many people enter private practice work-ing as "lone wolves." A therapist working in an organizational setting may desire the freedom from agency guidelines and pri-orities and seek the case control available in a private practice setting. The therapist then contracts to use space on an hourly basis, prints up cards, and agrees to see a family or two, usually at less than the going rate. Few of us will ever forget the anxiety of the first time we received *direct* payment for our services. If you do not produce a dramatic cure in the first session, you in-stantly want to give the money back! And yet your friends and colleagues, knowing how desperate and vulnerable you are at this juncture, send you all their most difficult families. One of my first was a family with a pregnant, suicidal young adult daughter with a drug abuse problem and a job history that would rival Ko-Ko's list from *The Mikado*. Nevertheless, we all cut our teeth on these families, survive them, and generally even manage to put a dent in them by sheer force of determination not to fail with our first few "private-practice cases." Never fear, your turn will come to refer similar cases to other friends and colleagues who follow in your footsteps.

It also does not take long for two related changes to come to pass. The first is that you stop feeling bad about the money you charge. The reason is the second—you rapidly realize that you cannot survive for long without answering services, bookkeeping services, secretarial services, malpractice insurance, a larger waiting room, a new set of captain's chairs, a coffeepot, and a Coke machine.

Collegial Affiliation. The "lone wolf" experience usually leads to stage two: association with colleagues or other professionals. Sometimes this occurs purely for financial and pragmatic reasons, such as a desire to share operational costs. At other times it is spurred on by a desperate longing for someone to talk to about your cases. Anxious "lone wolf" therapists develop a chronic habit of talking to themselves. Each person has his or her own private and sacred spot for obsessing anxiously about the day's interventions and the new handwashing compulsion case that is coming in tomorrow. Mine was the tub; others have confessed to the car, the john, and even church services. The desire to share the burden of therapeutic responsibilities often leads to a search for colleagueship. A third reason for pursuing colleagues is to develop a more predictable referral base and sometimes to enter an interdisciplinary practice that increases the likelihood of third-party coverage for services.

The quest for affiliation often leads to a hidden hazard for many family therapists, one that can profoundly affect their treatment effectiveness. Often the affiliation found will provide the shared financial and practical benefits but will not provide a supportive context for systemic work and thinking. The family therapist often joins a group of therapists with a primarily individual or intrapsychic or medical-model orientation. They may often be very positive about family and couples therapy and may welcome the family therapist as providing these additional resources. However, these colleagues often view family and couples therapy as an adjunctive therapy or as a set of techniques. There is often little recognition of the family therapist's systemic epistemology and the radical difference in underlying assumption between the family therapist and his or her associate. Several potential predictable problems result.

One of the most critical aspects of doing strategic and directive family therapy is a sense of confidence in one's reframings or tasks. Doing strategic and directive therapy, particularly with a clear symptom or problem as a crystallized family metaphor, involves pushing on that point in the system to enable the system or sequence to break loose and change. At this point, the system of family (or client) plus therapist is very intense. Anxiety is often high for both family and therapist, and crises and pressures from the family that test the therapist's resolve are frequent. It is critical whether the therapist will be inducted or engulfed by the system with which she or he has joined or will remain connected and outside long and powerfully enough to pull it over the edge to change. It is at this point that the strategic therapist must stand, face to the wind, in the bow of the ship, saying to himself or herself, "Damn the torpedoes, full speed ahead!" If the first mate or, worse yet, the owner of the ship mutters thoughtfully at that moment, "Have you considered the possibility that the ship's bulkhead is cracked?" it can take more than a little wind out of your sails at a critical moment. Such a comment or observation may be made formally at a staffing or informally over the coffeepot; it has, nevertheless, the same devastating effect on the therapist, who must continue to push or mold the reframing or directive, to hold ground with the family until the desired change can be secured.

The strategic and systemic viewpoint places an emphasis on a belief in change and in what is possible. It is an optimistic perspective that comes down heavily on the side of the forces and potential for health in an individual or a system. Many more-traditional models of therapy are based on nosological systems that focus on identification and treatment or management of pathology. When a crisis occurs, these differences in perspective lead people to see the same data in dramatically different ways.

Such crises often involve a temporary increase in symptomatic behaviors and the threat of such extreme behaviors as divorce, suicide, panic attacks, psychotic manifestations, or running away. These escalations are usually read by less systemic therapists as confirmation of the depth of the individual pathology in the identified patient, and then often lead to recommendations for more long-term and drastic treatment measures, such as hospitalization, medication, and a return to in-depth individual treatment. The situation is often isomorphic with the anxiety of the family system that the identified patient really needs help and the anxiety that the family cannot handle the crisis and subsequent change. The strategic family therapist with pressures and doubts of his or her own is particularly vulnerable at this point to the comments of well-meaning colleagues that emphasize the pathology of the identified patient and the seemingly more conservative measures of traditional treatment. Thus, a collegial network can clearly become a significant part of the therapist/family system and have a profound influence on the resolution of the crisis.

A couple were referred to treatment for a long-standing compulsion of the wife's. The compulsion took the form of a "wiring phobia." The sight of appliances in her home or electrical wires on the street would precipitate an extreme feeling of panic that the wires were loose or damaged and that someone would be seriously injured. Indeed, her brother had been almost killed by touching a live wire in childhood. The symptom and case history were clearly a classic case from an analytic perspective, but several years of therapy with several excellent individual therapists had failed to produce a change in her phobia. She was referred for brief therapy with the admonition that she was severely disturbed and a very chronic case. She was seen with her husband, who was very involved in the symptom and eager to help. The symptom was most severe in his presence. When the panic took over, the wife would ask her husband to inspect the wiring and reassure her that everything was okay.

Only after his inspection and reassurance would the panic begin to subside. The client's mother had a history of "nervous breakdowns," and the client feared this would be her fate also. As the present system emerged, it was discovered that the husband, a very bright young lawyer, had a severe problem with chronic procrastination. This had resulted in his previously failing the bar several times before passing and currently in his being six months behind in his paperwork. The household was consequently under constant pressure of fear of financial and occupational catastrophe.

After several months of joining, collecting data, and first-order probes and interventions, a major use of symptom prescription seemed the appropriate intervention. The husband and wife had been keeping track of "wiring" episodes for several weeks. The therapist made the observation that the husband's procrastination was something that, despite all attempts, the wife was unable to influence. This clearly caused waves of panic, anger, and helplessness from which she had no recourse. The husband, likewise, felt helpless in the face of his procrastination and the distress it caused his wife. This clearly was a concern for both of them, but one in which the expression of concern and offering of reassurance seemed futile. However, the financial uncertainty was of daily concern to the wife, who did not wish to nag and make her husband's burden heavier, since she knew he was trying.

I asked the husband and wife whether they would be willing to try an experiment that might give them some comfort and might even reduce the "wiring phobia" somewhat. They were willing to agree to almost anything. The wife was asked to perform a task several times during the coming week when she was upset about the husband's procrastination. On at least three such occasions, she was to *pretend* to have a "wiring" episode and, as always, to ask for her husband's help and reassurance about the wiring. She was not to tell, nor was he to question, whether any attack was a "real" or a "pretend" episode, but he was to check the wiring and reassure her as always. I insisted that this was a way for the wife to allow the husband to feel useful and reassure her when she was anxious without nagging or undermining him. I wasn't sure what, if anything, this had to do with the symptom, but at least it was a way to make use of an otherwise annoying and frustrating problem. The couple finally agreed to the task and were told to try it for two weeks and come back. During the next few days I received several highly emotional phone calls from each spouse. The wife's anxiety had escalated to almost uncontrollable proportions; maybe she should be hospitalized. I consulted the referring psychiatrist, a colleague, because of the intensity of the client's affect. He reaffirmed the poor prognosis and talked about an underlying psychosis. Perhaps hospitalization at this time would be necessary. I asked the wife whether she had done the task. No, she had been "too anxious," she replied. I said I felt the task was really important, more now than ever, and pushed the wife to do the task. She was furious that I was pushing her to do the task when she was fearing a nervous breakdown. I wavered. "Perhaps," I thought, "I really need to hospitalize." Teetering on the brink, I found a final toehold. "If you will do the task, I will get the psychiatrist to prescribe some medication that may help," I replied. The bargain was struck. Ten days later, the couple came in for their scheduled appointment. The wife had seen the psychiatrist and had both taken the prescribed tranquilizer and done the prescribed task the same day. She had repeated the task on several other occasions. She had begun to get angrier with the husband and less anxious about the wiring and had applied for a new job with a higher salary. The husband had begun to get fed up with the wiring phobia and was making noises about refusing to check up and reassure the wife about it in the future. Besides, if he was going to catch up on his paperwork, he needed to stay late at the office some evenings and couldn't hang around the house reassuring his wife all the time. After several weeks the couple terminated therapy, and the wife started a new job.

This sequence seems a good illustration of the influence of epistemological differences at a critical moment. Of course, we will never know the relative impacts of the task and the tranquilizer. It is likely, however, that to have hospitalized the identified patient at the critical juncture of change would have fulfilled her own catastrophic fear, reinforced her as the "sick" one, and precluded any likely job change in the near future.

Having worked in several more traditional interdisciplinary settings for many years before having the supportive context of a family therapy institute in which to practice, I can assure you that the task is at least several times more difficult in the former situation. It is like swimming against a slight current, as opposed to going with the current. The current may be so slight and so constant that one is not even aware of its pressure until it is gone.

Such an influence can be particularly devastating to young, less experienced therapists who do not have a backlog of experience to give them confidence in the rightness or timeliness of their interventions. At the same time, it is these same young therapists who are most likely to find themselves in this situation.

Another problem for the family therapist in private practice is learning when and how to work with cases in which another therapist is already involved. This is a common situation because when there is a family with a problem, one or more family members are likely to be already working with a therapist.

One influence that increases the likelihood of multiple therapists is the tendency of many individual therapists to view couples and family therapy as an adjunctive treatment. Consequently, many therapists will continue individual therapy with an adult parent or spouse while referring the family concurrently to a family therapist for a child or marital problem. This problem can be particularly thorny with remarriage or blended families in which a child is still triangled between ex-spouses. In these cases, when the dyad has already become adversarial at both a personal and a legal level, it is very easy for a therapist to get into a coalition with a patient in individual therapy and to become inducted into the adversarial system. Under these circumstances, I have had at least one occasion to work together on a case with another therapist who was both a friend and a colleague and was someone who thought systemically. We found our attempts to communicate with each other professionally about this case strained at times under these, the best of circumstances. The complications added by feelings of professional competition, differences in professional affiliation (that is, psychiatrist, psychologist, social worker, marriage and family therapist), or differences in epistemology only make the task more delicate. As a systemic therapist, you have the responsibility of finding a way to join with the other therapist "at his or her view of reality" and, from there, to try to move toward a middle ground.

I do not want to suggest that well-meaning, mutually respecting therapists, even of different theoretical bents, cannot collaborate successfully. But there are hidden dangers of therapist pride and competition or unrecognized conflicts in epistemology. These can lead therapists to triangulate the client or family.

A family therapist armed with an enthusiasm about brief therapy and strategic reframing and interventions may charge into a family or couple, assuming it is safe to ignore the fact that one member of the family is in individual therapy. Often the person in individual therapy is not a peripheral family member but is the identified patient or the person most invested in the problem—that is, the overinvolved parent or the dissatisfied spouse. Failure to regard the other therapy and therapist as a part of the system and to evaluate it and work it through before initiating therapy is a serious error. Often the other therapist comes from a background that regards long-term, in-depth insight therapy as essential for change. Or the therapist may come from an orientation that emphasizes the communication of feelings as the source of change. Whatever the therapist's epistemology, it will have been transmitted to the client in some degree. A more problem-focused family therapist with differing ideas about the nature of change and the rate at which change can occur may readily triangulate or polarize the system, leading to a stalemate. A sense of frustration and failure for the family therapist or overt or covert conflict in some part of the system may result. The system of the two therapists and family may duplicate the pathological triangle created by two parents in conflict over the nature and solution of a problem in a child (Haley, 1980).

For example, Johnny and his family come in with a bedwetting problem. The parents agree that Johnny has a problem, but they disagree about its cause. Mother thinks Johnny is anxious and insecure because his father is too harsh and critical. Dad thinks Johnny has the problem because his mother babies him too much. And so they go round and round until a therapist arrives with a perspective that is "meta" to both of their epistemologies and comes up with reframing that can include both of them.

Likewise, two therapists may agree that a family member has a problem but disagree about the cause of the problem and the kind of therapy indicated. The family can thus become a conflict-detouring mechanism and be placed in the traditional bind of having two authority figures in conflict over alternate realities. Since this situation often makes people act crazy in families, we can assume it might have similar effects in the therapeutic context (Haley, 1980). Again, this kind of error is most likely to evolve from the tendency to regard family or strategic therapy as a set of techniques rather than an integral part of an underlying systemic epistemology. Thinking systemically means you must think about all the systems involved, including other therapists, not just the family system.

A couple were referred to a family therapist because of the wife's dissatisfaction with their sexual relationship. The husband was very invested in making the marriage work and was most willing to come to therapy. The wife was in analytically oriented psychotherapy. She had sought therapy originally because of a series of sexual affairs. Her therapist had indicated that this was a deep-seated problem rooted in a poor resolution of her relationship with her father. A course of long-term, in-depth therapy was recommended to resolve the underlying conflict. Her marital dissatisfaction and the subsequent affairs were disclosed to the husband after individual therapy was well underway, and it was at this point that the couple were referred to me to work on their sexual problems. What evolved was an irresolvable impasse created by the two therapies and an underlying conflict in the assumptions about how the problem might be resolved. The husband was angry and indignant about the affairs but had to be understanding, since they were a "childish"

manifestation of an underlying conflict over which the wife had
no control. He wanted to work on their sexual problems but
felt angry and inadequate because of the affairs. He vacillated
between being dogmatic, judgmental, and critical and being
understanding and loving, much as the wife's father had done.
The wife could not find the husband attractive because he·was
too much like a father. She was subsequently unwilling/unable
to commit to giving up the affairs. If she did, there would be no
reason to continue individual therapy, since that was the presenting problem. She felt that the individual therapist understood her better than her husband did, and she was not willing
to risk giving up therapy. The continuation of the affairs in
spite of the marital/sexual therapy reinforced the individual
therapist's hypothesis that the affairs were unresolved problems from the past. Although interventions by the family therapist produced brief islands of respite in the marital and sexual
relationship, these changes could not be maintained and solidified because of the impasse with the affairs. The wife became
more convinced that analysis was the solution. The husband became discouraged, and I suggested that perhaps I could be of
more assistance when the analysis was complete.

This situation of conflicting therapeutic epistemologies
created a double bind for each person in the system. Although
the sequence can be punctuated in many ways to produce dif
ferent linear hypotheses about the "real" problem, the dilemma
is precisely parallel to that of the two parents who disagree over
the cause of, and solution to, Johnny's bedwetting problem. In
the absence of an intervener at a meta level, there is an irresolvable repetitive sequence.

Clearly, one of the most direct solutions to such an impasse is for the therapists involved to be able to metacommuni-
cate beforehand and to arrive at a definition of the problem and
a resolution agreeable to both. They may agree that one or the
other form of therapy should be followed. They may agree to
try brief therapy with a break from individual therapy. They
may agree that the long-term analytic therapy should be pursued as the sole solution and that family therapy would not be
helpful, since the real problem is with the wife. It will often be

incumbent on the systemic therapist to develop a reframing of the therapeutic tasks and goals with the other therapist that allows each of them to function effectively in a particular arena without working at odds with the other. This often requires considerable creativity and skill on the part of the systemic therapist. Still, it is often possible to carve out an area of concern that may be pursued in individual treatment with the understanding that other things can be worked on in marital therapy while not changing the "core" problem being dealt with in analysis. (Reamy-Stephenson and Greiner, in Chapters Three and Nine, also discuss ways of doing this.)

A wife came to a family therapist saying there were real problems in her marriage. One of the conflicts was that her husband, a scholar, had great difficulty getting his work done and was in analysis for this problem. Both husband and wife believed in analysis, but she feared the marriage would not last as long as the analysis. The husband agreed that he could try to make some small, superficial changes while working on the "core" of the problem and felt that couples therapy would help her survive in the marriage through the analysis. Both husband and wife saw analysis as important to the creativity and depth of his scholarship. The analyst agreed to the husband's attending couples sessions with the wife on occasion to deal with pressures in the marriage caused by his problems. The problems with work initially touched on almost every aspect of their lives together. The family therapist was able to gradually block off their talking about his "problem with work," since that was now the purview of the analysis. Having done this, they had to talk about money and time management problems in many other ways. Gradually, many of the marital conflicts that had originally been defined as related to the husband's "problems with work" were reframed in other ways and resolved. The old vicious triangle and unpleasant complementary relationship sequence created by the wife's trying to "help" the husband with his "problem with work" were eliminated by the boundary created with the analyst. The marital relationship greatly improved, and the husband continued his analysis regarding work.

Reframing and boundary setting are probably the most

helpful tools at the systemic therapist's disposal for creating a context in which collaborative therapy can be done successfully. Another useful approach is the "illusion of choice."

A couple were referred to a family therapist. Both were Ph.D.s in an academic setting, and both had been in individual analytic therapy for several years. Analytic theory was highly congruent with their world views; however, they frequently got into a symmetrical escalation that bordered on violence in their marriage. The therapist of one spouse became sufficiently concerned and referred them for couples therapy because of the chronic marital conflict. Neither spouse and neither individual therapist had any thought of stopping or interrupting the analytic treatment. In the couples sessions, discussions of routine conflicts and decisions rapidly moved from which movie to see that night to analytic mudslinging, with each spouse offering cogent interpretations of the other's behavior. Very close to the dialogue from *Who's Afraid of Virginia Woolf?*, this quickly escalated to frightening proportions. Numerous attempts at straightforward, first-order interventions failed miserably. I finally proposed the following "illusion of choice":

Your attraction in your marriage is clearly enhanced by your selection of each other as working opponents. The absence of competition and conflict in your marriage would clearly be boring to both of you. You can, of course, continue with your present path of seeing who can come up with the most telling and devastating analytic interpretation. In fact, you could each increase the frequency of your appointments to gather more ammunition. Of course, this often leads to a fear of violence, and it could get very costly. I do have another idea that you might want to try, but you would have to agree ahead of time to try it before I tell you what it is.

After thinking it over for a week, both agreed to try the other task because of their increasing fear of loss of control.

They were instructed to go home and prepare a number of small strips of paper and to put a supply of plastic straws in their desks in the office they shared at home. The next time they found themselves in their usual escalation, the husband was responsible for stopping and insisting they retire to the office to continue their fight. There, both were to write their most vicious interpretations of the other's behavior, family, and character structures as fast as possible on the strips of paper for ten minutes. Then they were to load their straws with the first interpretation and commence firing in a spitball fight. They agreed to follow this procedure for a month. In the first trial, they both ended up laughing so hard they couldn't fire a spitball and decided to go out for a walk. The use of analysis as a weapon dropped out, and couples therapy continued for a short time, producing some resolution of some old conflicts in their families of origin and in their marriage.

Often with a difficult child-focused case a therapist will run into difficulties midstream in therapy, and one or another family member will recruit another helping professional. Such an addition runs the risk of endangering or sabotaging a treatment strategy in progress and must be dealt with carefully and by using the system rather than in a reactive or confrontive manner.

A family were in treatment because of their eighteen-year-old anorectic/bulimic daughter, a student at a college over 1,000 miles from home. The family first brought Edie in when she came home for Christmas vacation weighing eighty-two pounds. An initial intervention of requiring the daughter to leave the bathroom door open when vomiting reduced the bulimia from two or three times a day to two or three times a week. The three or four weeks Edie was home on break were then used to set up a treatment strategy to put the parents in charge of her symptomatic behavior when she went back to school. The following is a transcript of the reframing done with the family to get both the parents and the identified patient to agree to the treatment program.

Therapist: Well, it seems to me that getting angry is perfectly normal. Normal adolescents get angry with their parents, and they get frustrated and don't want to listen.

Edie: It's not that I didn't want to listen, it just wasn't fun conversation, and I was just sick of it.

Ther.: Perfectly normal feeling. Most adolescents feel like that when they have to sit down and talk with their parents. [To parents] Usually that comes about because they have done something that forces you to come in and take care of them, and Edie does that. They don't make the right decisions or aren't old enough to make those decisions or can't handle those decisions, and then you have to come in and exercise some authority until they can prove they can do that themselves.

Dad: Makes sense to me.

Ther.: I think it may be that you really have to, both of you, be more active in checking up on Edie, because she sends you a lot of signals that she wants you to stay involved in helping her make decisions and things.

Mom: Should we?

Ther.: But it's almost impossible not to. One way is for Edie to continue to pull you in. Another way is for you two to be more active in checking up on her. Rather than waiting to be pulled in. How do you feel about doing that?

Dad: Well, it seems to me what you are talking about is a program where we would be more active, and I think that could be helpful.

Edie: I don't understand what y'all are talking about. You were telling me yesterday I had to grow up, and now—I don't understand.

Ther.: Well, that's a decision you will have to make. You will have to tell them to get out of your life. Right now you're having to pull them into your life.

Edie: I don't understand.

Ther.: Well, it is very simple to get them out of your life by handling your own problems. You know how to get them out of your life if you need to. And I'm sure that if you start gaining weight and doing okay in other things and having normal problems but not getting really upset, that they'll back off.

Edie: But I don't really want them out of my life. Do you understand that?

Ther.: Yeah, that's what you're getting, you're getting them back in your life, so when they leave—

Edie: You're not listening to what I'm saying.

Ther.: Okay, all I'm saying is that the two of you need to work out a program of checking up on Edie regularly.

Edie: I still don't understand what you're saying. When you grow up, your parents are still there, right? I just don't understand what you're saying at all.

Ther.: Basically, I'm saying your folks need to stay involved with you. And it's better to do that systematically and then—

Edie: I don't understand.

Ther.: Well, the other thing is, I'm not sure it's important for you to understand. If you were an adult, that would be different. Part of growing up is that you don't understand a lot of things.

Edie: So it's just going to happen?

Ther.: Well, this is an issue to be decided by your parents, and I'm not that concerned if you understand it. On the other side of this, you may understand, because that is what growing up is all about. Your folks do understand some things that you don't.

Edie: It's hard for me to trust in something I don't know about.

Ther.: [To parents] You know, I think part of the problem is, Edie is real good at being twelve years old or real good at being thirty-five years old, but she is not real good at being eighteen years old, and, ah, for the time being you've got to deal with her adolescent behavior. One of the things that is most important is to make plans for when she goes back to school—what kind of guidelines you want to set up, when you want her to come home, whether you want to go up to see her—

Edie: I don't think that's such a good idea.

Ther.: Yeah, but at this point that's not your decision. I would like for the two of you to work on coming up with some guidelines we can discuss at the next session.

The parents returned the next week with the following list of rules:

Rules for Edie Returning to College

1. Edie to come home for regular planned visits.
2. No eating meals alone.
3. Replace clothes as soon as they are too tight.
4. Parents will call Edie daily when they can talk to her jointly. Any emergency calls, parents will get together as soon as possible to return call.
5. Should accept *all* social invitations unless there is a very substantial reason to decline.
6. Weigh in weekly with nurse at infirmary and report weight to parents without prompting.
7. Honesty with parents about eating and throwing-up habits.
8. Dressing appropriately for cold climate.
9. Check out money decisions with parents.
10. Edie to come home immediately if weight falls below 85 pounds.
11. All rules from parents in effect until weight reaches 105.

One of the most critical interventions was that the parents (who were in constant conflict because they never had time together) agreed to find a time each day when they could talk to the daughter long-distance together. Whenever they spoke to her separately, they got different pieces of information about how she was doing and got into conflict. The system was working very well for several weeks. Edie was vomiting several times a week but could now usually relate these incidents to specific stresses in her academic or social life and was gaining weight gradually. At this juncture, the nurse at the infirmary where Edie had to weigh in began talking to Edie about her feelings and her problems. The nurse quickly pathologized the situation and started pushing Edie to get into intensive individual therapy. Edie, who was now being a rebellious adolescent about her parents' daily intrusiveness, seized the opportunity to press the parents to change course. The parents' anxiety was further heightened because they had each just received a letter from the daughter. In a perfect parody of the therapist's injunction against communicating separately with her parents, she had written a letter to both of them, cut it in half, and mailed one half to each of them. This combination of events was enough to resurrect the parents' old anxieties that, indeed, this child was deeply disturbed. The therapist conceded that perhaps that was true, although the girl was steadily gaining weight. Perhaps the program should be discontinued and a psychiatrist found at school to treat her individually. Given a forced choice, the parents acknowledged that actually treatment was going well and they could always find a psychiatrist later if things got worse. The parents were put in charge of calling the nurse and informing her of the treatment program. They told the nurse they felt things were going well and asked her not to discuss the problem with Edie any further. The nurse was thanked for her concern and interest and encouraged to talk to Edie about any *normal* problems she might be having at school. The nurse was also asked to call the parents or the therapist any time she became concerned about Edie's progress. In this way, the nurse was validated for her conscientiousness and concern and was made a part of the therapist/parent coalition and blocked off from a cross-generational coalition with the daughter. Thus, she became an effective member of the treatment team.

As with so many decisions in doing therapy, the easiest solution is a rigid rule that says, "I won't take the case unless the whole family comes in," or, "I won't take the case if someone is in therapy with another therapist." This is the safest and most conservative approach and is probably a good rule of thumb for the beginning therapist who wants to reduce the complexity of the task. However, a clear understanding of the need to think systemically and the ability to be creative in working with all the elements in the therapist/family system can lead to helpful and therapeutic interventions that are mindful and respectful of all the epistemologies concerned.

Family Institute or Group Practice as a Model. Sophie Tucker is supposed to have said, "I have been poor and I have been rich. Rich is better." Well, I have had nonsystemic colleagues and I have had systemic colleagues, and systemic is better!

For over five years I have worked with a group of colleagues who have various areas of expertise but share a systemic epistemology. We have evolved some very useful practices. As

Peggy Papp has pointed out, systemic therapy is not the kind of therapy in which patients give Christmas or Chanukah presents. Rather, it is a therapy in which often you work very hard to give credit to the family for the changes that take place. Having a "cuddle group" of colleagues who appreciate and validate your work is one of the great rewards of "working this way." Using a metaphor or story or indirect intervention and having a family return the next session and unfold to you the working through of that input is a great joy. But the icing on that delicious morsel is the intellectual pleasure and satisfaction of describing it to a supportive and appreciative colleague. Therapists feed people all day, and we need to be fed ourselves. This sharing of success and failure, hope and frustration, as well as occasionally being able to laugh at ourselves, is essential in avoiding burnout.

Another concrete advantage of a group practice of systemic therapy is the opportunity to work or consult with colleagues as a team on difficult cases or as part of the evaluation process. The staff at our institute have evolved a practice of asking one colleague to act as a consultant behind the mirror on an initial session. This is more practical financially than using a team on an ongoing basis. It does, however, give the advantage of a bicameral view of the system (Berger and Dammann, 1982) and facilitates early formulation of an overall strategy. Such a consultation may also be requested for a family with whom a therapist has got stuck.

Although the family systems institute or group practice provides the most supportive context for systemic therapy, it is not without its pitfalls. Family therapy is still a new field. Pressures within the group for orthodoxy can suppress the development of new ideas as well as the development and integration of the personal style of each member of the group.

Institutes or practice groups, like families, are usually not totally democratic associations among equals. There is usually a hierarchy based on seniority or administrative structure. Failure to recognize the impact of official or unofficial hierarchies can produce confusion for groups that attempt to work together as teams or in cotherapy models.

In the absence of a group practice or institute, many systemic therapists form peer supervision groups that meet regularly to provide support for their work. Doing systemic therapy in isolation is a lonely and frustrating experience. It is like speaking a foreign language and having lots to say but no one to talk to. Workshops and national meetings and reading lots of books are often the only outlets for therapists in such a setting. Possibly, finding a similarly lonely pen pal and swapping audiotapes would provide some respite.

On the Joys of Private Practice

I am sure being in private practice has a life cycle like everything else. I remember visiting Milton Erickson in his later years and being struck by his consummate skill in using all the artifacts in his office to engage and move people therapeutically. He knew the people and environs of Phoenix so intimately, having learned it not only through his own experience but from many years of knowing it through his patients and their families, networks, and experiences. He used his knowledge of his environment in each task he prescribed, each image he developed.

Having been in private practice for over ten years now in the same place, I am beginning to have a sense of those resources in my work. Knowing my terrain and my community, being a part of that community, I find myself no longer "doing therapy" but "becoming a therapist." In private practice, therapy is a relationship between people rather than agencies or professions. As a therapist, you will see families for whom you become a celebrant for significant life-cycle events. You will be invited to weddings and brisses and told of funerals or sent notices of such events. At times like this, I know that I follow in my family tradition of preachers and teachers and small-town doctors. As time goes on, being a family therapist becomes less a profession and more an identity.

The therapy of change involves not only the dramatic six-session intervention but much cleaning up of the corners and tacking down of the edges between the major shifts. Indeed, there is the occasional family with a clear-cut symptom that requires no more than a six- to ten-session treatment, but many families get beyond the initial symptom and stay to work on several other issues—marital, sexual, in-laws, or family of origin. Often families reach the end of their present concerns or goals and leave therapy. Sometimes I suggest a recess with an open invitation to return whenever and for as long as they choose. Many families do return over the years, for a divorce, a marital problem, children leaving home, or coping with aging parents or death in the family. Families seldom return with a problem of the same level of seriousness as the first time. They may come back for one session or stay longer in therapy again. They clearly learn to think more systemically over time, and as I said earlier, I become something of a celebrant in these families.

It is easy to get lost in the world of families with problems and to lose one's perspective on the real world. A good and well-balanced personal life is essential both to avoiding burnout and to being a good therapist who knows something about "normal families." One of my colleagues once said he knew he had confidence he could learn something from me when he heard I played on a women's soccer team and was vice-president of my kid's PTA.

Strategic therapy often involves pushing or stressing points in a sequence to get the system to change. This is done by reframing the way family members perceive the meaning of a sequence or by giving tasks or directives to family members or by restraining various members from changing. For this reason, strategic therapy is often viewed as manipulative and/or dehumanizing. Obviously, if it were, strategic therapists would not last long in private practice unless they had a wealthy grandparent or a generous patron.

In truth, no therapy, and most especially strategic therapy, can occur except in the context of a very powerful relationship and one in which the perceived intent of the therapist is basically benign. The part of strategic therapy least often described or shown on videotapes is the hours of mundane relationship building or the hours spent patiently coaching someone through a crisis over the phone. The process of pushing family members to change involves lots of getting to know each other and lots of emotional support to family members under stress at a given moment.

Family therapy developed from an exciting set of new ideas that were a radical departure from established epistemologies about treatment. The emphasis in the early development of the field was on these differences, often in a way that disaffected many of our professional colleagues. The private practitioner's reputation and livelihood depend heavily on the goodwill and mutual respect of the larger professional community. We have struggled to develop our skills in joining families at their "view of the world" in order to help them change. We must learn to expand our sensitivities to include similar tact, mutual respect, careful communication, and time invested in working with our professional community. More than any other, the context of private practice provides a crucible for interdisciplinary collaboration and creative integration.

3 Michaelin Reamy-Stephenson

Psychiatric Inpatient Units

Private psychiatric hospitals began to emerge in the United States in the latter half of the nineteenth century. To a family of "means" these private hospitals offered some relief from the disgrace and humiliation that accompanied commitment of a family member to a state insane asylum. Earlier in the century, state institutions had emerged to treat "distraught" persons, who began to be perceived by the professional community as sick and amenable to treatment and therefore to be separated from the delinquent and indigent (Hollingshead and Redlich, 1958).

During the past decade private psychiatric hospitals have mushroomed. The increased demand for these institutions seems related to three factors. Of primary importance was the nationwide trend of releasing patients held in state institutions, as a result of court decisions establishing patients' rights to mental health treatment in the least restrictive environment possible. A second factor is perhaps a greater level of acceptance of mental health treatment by the general public. Another possible factor is that private psychiatric hospitals, owing to relatively low construction costs, offer incentives for investors over general care hospitals.

A number of private facilities offer elegant surroundings, creating the aura of an idyllic vacation spot for the wealthy. Certainly substantial means and/or good insurance coverage are necessary prerequisites for private psychiatric hospitalization. As a general rule, when a private patient's resources are exhausted (or insurance coverage ceases), the patient is discharged or transferred to a state hospital. It is not unusual today for families to exhaust all possible means and incur tremendous debts in order to maintain a family member in such a facility.

The focus of this chapter is not whether psychiatric hospitalization is the treatment of choice. Certainly, studies conducted by the Denver group (Langsley and others, 1968) indicate that family crisis therapy is a more economical and less stigmatizing form of treatment than hospitalization. However, psychiatric hospitals are very much a part of traditional mental health care.

In our culture the physician is widely perceived as having the keys to life and death, as the "font of all wisdom." The psychiatric hospital staffed by numerous psychiatrists and allied staff could be described as a "collective doctor." Such hospitals represent the end of the line, the ultimate authority on a person's mental state. One might say the mental hospital functions as the "supreme court" in determining the belief system of patients and families about themselves and each other. Most typically, these institutions are based on a linear, monadic epistemology rather than an ecosystemic epistemology. Problems are seen as inside a person's head rather than as in the interrelationships between and among persons. The linear epistemology combined with the power of this "collective doctor" can contribute greatly to the undermining of families. If the patient is not to blame, then the family members must be. This same linear thinking is applied to staff. If morale is low and burnout high, the tendency is to blame particular persons—the administrator, the director, the social worker, the charge nurse.

In the following pages I will describe my experience developing and practicing family therapy in a private psychiatric hospital. I found my involvement with the hospital system strikingly analogous to the journey one follows with families in therapy. Changing belief systems and clarifying hierarchies were central to my work, as were joining, assessment, developing strategies and interventions, dealing with resistance, and experiencing the personal exhilaration that comes with significant change. The journey was complete with anticipatory enthusiasm, mountain vistas, treacherous passes, bursts of sunlight, and boundless opportunities for learning.

The Therapy/Work Setting

The Context. I was hired as a social worker "with family and group therapy skills" for a twenty-four-bed adult treatment unit (for men and women aged eighteen and up) at a private psychiatric hospital located in a fast-growing county combining Bible Belt rural and small-town life with rapid suburban development. Having long been one of the few alternatives to state institutions, this private psychiatric hospital was still perceived locally as a place for "crazy folks" and alcoholics. Adult patients typically carried diagnoses of schizophrenia, various affective disorders, and borderline personality.

The new unit director, Steve Howard, had, within the last three months, done a remarkable job in converting the unit from a custodial care "attending" model to a therapeutic community. The therapeutic community was directed toward using the social milieu to augment change through peer pressure, group process, and a level system. The level system gave patients the opportunity to earn degrees of freedom based on degrees of responsible behavior.

Although the director had some experience in family therapy, the demands of his position left him little time for seeing families. The interdisciplinary treatment team was made up of the director (psychiatrist), social worker (myself), rotating nursing staff (charge nurse, R.N., three psychiatric assistants), psychologist, and activities therapist, as well as the patients' attending psychiatrists. Patients were divided into two groups for group therapy led by the director and me as coleaders as well as one or two rotating members from the nursing staff. A community meeting for all patients on the unit was held once a week to discuss level changes and "therapeutic passes." Treatment planning was held weekly. The attending physicians attended treatment planning, but they did not participate, as a rule, in group therapy or community meetings. Thus, they were considerably more peripheral. Their interactions with the patients were primarily on a one-to-one basis for individual therapy.

Early Observations. Very little family therapy had been carried out on this unit during the previous years. The little that had been done appeared to have been typically directed toward helping the family adjust to having a schizophrenic member. When I arrived on the scene, I was eager to begin family therapy; however, I put some reins on my fervent eagerness. Having once experienced a concussion from diving into a lake without knowing what I was getting into, I moved slowly. I had made a study of change theory in graduate school, which reminded me again of the importance of moving slowly and of involving others in the change process.

I purposely spent a lot of time observing—gathering information with my eyes and ears while I participated in group therapy, community meetings, and treatment planning. One of the first things I noticed was that it appeared difficult for staff (particularly day-shift staff, who were not present during visiting hours) to see the patient as an active part of a family system. It is interesting that family therapy was a required part of the adolescent treatment program. It appears more difficult for many professionals to see the relevance of the family to the treatment of adult patients. Being caring people, the staff often became emotionally involved with the patients. This involvement sometimes became operational in a cross-generational coalition, with the staff member joining a child against the parents or an adult against the spouse. The situation was ripe for coalitions—patients rarely entered the hospital unless some kind of family conflict was involved, such as an overdose following the threat of divorce or "uncontrollable behavior" of a spouse or child.

Patients would complain in group therapy and in unstructured time about their spouses or parents. Accepting the patients' perception as the "objective truth," fellow patients and, perhaps more subtly, staff members could easily come to perceive (ˆ ɪd sometimes treat) family members who telephoned, wrote letters, and visited as somewhere high on the "monster continuum." (Understandably, when I did begin to contact families, I often found them feeling blamed and alienated from the patient and the hospital.)

In retrospect, in the beginning I think I was called on to "bring in families" for one of three reasons. The attending psychiatrist (and sometimes the nursing staff) was feeling helpless in dealing with environmental stresses described in the social history as related to hospitalization, such as loss of employment. As a social worker, I was a natural for this task. Second, some families had become problems for the psychiatrist and the hospital. Typically, an overly involved mother would be calling the psychiatrist and nursing station constantly to check on her son's medication and offer advice. I remember one case in which the father was particularly vocal about the dust under his daughter's dresser. Here still, staff seemed to be concerned about taking care of the family so that treatment could proceed efficiently, rather than thinking that changes in the family would have much to do with alleviating the patient's symptomatology. It seemed that unless the family was being intrusive or disruptive, the assumption was that the patient had a "supportive" family. (I soon saw that what these supportive families were usually supporting was the patient's role as identified patient.) Occasionally I was asked to "see a family" as a last resort if the patient was not responding to the treatment program involving individual, group, and activities therapy and often psychotropic medication.

One of the most memorable requests for "bringing in the spouse" was during the period when I was doing a lot of observing. The request followed this episode: The identified patient was an attractive, flamboyant woman in her early thirties who had become infamous in the hospital circuit. The rumor was that staff members had even been fired at other hospitals because of conflicts about her treatment. She was loud and exceedingly disruptive on the unit, constantly trying to convert patients, staff members, and visitors to her faith. She would enter other patients' rooms, open their drawers, and get into their private belongings. However, in time she gradually responded to peer pressure and natural consequences, and her charm began to win out. In group therapy and on the unit she complained bitterly about her very stingy husband, who locked up their checkbook and financial records and spent all the time in the basement looking at dirty pictures. Word spread among patients and staff. She found some young males (from the adolescent unit) particularly sympathetic to her plight. When her husband came to visit, he was met with suspicious looks and sometimes glares. One night he came to visit and refused to honor his wife's request for money. The patient ran over to join the adolescents, and her husband left in disgust. As he left the hospital, the adolescents leaned out the window taunting him. One young man shouted, "Pervert!" The husband then stormed up the stairs and slugged the adolescent, confirming everyone's belief that he was the villain.

It was time for family therapy. I had a hunch there might be another side to the story. There was. The husband claimed his wife had 450 outfits. The space under every bed in the house was stuffed with shoe boxes (as there was no room in the closets). He claimed the patient had been running up $300 phone bills each week (to her family) from the hospital pay phone. Until recently, he had been "walking on eggs," not setting any limits. He said he had been responding to a former doctor's advice not to put his wife under any undue stress. He had even been paying for the local dry cleaner's to do all the family laundry. Recently, on the verge of bankruptcy, he had "got fed up" and started clamping down. That case was an eye-opener for me and the rest of the team.

The Hospital Belief System. I began to study the hospital system in the same way I had learned to study families: focusing on the issues of belief system and hierarchy; training my eye to pinpoint dysfunctional sequences. I found an interesting mélange of belief systems. Certainly the medical model, with its assumptions of linear causality and focus on pathology, was most prevalent among the attending psychiatrists and some of the members of the nursing staff. However, some key members of the nursing staff, inspired by a young and charismatic psychiatric assistant (skilled in Gestalt therapy), shared the assumption that people could change. Critically important, the director of the unit held this belief. His arrival several months before had given a fresh perspective and a "shot in the arm" to the belief system on the unit. Staff were far more likely to see patients experiencing their first hospitalization as capable of change.

And then there were the "lifers"—those patients who were there to get stabilized through medication and hospital structure, with the expectation of their families and staff that they would be back again. These patients were seen consistently as sick or crazy. And assuming that "what you look for determines what you find," they provided many grounds (hallucinations, delusions, bizarre behavior) to qualify as having schizophrenia. Particularly distressing, I began to see how easily first-time patients could move into the ranks of the "lifers." Just a month or even weeks before, they had been sent home with the support and good wishes of the staff and community. They had earned their way up the level system by attending activities and being responsible group members. They had often done a lot of "growing," having, among other things, learned how to ask for what they wanted. Yet, I saw a number of them returning to the hospital, having regressed to their state before the previous hospitalization.

I thought I detected amid the more visible signs of frustration and hopelessness a glimmer of self-satisfaction and perhaps revenge on the part of the parents or spouse. It was as if by their expressions they were saying, "See, he (or she) is the problem, and you haven't cured him (or her)." I began to see that perhaps the only way they could compensate for feeling blamed and a failure as parents or spouses was to prove that the hospital had not succeeded where they had failed. And very quickly the pattern became established within the family, and between the family and the hospital, that when the going got rough on the outside, it was time for the fragile and vulnerable identified patient to return to the hospital.

The Hierarchy. The hospital hierarchy was complex and inherently confusing. There were essentially two formal hierarchies as well as the inevitable informal one. In the primary hospital hierarchy each member of the adult treatment team reported to the hospitalwide director of the department representing his or her particular discipline (social services, nursing, and so forth). The second formal hierarchy consisted of individual team members who, as peers, reported to the unit director. Staff members wore two or perhaps three or more hats. Several of the physicians who held positions in the formal hospital hierarchy (medical director, director of admissions) were themselves attending psychiatrists. To further complicate matters, there was the inevitable informal hierarchy among attending psychiatrists. There was also an informal hierarchy among adult team members, defined by clinical expertise and demonstration of leadership.

In a very general way, the primary formal hierarchy was defined through decision making on a myriad of administrative issues such as supervision of the stringent documentation needed to maintain hospital accreditation and third-party payments. The second formal hierarchy was largely defined through decision making and supervision related to clinical work.

In respect to formal hierarchy, the hierarchy concerned with hospitalwide issues was the most powerful. Attention to documentation (for example, ensuring the presence of a social history and progress notes in each chart) had to be top priority. Meeting hospitalwide responsibilities at times meant missing group therapy or rescheduling a family session. If the responsibilities defined by the primary hierarchy were carried out conscientiously, one's clinical work defined by the second hierarchy could be carried out with a minimum of disruption from the hospital administration. In my case meeting my responsibilities in each of these intertwined hierarchies necessitated fifty- to sixty-hour work weeks. Willingness to put in considerable extra unpaid hours appears to have minimized the inevitable pull between my clinical responsibilities on the adult unit and my hospitalwide social service responsibilities. If I had been unable to devote the extra time needed to meet these dual responsibilities that observations of others caught in this "tug-of-war" suggest, conflict would have been considerably more frequent, and time for clinical work (particularly family therapy) would have been sacrificed (compare Chapter Nine).

I found the hospital a fertile ground for cross-generational coalitions. Haley (1980) has noted the possibility that the more cross-generational coalitions an identified patient is involved in, the more extreme the symptomatology—in this case, the "crazier-acting" the identified patient. Having a treatment team that is ostensibly responsible for treatment as well as attending psychiatrists who have primary responsibility for their patients makes a confused hierarchy inevitable. Most of the attending psychiatrists saw their patients individually three times a week and had contact with the team only once a week, at treatment planning. Triangles between attending psychiatrist, treatment team (or members of the team), and patient seemed to me more easily avoided if attending physicians saw themselves as part of the team and attended daily staff meetings. If a triangle did develop, the attending psychiatrist inevitably tended to fill the role of the good father or mother who dropped in periodically while the active team members (director, social worker [myself], and nursing staff) were responsible for setting limits.

Other triangles involved the patient, day nursing shift, and evening shift (or members of these shifts). Most of the structured activities therapy took place on the day shift. Acting out on the part of patients tended to occur in the evening hours. Often a patient who had preferred status and was seen as doing well by the day staff was seen as a troublemaker by the night shift. Staff members had differential investment in patients, which predictably led to further triangulation. These triangles became particularly visible at times when patients were in conflict with one another or were requesting level changes and therapeutic passes.

I remember one case in which these coalitions were particularly evident. Linda was a woman in her early twenties, diagnosed as schizophrenic. I had conducted a few family sessions and saw the problem as a severe leaving-home issue (Haley,

1980). Linda had been "overinvolved" with her father, in coalition against her mother. When she was about twelve, her father had been drafted into the Army and sent overseas. She had responded by curling up in her bed, refusing to move until the Army released her father. And it did. I had become increasingly fascinated with an observation that when an identified patient is hospitalized, the same patterns that are dysfunctional at home tend to be continued over the telephone, during visiting hours, and on passes. If Linda demanded six quarts of soda delivered to the hospital doorstep immediately, her father would bring it. In addition, the patterns appear to be replicated on the unit. In this case "walking on eggs" was the general response of staff and patients alike, as Linda was perceived as especially fragile. This was particularly ironic to me in light of this young woman's competence. Not only had she survived three years as a chef for a fast-food operation, but she had fought the U.S. Army single-handed and won. Periodically, just before community meetings (when there was a high level of tension on the unit), she would curl up on her bed. Her nursing staff psychiatric assistant, Tom (who had been assigned to her at the request of her attending psychiatrist), would attend to her anxiously. Other staff members (replicating the role of her mother) would be furious that she was getting special attention; however, they were hesitant to be firm, as there was a subtle threat of disapproval from her attending psychiatrist. As time of discharge from the hospital approached, Linda became unusually mad. I began looking at hierarchy and found seven cross-generational coalitions readily apparent: Linda and father against mother; Linda and mother against father; Linda and attending psychiatrist against father; Linda, attending psychiatrist, and nursing staff counselor against the team; Linda and nursing staff counselor against the rest of the team; night nurse and Linda against the day shift; Linda and the director of nursing against staff.

Conduct of Therapy in the Setting

Introducing an Ecosystemic Therapy. While gathering the observations just described, I was, of course, participating as a staff member and as coleader of group therapy and the weekly community meeting. My observations led me to "chomp at the bit," wanting desperately to advocate for the virtues of strategic family therapy, to point out my (as well as other staff members') participation in dysfunctional sequences in an attempt to clarify the hierarchy. I saw the importance of family systems therapy for virtually all the patients—not just for those whose families were being disruptive to the hospital system. In spite of attempts to rein in on my enthusiasm, I was pushing, and the system resisted.

For example, just after I had joined the unit, a triangle developed between the admissions social worker, the nursing staff, and me. My positive belief about the patients and interest in the importance of family therapy were apparently coming across as blame to the nursing staff. They complained to the admissions social worker that I sat in my private offices and had no idea what it was like working all day on the unit. They accepted my offer to try to "walk in their moccasins" for a day by serving on the nursing staff, and I did so. This experience had the effect of breaking up the triangle and giving me another view of patients and the reality of the nursing staff. I learned a lot from it. For example, while carrying out patient-centered duties such as individual charting and taking of vital signs, I found myself focusing more on the identified patient and less on interactions of patients and staff. A felt sense of lack of private space emerged immediately. I was more readily irritated in my interactions with patients. I believe this experience led to my later becoming an advocate with administration for expressions of appreciation and improved working conditions for nursing staff.

I found it increasingly helpful to use with the hospital system the same assumptions about avoiding resistance that worked with family systems. I toned down my enthusiasm. Like Johnny Appleseed, I started small, "seeding" ideas—for example, sharing with staff members the husband's side of the story to contrast with the wife's claims of his stinginess, seeding the idea that there was more than one view and that the husband's and wife's behavior fit into a pattern. I made an effort to connect what was being seen by the staff with what I was seeing in the family.

Essentially all my interventions were directed toward finding commonalities between myself and various members of the hospital system. This was the pattern I followed in my own family of origin, and so it felt quite natural. I spent time joining with different levels of the hierarchy—getting to know people on a personal level. I worked very hard to avoid becoming part of cross-generational coalitions among staff members. My belief in nonobjective reality stood me in good stead. I saw other staff members as having another perception, not as needing enlightenment. I worked hard to find a common language. There were many opportunities for reframing, particularly during treatment planning. I didn't make an issue out of calling an overinvolved mother and child a "cross-generational coalition." "Symbiosis" would do. It was helpful to use Gestalt or Transactional Analysis (TA) language, with which some of the staff were familiar. Interestingly, over time, staff began to use systemic language.

It was particularly important to acknowledge to myself that there was a lot I did not know and a lot I could learn from others. Not being afraid to ask for help was important. It was essential to try to get beyond my own need for success, for a pat on the back, and to give others credit for their contributions. As with families, avoiding blame was central. It was important to respect the hierarchy, to acknowledge that the admitting psychiatrist had official case control even if our belief systems and approach differed drastically.

I took special care to take developing interests and amplify them. The admissions social worker (who was responsible for social histories for my unit) had had some exposure to family systems theory. Her increased interest led to more and more notes in her social histories pointing out dysfunctional family sequences, which I believe led to more referrals for family therapy. I appreciated this and expressed my appreciation.

I knew that if change was to occur (if family systems therapy was to become an integral part of treatment), staff at all levels of the hierarchy had to be involved in the change. Bringing in key members of the nursing staff as cotherapists in family sessions proved worthwhile in this endeavor. As interest in family systems increased, I received a request from the hospital's staff development coordinator to do an in-service on family therapy. Using a recent difficult case (in which we had successfully combined treatment on the unit, individual therapy, and family therapy), I developed a role play, asking team members from all levels of the hierarchy and departments to participate. Personal letters of invitation were sent to the medical director and attending psychiatrists.

In summary, no matter how valuable a modality family therapy was and no matter how much support I had from the director, it was important to move slowly and to work at all levels of the hierarchy, involving as many staff members as possible in the change process. Strategies for introducing family therapy were based on the assumption that resistance lies between people, not in a resistant client or colleague.

Danger and Opportunity. It seemed clear to me that we, as staff members, were often caught up in dysfunctional sequences with identified patients, as were family members. That is, we were repeating "attempted solutions" that were further exacerbating the problem, and as a self-fulfilling prophecy we were underlining the belief system that the identified patient was sick and hopeless.

I remembered the Chinese sign for crisis (composed of two parts, the words for danger and opportunity) and Milton Erickson, who consistently utilized what could appear to be an insurmountable liability and turned it into a force for change. It occurred to me that there might be a powerful parallel process— a synergism that could result from working with family and hospital unit in a parallel way. I shared my thoughts with the director, who had similar ideas. In sharing commonalities from his rich background in group therapy and organizational systems and my experience with strategic family therapy, we found ourselves more and more speaking the same language. In working together, we found that we shared a belief in the possibility for change in even the most seemingly "hopeless" individuals. With the increased involvement of other staff members, we began sharing our thinking more with the team. Everyone on the team had something to contribute, and there was much energy and excitement.

The developing focus became twofold—changing the belief system and clarifying the hierarchy. Assuming that how you define a problem determines how you go about solving it, *changing the belief system* of the hospital staff as well as the patient, his or her family, and other interfacing systems was critical. The longer the individual had been defined as the identified patient (and the more hospitalizations), the more other systems such as the extended family, neighborhood, or work settings had to be involved. With a few shared successes the belief system of the team was beginning to change. I had a hard time containing my enthusiasm with the team. I got a lot of teasing. The charismatic young psychiatric assistant playfully called me "God's advocate." The director reminded me, "Not every cloud has a silver lining; some are lined with cheap Dacron and polyester."

The second focus was on *clarifying the hierarchy* within the hospital, within the family, and between these systems. As described earlier, accepting as a "reality" the first formal hierarchy—the hierarchy describing hospitalwide department duties —as the primary hierarchy and giving careful attention to the duties prescribed by this hierarchy did much to reduce the inherent tug-of-war between my responsibilities to the hospitalwide social services department and my responsibilities on the adult unit (compare Chapter Nine).

Particularly helpful was the assumption on the adult unit from the beginning implementation of the therapeutic community that a clear hierarchy between patients and staff should exist. As in functional families—and against common therapeutic community ideology—there was no pretense that this was a true democracy. Patients had freedom to the degree that they showed responsible behavior and self-control. When they did not, the staff took charge. Our work on the adult unit was directed toward avoiding the kinds of cross-generational coalitions described in the case of the competent young woman whose behavior had brought her father home from the Army. Essentially, we worked toward developing a united front among staff members. A number of changes were made. A daily early morning team meeting was instituted in which information could be shared from family sessions, nursing report, and individual sessions. Here strategies for the day were developed. Attending psychiatrists were invited to these meetings. An emphasis was placed on involving the attending psychiatrists in treatment planning. This emphasis often meant being flexible to fit their schedule and being more sensitive to their possibly feeling "pushed out" by the team. Several changes were instituted to avoid conflict between nursing shifts. For example, treatment planning was moved later in the day to accommodate individuals from both shifts.

Several procedures related to family therapy were instituted. Inviting attending psychiatrists and key nursing staff members (who held prominent positions in the informal hierarchy) to act as cotherapists or "sit in" for part of a family session helped maintain a more united front. The referring psychiatrist was given credit for recognizing a family problem. In a parallel way, nursing staff were given credit for recognizing dysfunctional sequences among family and staff at visiting hours.

Our attempts to create a united front among staff, though not completely successful, cut down substantially on coalitions that crossed hierarchal levels. Having a vehicle (a regular staff meeting) for processing staff conflicts often facilitated the breaking up of coalitions before they became rigid.

Use of Medication. The unit director's belief was that psychotropic medication should be used to relieve symptoms of depression and anxiety, in amounts that would facilitate, rather than block, positive learning and behavioral change. His further assumption was that, ideally, the medication would be gradually reduced through the period of discharge and eventually eliminated when the patient had demonstrated a period of well functioning in his or her natural environment.

However, control of medication rested with the patient's attending psychiatrist (compare Chapter Eleven). Although, as a rule, the director was more conservative in his use of medication than the other psychiatrists, he chose to deal with issues of medication indirectly. He recognized that medication is often prescribed as a means of reducing acting-out behavior disruptive to the hospital system. He therefore concentrated on developing a highly structured program with prescribed limits and natural consequences for behavior. Interestingly, as this structure became well established both on the unit and within the patient's family, acting-out behavior declined. At the same time, the prescription of medication by attending physicians dropped substantially. Exceptions occurred when the team had joined poorly with an attending psychiatrist who, feeling excluded from the change process of his or her patient, appeared to cling to the prescribing of medication as some vestige of control.

Parallel Process with Families

If it is important for staff members to be a part of changes while a patient is on the unit, it is infinitely more important for the family, the primary social system (from which the patient came and to which he or she will return), to be part of the change. As a general rule, I found, the longer the person had been labeled as an identified patient and the more hospitalization, the more interfacing systems needed to be involved (for example, extended family members, employee assistance, fellow employees, and even employers). The critical factor here appears to be the belief system. If a person is perceived as "crazy," he or she will be responded to as "crazy" and, in turn, will act crazy. The more people see the patient as crazy, the more the problem is perpetuated.

One of the first things I did as I began to see families was to search out themes in the ideology of the therapeutic community that were consistent with moving toward better functioning of the family system. There were a number of "group norms" that were indeed consistent, such as balancing belonging and autonomy, providing natural consequences for behavior, encouraging initiative, avoiding "family secrets," normalizing life-stage logjams (leaving home, empty nest, retirement), and believing in change. My position of leadership in group and community meetings (and, of course, family sessions) provided many opportunities to amplify these norms—and opportunities to ignore or downplay norms that were less helpful. For example, I have seen the norm of "me first" (which seems very prevalent in therapeutic communities), symbolized in the song *I Did*

It My Way, wreak havoc in marriages and families. If the family were not involved in therapy, it was a sure disaster. Typically, the wife would go home on a pass, "tell off" her husband, and receive accolades from the group on her return. If she had indeed been behaving like a doormat in the past, the husband (and often his extended family) would respond to this change by focusing even more on her "craziness." Often the wife's demanding that her needs be met above all else was part of the very behavior that was the problem.

Working with the family within this context had some constraints not operating in outpatient therapy. Interventions directed toward a drastic unbalancing of the system were not appropriate. Not only would this not be tolerated by the conservative hospital system that typically responds to crises with medication and restraints; but also, the patient is, of course, confined in the hospital. A step-by-step process that worked analogously to the therapeutic community's level system seemed to work best.

Taking Referrals. Referrals were taken only directly from an attending psychiatrist. I found that the degree of success of my work was integrally related to the belief system and behavior of the particular attending physician with whom I was coordinating treatment. The most critical factor for a positive outcome seemed to be the physician's tendency to focus on the "core of health," the strengths and assets of the individual and family, rather than on pathology. An attending physician with whom we shared the most "successes" had a sampler on his office wall that read: "A ship in a harbor is safe, but that is not what ships are built for." These collaborations also worked best when the attending physician (or family therapist) was interested in a team success more than a personal triumph.

There was far less success when I was working with an attending physician who seemed alienated from the team. Predictably, in such cases the patient became triangulated between the attending physician and the team. Unfortunately, the resulting battle could involve an attending physician's clinging to a focus on pathology as we focused on strengths. This split often replicated splits in the family. An attempt by any therapist to "re-raise" a child, to replace the natural parents of a patient, under-mined the family system. The most difficult situation for me personally was working with attending physicians who, with the best of intentions, nurtured dependency, weaknesses, and pathology in the patient. I found these physicians often to be compassionate and conscientious and to have the highest ethical standards. This often meant they spent more time with their patients, which, ironically, made my work far more difficult.

Initiating Family Therapy. After the referral was made, I first contacted the patient, normalizing the feelings of anxiety about meeting with his or her family that were often present. Through experience I found it important to clarify the differences between family therapy and other forms of therapy the patient had experienced—specifically, to note that family members (including the patient) would not be asked to "bare their souls." Often the patient's anxiety seemed related to a feeling that he or she was responsible for directing the outcome of the family session. (Certainly many identified patients seem to have an inordinate sense of responsibility for other family members.) I made it clear that directing the session was my responsibility.

In working with a multitude of inpatient families, I essentially never saw a family that did not have flagrant cross-generational coalitions. The most destructive ones appeared to be covert and less obvious (Haley, 1976). This observation led me to establish structure from the beginning phone contact. If the patient was married, I would contact the spouse and arrange to see the couple without their children, to underline that subsystem. I found the spouse typically very protective of the children and reluctant to bring them to the hospital environment. After joining with the spouse and developing a more normalized frame, parents were usually willing to include their children if that seemed appropriate. If at all possible, family sessions were held at an outpatient clinic adjoining the hospital rather than on the unit. Even if unresolved marital conflict appeared to be the issue, I found that meeting with the entire family, with a focus on relieving the children from predictable feelings of responsibility, was an important preventive measure.

If the patient was a dependent child, I took great pains to

speak to both parents (together if they had an extension telephone) in setting up the initial session as well as in future contacts. This procedure was especially productive if one parent
was involved and one peripheral. An implicit message was communicated—that the two were equally important in their child's
treatment and life. In one case of this sort, an overly involved
mother (who had been harassing the nursing staff with constant
phone calls) showed up alone for the first session in spite of my
having contacted both parents. I saw her for a brief fifteen-min-
ute session, explaining that I would also need to see her husband for fifteen minutes before the first family session could
commence. After that they both came to sessions without further interventions on my part.

It seems important to clarify that a "dependent child"
could be eighteen or thirty-five. An assumption of dependency
was based not on physical proximity but primarily on financial
dependence. If a thirty-year-old patient was living on his own
yet was financially dependent on his parents, it was assumed
that leaving-home issues were involved and that it was appropriate to involve the parents in family therapy. (Certainly there
were circumstances in which a patient was financially independent but involved in recursive sequences with parents in which
it was still helpful to involve the parents in the therapy.)

A perennial problem in family therapy is getting the family to come in in the first place. In the private psychiatric hospital context, the therapist usually has a "lever," as family therapy
can be easily framed as reducing the length of hospitalization. However, this lever is not enough. I found it most helpful
to "feel into" the family system at that point in time—to anticipate that family members would be feeling blamed, hopeless,
and angry at the identified patient and past therapists and
would be experiencing fears about finances (usually in direct
proportion to the number of hospitalizations). Above all, it was
helpful not to label the problem a marital or family problem
(that, for the layperson, is synonymous with bad parenting). I
learned that resistance can often be prevented before it develops. A good admissions social worker can help immensely with
this process through a nonthreatening, nonblaming attitude. My

focus was on asking for help, stressing how important family members were as resources, how much they knew that I didn't know. I seeded the possibility of breaking the revolving-door cycle of hospitalization that had been such a burden to the family. In my position as social worker for the hospital, I offered to help with any liaison problems they were having with the hospital. I remember one spouse who sat anxiously preoccupied for two sessions until I realized that she had been waiting to receive an overdue letter from the hospital that was necessary for her husband to continue receiving his salary. This was a rich opportunity for an enactment for a couple who had difficulty advocating for themselves. With my support they went to the appropriate office and requested the necessary document.

The best time to schedule the first session seemed to be early enough to prevent further alienation of the family but late enough to assure some "progress" (to give credibility to the therapist as a representative of the hospital). Any observed progress was credited to the parents or framed as indicating strengths in the individual and family.

Most people like to know what to expect. The nature of the hospital context and the state of chaos of these families perhaps makes it even more important to make clear what will happen in therapy. Levels of anxiety seemed to be visibly reduced when I described the problem-solving nature of therapy and made it clear that I was not interested in "pointing fingers"— that not only was that destructive, but also I had found that things were not that simple. Clients were given a chance to ask any questions or express any concerns (to me or to the attending physician if present). I then explained that I would be asking each of them questions and proceeded with the assessment model developed at the Mental Research Institute (MRI) in Palo Alto (Watzlawick, Weakland, and Fisch, 1974), involving a description of the problem, the attempted solutions, the outlining of goals, and the determination of the world view of family members. I found it most helpful to predict that they would naturally have different views of the problem and, understandably, feel uncomfortable when someone else was expressing his or her view.

Setting appropriate goals—the least amount of change that would be considered progress—was one of the more difficult tasks. Typically, client families seem to expect too much or too little. A typical unreasonably high goal of a husband for an apparently profoundly depressed wife would be "It will be progress when she's at home, doing all the housework, taking care of the kids, fixing my meals, and smiling like her old self." At the other extreme, I have seen a mother so stuck in her belief system about her "helpless, incompetent" son that she would define goals that he had already reached during the first two weeks of hospitalization. Family members were nudged toward developing measurable goals that were workable within the hospital context.

A central focus of the first session (though carried out by indirect means) was creating a sense of a "new beginning," the idea that this time things might be different. The possibility of change was seeded, often using the language of change—for example, commending the family for the first "giant step" their son had made in making a level change. I often used a task such as giving various family members a small slip of paper as they left the session on which I had written, "When you look at your wife [husband, son, daughter], can you tolerate the possibility that things can get better?" I warned them that they would have a tendency to answer the question too quickly.

Bringing Information Back to the Team. The information provided through the MRI assessment model was then shared with the team during treatment planning and morning staff meeting. On the basis of this information (and observations of the patient interacting on the unit) a working frame was developed. Some form of developmental frame usually worked well for young adults within the hospital context, based on level systems and the "letting out of reins." An "illusion of choice" was used. For example, a choice might be given between seeing Susan as a fourteen-year-old girl in the body of a twenty-five-year-old woman who was in desperate need of fourteen-year-old experiences (setting of parental limits) *or* as a chronic mental patient resting at a comfortable way station en route to the state hospital. This approach had the advantage of avoiding resistance by offering choice plus defusing inevitable "double messages," knowing that certainly some of the staff and perhaps the attending psychiatrist saw the patient as chronic. This illusion of choice was used in the family as well as on the unit. If the patient had a temper tantrum and stormed out of group therapy, this behavior could be used to confirm that he was a fourteen-year-old—or perhaps a two-and-a-half-year-old.

As a team, we became quite efficient at comparing the "attempted solutions" of the family with our own—determining from the family what was not working. I remember one case involving a forty-year-old woman who was considered profoundly depressed (she had been lying at home staring at the ceiling, ignoring her domestic responsibilities), who continued to go downhill in the hospital. She moved into what her attending physician feared was a psychotic depression. Several medications had been tried, to no avail. I was asked to bring in the family as a last resort. It became readily apparent that we as staff members (in individual and group therapy) were essentially applying the same solution as family members. In some shape or form, we were all trying to get her to "try harder." We apologized for a "misunderstanding." We acknowledged that we had not realized that, if anything, Mary had been trying too hard. We prescribed a week's vacation for Mary. My (psychiatric assistant) cotherapist suggested that she work on a suntan. During her "vacation" her only visits and phone conversations were to be with her husband. (This had the effect of strengthening the marital dyad and cutting off an older sister's constant "try harder" demands.) In group therapy, staff members made their apologies to Mary and stopped pursuing her. In two days her husband reported seeing the glimmer of a smile for the first time in several months.

As described above, "small-step goals" were defined by family members (with particular attention to the goals of the adults involved). Often parents complained that their son or daughter was irresponsible about money. The child was constantly "totaling" cars (which were promptly replaced) and abusing the use of credit cards (which were generously offered). Having the parents and child develop a budget for spending money on the unit, to include snacks and outings, was the first step toward learning financial responsibility. Sometimes a young person began work toward the grade equivalent degree (GED) while in the hospital.

Staff members often had their own ideas about goals for patients. It was usually possible to link an important treatment goal of the team with the value system of the family to make it viable. A very common situation involved a woman in her forties whose last child was reaching adolescence. Having married young, Sarah had typically centered her whole life on her husband and children. She found herself losing interest in cleaning house and cooking for a family who were scattered in many directions. Her husband, Bob (living and breathing "the work ethic"), perceived her as slacking off on her responsibilities and constantly complained about the state of the house. The situation peaked with Sarah taking an overdose and being hospitalized. Team members (as well as other patients) saw the importance of Sarah's developing some leisure activities or perhaps a part-time job to give her life some complexity. We were able to link Bob's work ethic with Sarah's "hardworking attempts" to learn to advocate for her own needs, which might mean some time for leisure activities after she got her housework completed. Bob was willing to accept this plan (as his own). Sarah was given an interest inventory by the psychologist; explored leisure pursuits with the activities therapist; and began using therapeutic passes to look for part-time employment. Thus, the treatment goals of the team were linked with the goals emerging from family therapy in support of relevant life tasks (Stanton and Schwartz, 1954).

Using Rituals of the Therapeutic Community. The rituals of group therapy and community meetings were valuable opportunities for reframing, "tacking down" frames, amplifying strengths, and gently nudging the group norms in a direction consistent with progress toward well functioning (Berger, in press; Dammann and Berger, 1983). Both the director and the psychiatric assistant (the staff members most involved in group therapy) had been well trained in Gestalt therapy. Their emphasis on gaining closure combined well with my interest in avoiding family secrets. Together with the other team members, we developed some general guidelines for group therapy. Consistent with my observations of family communication patterns, many patients spoke "about" someone in the group. (Rather than saying, "Tom, I think you're spending too much time in your room," the patient would say, "I think Tom is spending too much time in his room.") We spent a lot of time emphasizing direct communications in group, and these communication experiences seemed to have an effect on family communication (and vice versa). Consistent with the developing norm of valuing direct communications, patients in marital therapy were discouraged from discussing their marriages outside the session— that is, in group therapy or in the community.

The ritual of the community meeting provided an opportunity for reframing patient behaviors, as in the following example. Simon, a man in his late twenties, was diagnosed as schizophrenic. He could be seen as a throwback to the 1960s hippie generation. Dressing in a bohemian fashion, he carried his belongings in a leather backpack to the dining room. This behavior, combined with his disheveled, unwashed appearance, became a negative focus for the community, made up of primarily rural or suburban, middle-class, Bible-belt folks. Simon ignored other patients' critical comments and became more and more alienated from the community, often disrupting group with long, amorphous monologues. Simon had some assets that were not being tapped, such as his extensive experience in drama and filmmaking. It seemed clear that until Simon joined the community, peer pressure would have little effect on his behavior. Michael Berger, one of my consultants, suggested the following intervention: At the next community meeting Simon began his intolerable monologue. Instead of sitting through the usual painful period of "walking on eggs" followed eventually by Simon's expulsion from the group, I looked squarely at him and said, "Simon, it's such a shame you insist on being so ordinary, bourgeois, hospital crazy when this community could really use a little artistic craziness." He stared at me silently for the rest of the meeting. It may have been a coincidence, but two weeks later he was busy using the hospital video equipment in filmmaking. Patients were heard expressing their appreciation to Simon for sharing a Russian play and a multilingual Bible that he had stashed away in his knapsack.

One of the most difficult tasks was coordinating a homework task given at a family session with the granting of a therapeutic pass, which was the prerogative of the community. (Passes and level changes required the backing of at least one staff member and the majority of patients.) Here it is perhaps particularly obvious why good staff coordination was critical to the working of family therapy in this context. A team session before the community meeting helped by giving staff the opportunity to discuss the timing and parameters of passes. However, there was never enough time for all the processing needed. Therefore, much of the nudging and maneuvering had to be done in the actual community meeting. For example, one of the group norms (for women) that was not always helpful was that the patient should go home on the first pass and not do anything—just relax and be a guest. However, many of these women came from "all or nothing" households. They either did all the housework or came to the hospital letting their resentful husbands take over all of it. I remember one community meeting where the group accepted my modification (decided earlier in a family session) that Annie could do (only) an hour and a half of ironing, which would allow her husband to spend a comparable amount of time on his neglected woodworking.

There was one group norm that I worked particularly hard to change. One of the most recurrent themes expressed by patients (and often staff) was "I'll vote for your pass only if you promise that if things get bad, you'll come back [early] to the hospital." This norm gave me the horrors. I could see how we were participating in the development of the very internal map that guided the "revolving door" pattern of returning to the hospital after discharge. I worked on gradually nudging that norm by saying repeatedly, "I'd prefer that you stick it out through some predictable discomfort."

The telephone, visiting hours, and therapeutic passes could all be used as opportunities to break rigid patterns and restructure the family. Homework tasks could be carried out during visiting hours. For example, a pursuing wife could be asked to distance from her husband, or a playful fight could be prescribed. Passes were used as an opportunity for job interviews and for renewing outside friendships and support systems (for example, returning to membership at a local church). This process was immensely easier for inpatients who lived within a reasonable distance of the hospital. For patients who lived farther away, homework tasks were adapted to larger, less frequent blocks of time.

One of the beauties of strategic therapy, based on Ericksonian principles, is that what could appear to be a liability or even a disaster can be turned into an opportunity. One case in which this principle was particularly evident was also an example of how, in finding myself spinning my wheels as therapist, I changed my view, and reality changed with it. Roger, aged fifty, had been hospitalized for an aborted attempt to kill his boss and himself. Roger had been fired by his boss, after twenty-five years of apparently loyal service, when he had developed a possible heart condition. Roger saw his chest discomfort as developing after heavy lifting that was not part of his job description. Roger was charming and charismatic and emerged as a leader in the community. I admired Roger, and suspecting that a degree of racism was involved in the firing (Roger was black, the employer white), I found myself furious at his employer. Roger was clearly under terrific financial strain; utilities were being cut off and the bank threatening to foreclose on the mortgage. Meeting several times with Roger and his physically disabled wife, Edna, I focused on helping Roger apply his mortgage protection insurance and seek worker's compensation funds and unemployment benefits while he pursued a new job. Just before discharge I had a sense that I was spinning my wheels, that I was perhaps pushing my goals on Roger and his wife.

One day I was walking from the hospital with Roger and Edna for our appointment to be held in the adjoining building. A pickup truck filled with people pulled into the parking lot. Roger explained, "Those are my kids, they're waiting to pick up Edna after our meeting." I was dumbstruck. At that moment I realized that my mind set about the problem had led to my completely missing a crucial step—I had never even asked Roger about his children! Shifting gears on the spot (and with Roger's and Edna's approval), I invited the children into the session. Within ten minutes I found that, of the six young adults (four children and two spouses), all of whom lived with Edna and Roger, only one had a job. Roger, in his eloquent way, described his family by stating, "It's like the engine has broken down and all the cars are lying around in the railroad yard." He then added somewhat apologetically, "Before I came to the hospital, I had planned to get my house in order." Plans were made for the children to look for jobs. However, at the next meeting, the cars were still lying around in the railroad yard.

The very next day was a community meeting at which Roger applied for Level V, the top level, given only to patients who had demonstrated great responsibility and leadership in the community. Patients and staff alike began to offer their support for Level V. I took my turn, stating, "Roger, you have indeed been a leader in the community. However, I feel your tendency, if anything, is to take on more than your share of responsibility. I will be willing to vote for Level V after you demonstrate that you can share responsibility by 'getting your house in order.'" The community supported my suggestion. That was Wednesday. On Monday, Roger returned from a pass proudly stating that all but one of his young people had jobs. This was a good example of how a therapeutic community and family therapy can be used in a collaborative way.

Middle Family Sessions. Ideally, by the middle of family therapy, the belief system has turned around; that is, the patient/family/community has chosen the more normalizing frame. Symptoms have subsided and the patient has made progress within the community's level system. Rigid sequences have begun to give way to new patterns, and the hierarchy has begun to be clarified (through work in family sessions and on the unit, homework tasks, and so forth).

I have found that, as a general rule, what is important to remember in outpatient therapy is even more important to remember in inpatient therapy. Thinking in terms of the protective function of the symptoms is usually very helpful (Madanes,

1981). For example, when patients have developed symptoms during the leaving-home period (Haley, 1980), the symptoms can commonly be seen as providing a focus for a dysfunctional marriage. Haley notes that symptoms appear to emerge just before the child reaches the point that, in that particular family, means "ready to be on your own." Thus, in one family the measure may be high school graduation, and in another graduation from law school. A wife's episodes of depression can be seen as protecting her husband from facing an "empty retirement" by giving him a new job in caretaking. Although I do not find a focus on causality particularly helpful, the protection metaphor is useful in giving symptoms (even those perceived as hostile) a positive connotation. In any case, the child's symptoms seem to "fit" with the dysfunctional marriage or the wife's depression with the husband's upcoming retirement. It appears to be a familiar pattern among all human beings that if we focus on one problem, other issues get put on the back burner. When a family has a (perceived as) chronic member, one can be sure that they have put a lot of issues on the back burner, and the issues may have sat on the back burner so long that they're stuck there. Generally, the longer issues remain unattended to, the more formidable they appear.

In an early session, with this assumption in mind, I usually ask each family member how much time he or she spends thinking and worrying about the problem. Often one or more family members will acknowledge spending every waking moment with this focus. I usually make a ritual around this question, in which the exact amount of time is calculated (Dell and Goolishian, 1979). This gives the therapist early information on which family members need to get busy in their lives so they will not slip right back into the more comfortable, familiar focus on the patient. I then ask family members, as a homework task, to determine just what they would think about doing with their time and energy if the patient were going on with her life and they did not have to worry about her anymore. I tell them that it is natural to feel uncomfortable when they try to answer the question and that they should not move too fast, just barely begin to think about it. Information of all kinds emerges, which provides working material for family sessions and gives family members their own tasks while the patient is working on her tasks in the hospital and on home visits. A husband may work on developing leisure pursuits in preparation for retirement; a mother whose son is leaving home may begin working part-time, shifting her focus from her son; and so forth. I predict that as family members begin to work on their individual tasks (and couple tasks), the identified patient, out of caring, will no doubt provide a focus by escalating his or her behavior, sensing their discomfort and not knowing that they can handle going back and picking up the pieces of their lives. *Predicting a backslide appears to be critical in these families.* If it does occur (after the therapist's prediction), family members appear to pursue their tasks with even greater resolve.

An identified patient can be seen as serving a protective function on the hospital unit as well as in the family (Haley, 1980). David Jennings, a nineteen-year-old "diagnosed schizophrenic," had had a number of hospitalizations throughout the city and was well known for his bizarre behavior. There was severe conflict between Mrs. Jennings and her husband's extended family, who perceived Mrs. Jennings as a terrible mother, stating that David would be fine if it were not for his crazy mother. Mrs. Jennings received no support in this battle from her husband. David's behavior could be seen as serving a double protective function: First, it gave his parents a focus other than the conflict with extended family. Second, if David proved he was really sick and not just misbehaving, then his mother might be let off the hook. David worked very hard at this. Relatives had found him standing in their garage wrapped like a mummy in masking tape. He had shown up at a mental health clinic near his grandparents' home, covered with mud, claiming he had been buried alive.

David had made considerable progress in the hospital. His parents had been involved in treatment and had begun working together in parenting David. Unfortunately, however, I had not been successful in recruiting Mr. Jennings' extended family. As David moved toward discharge, predictably, conflict began to rise between Mrs. Jennings and the extended family. David began acting mildly intrusive and disruptive on the unit. At that time there was a lot of tension on the unit and an inordinate number of cross-generational coalitions involving staff and patients. David quickly became the focus of the unit, and there was talk of a possible administrative discharge. Interestingly, two other equally disruptive patients were hardly noticed. A special community meeting was held to deal with the growing sense of turmoil on the unit. As the community began to gather for the meeting, I had a sense of attending a witch trial. David entered the room. Rather than taking a seat with the rest of the community, who were sitting in chairs arranged in a circle, David sat on the floor in the middle of the circle. His look of expectation all but said, "Dump on me." David, with insistence from the staff, finally took his place in the circle. Immediately the focus of the meeting became David's disruptive behavior. One patient stated with disgust, "Even when he's not around, he's bugging me, that's all I talk about, he's taking over my life!"

I asked the patients what they would be thinking and talking about if David were not on their minds. There was silence. One woman said, "I guess I'd be thinking about going home on Friday and whether or not I'll get along with my husband." A man said, "I'd think about how hard it's going to be going back to work." Two patients (the other disruptive ones mentioned earlier), continuing to focus on David, stormed out of the room. David jumped up and followed them as if to take the heat off them. After the three young men were brought back into the room, the meeting continued. We were able to frame David's behavior as monumentally caring, pointing out how he was willing to sacrifice his life to protect not only his family but other patients and staff from their pain. Patients supported this frame, agreeing to attend to their own tasks. To solidify the change, a contract was made among members of the community that no one would talk to anyone else about a third person for a week. (The exception was staff talking in treatment planning.) After the patients were dismissed, the staff asked themselves the same question. We came up with all kinds of things we were avoiding—for example, frustration with particularly difficult cases and administrative issues (Stanton and Schwartz, 1954). I was able to bring this proof of David's caring, self-sacrificing nature to the next family session. Significantly, David's behavior improved dramatically, and patients and staff got back to business.

After the initial assessment has been carried out and some progress has been noticed, I find it particularly helpful to complete family genograms. I make a ritual of the process, using a large piece of paper, which I tape on the wall. Particularly for more visually oriented individuals, this seems to facilitate the process of stepping back and looking at one's life. This is particularly valuable for blended families where a "shared history" can be created. The genogram offers an opportunity to define family patterns, to see how symptoms fit in, and to determine value systems and is, therefore, a rich source of information for reframing (see Chapter Ten).

While middle sessions are being conducted with families, work toward breaking dysfunctional sequences on the unit continues. Positive reinforcement (through the level system and granting of passes) and in some cases "restraint from change" are used. Thus both sides of the illusion of choice are covered. If the more normalized frame is chosen—for example, the patient is seen as a fourteen-year-old in the body of a twenty-five-year-old—then "growing up" and working one's way up the level system are appropriate. If the "sick path" is chosen, then the patient and family can be encouraged to take the easier path and commended for doing so (for example, by pointing out how the easier path will allow family members to avoid dealing with those unpleasant "back burner" issues and to comfortably settle into devoting the rest of their lives to caring for their "sick" family member).

The patient works on goals that have grown out of the family session (perhaps supplemented by staff at treatment planning). In the case of a child, parents have from the beginning begun to negotiate guidelines for the child that are in effect while the child has a pass. The inevitable testing of limits that occurs during passes is useful material for family sessions. The therapist has many opportunities to normalize the patient's "adolescent" behavior and to support and amplify the parents' competence. In a comparable way, an adult patient has negotiated guidelines with his spouse or living partners. By the time of discharge, guidelines for living at home have been practiced.

Discharge. My position of involvement with the family, attending physician, and team placed me in the best position to orchestrate the discharge process. The ritual of discharge is an important one (see Chapter Eight). Haley (1980) has suggested that parents decide when a young adult is to leave the hospital. I have found this to be feasible when the attending physician, team, and family have worked well together. If they have, I have found the deciding factor for discharge to be whether the parental guidelines for living at home have been decided and well tested. If the attending physician was alienated from the team or coordination of treatment was poor, a precipitous discharge often led shortly to readmission.

I found it extremely important to predict a relapse at discharge and to normalize how much more difficult living together full-time will be. (Relapses have also been predicted at points during hospitalization when the patient was progressing "too fast.") It is important to have some plan that extends into the future on which to work so that going home from the hospital is not the final goal. With a young adult, for example, the plan might mean having a job lined up or intending to enroll in college or vocational school—the preliminary work having been done while in the hospital. I have found that parents of "mad" young people typically will say, "He can start paying for his gas and contributing to room and board after he finds a job"— which could be two years with that kind of offer! I find it more helpful for parents to set a time limit (Haley, 1980). For example, beginning a month from discharge, the young person must contribute $25 per week toward family expenses or move out. Usually he or she gets a job.

Dealing with the predictable stigma of psychiatric hospitalization was an integral part of the discharge process. The widely experienced "walking on eggs" behavior (around persons who have undergone psychiatric hospitalization) of extended family members, employers, colleagues, neighbors, and other professionals was anticipated and discussed openly. This behavior of the general public was framed as awkwardness related to fears growing out of ignorance and archaic perceptions of psychiatric hospitals as insane asylums. Patients were framed as the well-informed enlightened ones whose task it was to put these persons (who knew of their hospitalization) at ease by initiating a matter-of-fact dialogue about the hospital experience and dispelling myths of their fragility. Practice role plays were helpful in this endeavor.

My experience supports the validity of Haley's (1980) emphasis on avoiding the first rehospitalization as of primary importance in preventing the development of a rigid "revolving door" pattern of rehospitalization. The longer an individual has been an identified patient (and the more hospitalizations), it appears, the greater the chances of any behavior (even the most functional) being labeled "crazy." This makes it particularly important to involve extended family members in the change process and to change their belief system about the patient. For example, in working with a fifty-five-year-old woman who had had fourteen hospitalizations, I involved her husband as well as sixteen assorted children and spouses of children. A few weeks after discharge, a sister visited from another state, and they went shopping. Sally picked out some yellow shoes. Her sister insisted she should buy the green pair. (The sister had apparently always made decisions for Sally in the past.) When Sally refused, her sister told her it was "time to go back to the hospital." Fortunately, there were enough people in the family who were taking the more normalized view, but this incident did shake Sally's own belief system a bit. It also underlined anew for me the importance of reaching other systems than the immediate family. I have occasionally, as a second choice, used the telephone to talk to extended family members at a great distance to seed the idea of a new beginning and have them share in a new frame.

We found that frequently patients had difficulty with endings and would avoid terminating from the therapeutic community in which they had been intimately involved. A ritual was made out of terminating from the group, again underlining the theme of a "new beginning." Staff could split in predicting continued progress or predicting a return to the hospital as a way of challenging the patient.

In the initial family session, the expectation was clear that the family would continue in outpatient therapy after discharge to help them through the transition. The average hospital stay was between six weeks and three months. Most commonly I met with families once or twice a week initially, moving to once a week during hospitalization and continuing at that frequency for about a month after discharge, then moving to twice a month and monthly rather quickly. It was usually possible to terminate families two to six months after discharge. For patients who had a long history of hospitalization, it was helpful to have follow-up "maintenance sessions" again at three months and every six months after termination. These postdischarge sessions appear to be critically important in "tacking down change," dealing with predictable relapses, and avoiding rehospitalization. When hospitalization was much briefer, family therapy was more concentrated during and after hospitalization. (Recent trends in Medicare and private insurance coverage toward reduction of dollar limits and lifetime days for psychiatric hospitalization are currently reflected in trends toward shorter hospitalizations.) Unfortunately, many psychiatric hospitals restrict family therapists who are part of the staff from working with families after discharge. This ruling interrupts support at a critical time for the family in making the transition from the hospital to the home environment (see Chapter Nine). A second alternative is making a referral toward the end of hospitalization and involving the new family therapist in the discharge process.

It seems to work far better if a young person with a leaving-home issue is discharged to his home, even if he is there only briefly (Haley, 1980). It seems to be all but necessary to return home before you can leave home successfully. I found a tendency of colleagues trained in other than systemic therapies to assume that if a young person was in conflict with her family, she should avoid going home—she should get her own apartment or go to a halfway house. What usually happens with this premature move is the young person fails at this level of independence, which underlines the old belief system that she is helpless and incompetent. Occasionally a halfway house is necessary if there is essentially no family of origin or other surrogate family system. I think these situations are rare in the private psychiatric population, and all effort should be directed toward working within the existing family structure. Halfway houses often, from my experience, seem to perpetuate the status quo. Minimal survival behavior seems to be expected, the occupants usually being perceived as incompetent and chronic. If the experience in the halfway house is focused on moving toward well functioning—for example, helping the patients find work or enroll in higher education—and there is an assumption that the occupants work toward more independence and "leaving home" (leaving the halfway house), this may be a viable second alternative. Joel Bergman (1982) has developed a type of community home very different from the usual halfway house. First, staff members are required to have had no previous mental health training—that is, no training in looking for pathology. A consistent frame, or belief system, is developed and is shared among staff and patients alike, which appears to lead to dramatic changes in the behavior of individuals who have been previously hospitalized for as long as twenty-five years. Bergman's experience again underlines my sense that the belief system out of which the patient and significant others (family, psychiatrist, social worker) respond is the critical factor.

Finding Support

I have long recognized and accepted that support and validation for my work are essential to my sense of integrity as an individual and to the continuation of expenditures of intellectual, emotional, and physical energy. I sought support both outside and inside my work setting. A search for outside support led me to the Atlanta Institute for Family Studies, where weekly consultation provided a distance that allowed me "meta-glimpses" of the work setting of which I was a part. I am also fortunate enough to have a husband who is a clinical social worker and who at that time had had a wealth of experience working in private psychiatric hospitals. Support inside the setting came from multiple sources. I cannot overestimate the importance of having the support and backing of the unit director. Without his backing I would never have been able to do my work. Since he and I both are driving self-initiators, we could have readily had a head-on collision. I think the key to the synergism we experienced was the continuing mutual validation and careful attention to boundaries and role definition. As noted earlier, this feeling of mutual support in time seemed to pervade the treatment team as a whole. Certainly, I felt considerable support from other team members. The unit director's studies in Eastern philosophies and martial arts, I believe, contributed to his decision to introduce the family therapy component of his program more indirectly. Even though he had hopes for a comprehensive family therapy program down the road, he did not at the time of my hiring announce "from the top" the beginning of a major change in the treatment program. Such an announcement could have devalued and threatened other team members and inspired massive resistance. Instead he introduced me as a clinical social worker who would be conducting group and family therapy. His approach fit well with my own Johnny Appleseed approach. Perhaps most important, he and I both valued the contributions of other team members.

Interestingly, the crucial support came, over time, from what is often considered the enemy—the hospital administration. As a member of the social service department (and especially after being appointed director of social services hospitalwide), I had many responsibilities beyond those related to my work on the adult inpatient unit. I believe, in retrospect, that careful attention to those responsibilities, such as preparing for accreditation by the Joint Commission on Accreditation of Hospitals (JCAH) and coordinating hospitalwide, ongoing social work support services, was integrally related to the administration's increased interest in and validation of my work with families. This support included willingness to allow flexibility in scheduling to allow for the continuation of work with families after discharge. If, out of my enthusiasm for strategic therapy, I had failed to attend to these other administrative tasks, I think my behavior would have had the effect of discounting the importance of tasks that were highly valued by the administration (and for which the administration was ultimately accountable). In that case, in turn, the administration's support for my interests would not have been forthcoming.

Conclusions

I have noted that the psychiatric hospital has the potential for facilitating change or perpetuating chronicity. Unfortunately, I believe the latter is more common. The stigmatizing effect of a psychiatric hospitalization cannot be overestimated. I have seen patients whose every effort has been undermined by a well-meaning therapist and well-meaning relatives and neighbors. I remember Larry, a young man with obvious assets. He was handsome, intelligent, and gifted in athletics. At seventeen he had "fallen apart" and had been diagnosed as schizophrenic. His father wrote a book about the heartrending experience of working with a schizophrenic son. The book sold out in the family's hometown. Several times Larry got back on his feet and got a job and a girlfriend. Each time, however, word would get out that Larry was the schizophrenic in the well-known book. Fellow employees would begin "walking on eggs," treating him as fragile, and his girlfriend would drop him. To top it off, his efforts to improve his lot were met with warnings from his former psychiatrist that he must learn to accept that he was a schizophrenic and would never get well. Each of these episodes had been followed by another hospitalization. If the family and hospital as a "collective doctor" see the patient as "crazy" and respond to him as such, it is highly unlikely that the patient will stop acting crazy. The hospital offers a myriad of opportunities to exacerbate the situation by underlining the belief system supporting the patient in dysfunctional sequences and cross-generational coalitions.

However, the hospital can use its power to change the belief system, interrupt dysfunctional sequences, and clarify the hierarchy in more than one context. If the "collective doctor," the experts on craziness, indicates that you (your son, your wife) are not crazy, that is indeed hopeful and newsworthy. The key to making this work appears to be cooperation among attending physician, team members, and family members so that the patient does not become a pawn in intrafamily, intrahospital, or family/hospital conflicts. Making this work takes a huge amount of time and energy. When it does work and a patient is able to break (or avoid) the revolving-door pattern of hospitalization, it is time for rejoicing.

There may indeed be unwanted consequences for a psychiatric hospital when an ecosystemic approach involving family therapy is introduced. Private psychiatric hospitals are private businesses. Keeping beds filled ensures that salaries and taxes are paid and a comfortable profit margin is maintained. Any therapy that works toward shortening hospitalization and breaking patterns of recidivism will at least initially lead to more empty beds (see Chapters Nine and Eleven). However, if a hospital could define its goal as breaking the revolving-door cycle and returning the patient to well functioning in the community, perhaps its referral base would expand considerably. Certainly this is a risk that few private institutions may be willing to take.

In addition, an ecosystemic approach in which family therapy is central to treatment certainly threatens the all-powerful position of the attending psychiatrist. Those psychiatrists who dare to change their epistemology and pursue training in systemic therapy (beyond their grueling medical training) are indeed admirable. Most of our failures could be perceived as being related to failure to enlist attending physicians as part of a cooperative team effort. The physician has expertise that must be acknowledged and validated (see Chapter Eleven). Ideally a therapeutic community could perhaps be set up in such a way that patients were admitted to the team (the team including psychiatrists), all of whose members were involved in the day-to-day activities on the unit. Combining an attending model with a therapeutic community is inherently problematic. Most typically, the attending psychiatrist who drops in periodically for individual sessions replicates the peripheral noncustodial parent, whereas the team (or some of its members) replicates the stay-at-home, limit-setting, grouchy parent—a pattern not uncommon in the families of these patients. The possibility of triangulation continues after discharge if the patient is involved in ongoing individual therapy. Again a good working relationship between the attending psychiatrist and the family therapist is essential. Ideally, an agreement should be made that a rehospitalization will not be carried out without prior consultation with the family therapist to consider other alternatives. Even with the agreement of the attending psychiatrist, this is often very difficult to implement, since a rotating "doctor on call" plan is often used for hospital admissions. I have found that client families at a weak or angry moment will call the hospital, and the patient will be admitted unnecessarily. One of my most frustrating (and at times rewarding) cases involved the fifty-five-year-old woman who picked out the yellow shoes. She and her family had done beautifully for two years, breaking a long-term chronic path. A backslide occurred after radical surgery and chemotherapy involving steroids. Being out of town, I was unable to help this family over the predictable adjustment period. As stress levels increased, the family began to regress to old, familiar patterns of behavior (Sally's husband distancing by spending hours with their grown son at a time when Sally needed his involvement and support). Her husband could not accept that Sally did not feel up to cooking on Wednesday, the day she underwent chemotherapy. One Wednesday evening when Sally's husband and son were involved in a project together, Sally, with her usual flair for drama, began to conduct a marriage ceremony between her husband and son. She then called the family to dinner and served boiling water in china soup bowls. The family packed her up and drove her to the hospital, where she was readily admitted on the basis of her bizarre behavior (seen out of context).

In another case, I was consulted and a readmission was intercepted. A young woman who was desperately fighting to maintain a positive belief system about herself had threatened to drink some household cleaning products. Having a good relationship with the parents and young woman, I was able to intervene on the telephone, trusting the patient's word that she would not do anything to harm herself before the next family session. Recently, I received a letter from the young woman, who has since left home, has enrolled in a master's program, and is being validated by her university community as a gifted artist.

My observations suggest that perhaps the attempted solution of return to the hospital has more to do with a person's becoming a chronic patient than depth of pathology does.

This chapter is not an overview. It is written with the assumption that there is a particular value to an in-depth study of one family therapist's experience within a particular context, as there is value in an in-depth study of one particular family in therapy with a particular therapist or therapists (Napier and Whitaker, 1978). Rollo May (quoted in Keeney, 1979, p. 122) has stated, "We don't investigate nature, we investigate the investigator's relationship to nature." Thus, I no doubt have presented a necessarily skewed view, having my own internal maps through which I process data.

Each family therapist's path will differ, as will each psychiatric hospital unit. As each family therapist and family interface in a pattern unique to them, so will each family therapist interface with the hospital system in a particular way. It will make a difference how the therapist enters the system and whether family therapy is already established as a valued modality. It will make a difference where you are in the hierarchy and whether you are a psychiatrist, psychologist, counselor, or social worker. Each family therapist has the opportunity to use his own personhood, his own strengths and assets. However, what does seem clear is that, no matter who you are or how you enter the system, *it is critically important to join with all levels of the hierarchy and to involve them in the change process.*

A major focus of my work centered on changing the belief systems of colleagues as well as patients and their extended families. In this process I discovered that the very same assumptions (underlying strategic/structural therapy) that work with family systems work with hospital systems. It was essential to "start where the colleague is at" (Weakland and others, 1974), to recognize colleagues' resources and assets, to ask for help, to work toward developing a common language, to accept that my own world view was one of a myriad of views, and to work toward a shared success. These general principles may have relevance that goes beyond my experience. More recent experience as a private practitioner conducting family therapy in inpatient settings has confirmed to me the workability of these principles for an outsider entering the system. Certainly the necessarily limited involvement in the hospital system that one has as an outsider reduces the possibility for the development and "tacking down" of comprehensive frames as well as the opportunity for ongoing monitoring (and interrupting) of staff members' participation with patients in dysfunctional sequences. However, taking time to develop relationships with attending psychiatrists and other significant staff members and attending treatment planning seem well worth the time and energy involved.

Perhaps what I am really talking about is not introducing and carrying out family therapy as a modality but, rather, introducing an ecosystemic epistemology and carrying out an ecosystemic therapy that involves a parallel process in families and within the therapeutic community.

In summary, I found working on an inpatient unit to be both exhausting and energizing, both profoundly discouraging and inspiring. I found the psychiatric hospital as "collective doctor" to be in a position to facilitate change or perpetuate chronicity. Difficult as hospital settings are to work in, they are too important (and the change possible within them too promising) to be avoided or ignored.

4 Douglas Carl

Community
Mental Health
Centers

The Mental Health Center Act of 1963 changed the course of public mental health in the United States. Before then the preponderance of public mental health "treatment" took place in large, centralized state hospitals. People were often committed to these hospitals for long periods; many were "warehoused" for the better part of their lives. The 1963 law established a mechanism for treating people with psychiatric problems in the community. It directed states to establish community mental health centers, with the help of federal money, to deal with as many psychiatric problems as possible on an outpatient basis. This represented a monumental philosophical change and raised difficult questions about implementation: first, what to do with literally tens of thousands of people who had become institutionally dependent and, second, what treatment model to establish in the community? The mental health professions rushed in with the best that they had available.

We have come a tremendously long way since 1963. Most of the large hospitals have been emptied, and all states have established operational mental health centers, although many programs are now threatened by dwindling federal funds. Still, we have succeeded in handling large numbers of formerly institutionalized people within the community. There is no doubt that the quality of life has improved for a great many. Yet some mental health professionals feel we have gone as far as we can go with the traditional treatment models that were patched together to answer that sudden call in 1963. Some also believe that, for all the good intentions, we have succeeded in creating a group of institutionalized outpatients to replace those institutionalized inpatients. We have a great need for a better treatment model.

Implementing a Family Systems Approach

The systems approach to change belongs in community mental health. It is the most pragmatic, effective way to tackle the myriad problems facing the community mental health worker. Yet practitioners as renowned as Jay Haley (1975) protest all too knowingly that family therapy systems intervention should not be attempted in public facilities. And in actual practice few mental health systems, public or private, have formally incorporated this approach. Why? Because for all the sound arguments for its adoption, and for all the miserable failures of other approaches, there are an equal number of practical obstacles built into existing mental health systems that defy implementation of change. It is this same defiance of change that so often gets handled dramatically and effectively through the innovative interventions of practicing family therapists. Family practitioners may need to learn to extend their intervention into systems outside the family itself.

To begin, let us look at the typical mental health system operating a network of community mental health centers and hospitals. The system has revolved around treating the individual as an entity unto himself or herself, with an individual diagnosis, a personal chart, and treatment within an operational division (adult, as distinct from child and adolescent, as separate from developmental disabilities or alcohol and drug). Everything makes it convenient and logical to treat an individual and difficult or cumbersome to tackle systems.

The existing systems have done an excellent job of learning to focus on the individual, to understand his or her motivations, to explain the causes of aberration. At the same time, this individual focus has helped little in understanding and promoting change. It provides no understanding of the context in which problems take place.

As with any bureaucratic system, one of the purposes of the community mental health center is to increase or at least maintain its own domain. Therefore, systemic thinking and the therapeutic work deriving from it must be presented in such a way that they are not threatening to the institution's resources and domain. Unfortunately, many mental health appropriations tie funding to head count, which means that the system becomes invested in keeping clients, not discharging them. The life of a typical chronic adult mental health client revolves around visits to the mental health center, short hospitalizations, and medication. The central events in life concern past hospital stays, schizophrenic breaks, and the specter of craziness. Sometimes we see a client, hospitalized once ten or fifteen years ago, whose life still revolves around that hospitalization and the prevention of a recurrence. Clients who "do well" may be given the opportunity to become volunteers at the program. As mentioned earlier, we have succeeded in substituting institutionalized outpatients for institutionalized inpatients, but we feel happy because they look better and they are "functioning" in the community.

A further obstacle comes from various segments of the community. Community members, too, belong to various systems of their own, all with the potential for resisting change. Chronic mental health clients often represent a community nuisance, which the community wishes would go away. Certainly the chronically mentally disabled are a problem to their own family systems. It is convenient for the family to have a community mental health facility willing to accept responsibility, often dealing with the problem without involving or bothering anyone else. Many times it is the client's family member who makes just such a request: "Fix him up, and when he's better, I'll take him back." The traditional model remains viable partly because it accepts the responsibility of caring for people for whom various community members no longer wish to care. The community as a whole may seem less concerned about change than about relief.

A final problem is that many chronic mental health center clients are diagnosed as schizophrenic. This diagnosis provides staff with an excuse for not changing the client, since schizophrenia cannot be cured. If the client does well, his or her schizophrenia is in remission. If the client does poorly, he or she is only following the expected path to decompensation. What is critical for the systemic therapist is that he or she cannot succeed with schizophrenia. Rather, one must be willing to step outside the traditional parameters, see this "disease" in a different light, and reconceptualize it as a problem that can be solved.

Why a systems approach for a mental health center? A systems approach is just that—an approach. Family systems therapy is not an "add-on" to be incorporated into an existing program as an additional treatment modality. The reason is that systems work represents a perspective for dealing with problems that is quite different from more traditional approaches, and a systems treatment modality is not compatible with intrapsychic, individual treatments in any workable way. In other words, if you add family systems work onto your traditionally oriented work system, you can count on conflict and frustration. (For creative solutions to this dilemma, see Chapters Two and Nine.) Whatever the divergence between private and public treatment in the past, the differences are becoming even greater today, as public mental health moves to focus primarily on the chronically psychiatrically disabled client. In actuality, though, the public sector has the best overall resources for dealing with chronic clients, and good work with the chronic client also has its rewards. Here are some advantages enjoyed by the public sector:

• Easy access to support systems not available to the private sector, such as foster homes, group homes, halfway houses, vocational rehabilitation, day programs, and sheltered workshops.
• Staff who work on salary rather than on an hourly fee, allowing "nontherapy" hours without loss of income. This should permit staff to perform liaison functions, home visits,

and follow-up difficult to justify financially in a private practice setting. (Caseloads in some mental health centers do not
permit time for anything really productive. A systems approach can alleviate this problem by helping to move people
through and out of the system.)

- A position as the only game in town. Mental health centers
  have leverage in that most clients have no reasonable alternatives for treatment. This should permit mental health centers firmly to prescribe and implement the treatment program deemed best suited rather than one dictated by a client.
  This is, however, an advantage most mental health centers
  do not use.

Another reason to think systemically in mental health
centers involves the way the mental health center often becomes a "substitute family" for the client or a significant system in his or her life. Many times in doing workshops people
say to me, "What you say is fine for clients who have families,
but what about clients who have no family at all?" My reply is
"All people have families or significant systems that function as
support." Often the "family" of the single chronic client is the
mental health center itself. The client spends days at the center,
in programs, with workers, in the waiting room, in center-linked
housing. Mental health workers become the client's significant
others. The system takes care of the client. He or she is, in effect, a child of the system. As in other family systems, the mental health center system and the client often develop a dysfunctional relationship that makes it difficult for the client to leave
his or her mental health center "home."

There is another factor to consider. Roles carry with
them very powerful attributes and expectations. Nowhere is
there a more powerful role than the role of chronically disabled
client. This client must act a bit crazy from time to time, or the
doctor and caseworker will have no reason to see him. This is
not to imply that a chronically disabled person consciously acts
out a charade. However, there are demands for role consistency.
How long would this client receive services if he came into the
center and had rational, assertive conversations with staff? Fur-

thermore, a chronic client in crisis has the capability of mobilizing an entire mental health center, receiving the intensive attention of mental health professionals.

In this way the roles of center staff complement the role of chronic client to maintain the status quo of the system. This description fits the family system of a chronic client just as well. Most public mental health centers, like most families of chronic patients, may be characterized as chronically disabled.

The concept of triangles is addressed in family therapy primarily in regard to the involvement of a third party in a two-party communication or dispute. Often the "involvement" takes the form of a symptom in the third party, which distracts the two warring parties (Haley, 1976; Minuchin, 1974). Murray Bowen (1978) has said that two-person interactions are unstable under stress and tend to bring in a third party. To this statement we need to add a corollary: Communication between two agencies or between an agency and a family will tend to be unstable under stress and bring in a third party (Carl and Jurkovic, 1983; Coopersmith, 1982; Clark, Zalis, and Saccho, 1982; Chapter Nine in this volume).

This idea is particularly relevant to mental health centers, since they routinely get referrals from the courts, from family and children's service agencies, and from mental hospitals. Often the referring agency has one agenda and the treatment agency another, and the family gets "triangled." Or sometimes the family is at odds with the referring agency and will "triangle" the mental health center. This is yet another reason for public mental health workers to have knowledge of systems and know how to deal with them.

Organizational Issues in Implementation

Systems therapists and theorists have shown a certain shortsightedness. Although some have argued for establishing a systemic approach in public mental health, we have almost universally ignored the need for assessment of the systems in which we want to institute change. Any family systems therapist worth his or her salt has a plan for change in a family based on an assessment of the interactions in that family. Yet we have avoided doing "assessment" of the mental health systems in which we wish to cause change. A family system knows how to circumvent ill-conceived therapeutic interventions. A treatment system proves no less resourceful. If you want to help families change, you deal with hierarchies, boundaries, sequences, and interactions in a way that the family can accept. We have been inept in dealing with those very things within treatment systems, neither identifying the crucial factors nor finding ways to make change palatable for the people involved.

Organizational psychologists provide some preliminary thinking in this area. Edgar Schein wrote: "These new systems models do not have the neatness or completeness of the classical concepts of organization, but they are a closer approximation of what researchers find when they actually study groups" (1980, pp. 187-229).

I think that organizational behavior can be explained satisfactorily using a systemic approach and that, in assessing an organization, we need to attend to such things as sequence, hierarchy, boundaries, roles, triangles, coalitions both overt and covert, and life-cycle issues, just as we do with families.

So when you return to your mental health center after attending a family therapy workshop or watching Minuchin work on tape or reading this chapter, all enthusiastic about doing family systems work at your place, go back to your setting mindful of the need to be a good systems therapist. Remember that big changes result from a series of little changes at opportune times and places. Assess the system and its complexities, and you will gain a greater understanding of when and how to implement a significant change in the therapeutic approach. You will greatly improve your chances that the change will stick.

Here are some general areas for scrutiny:

• *Hierarchy*. What is the hierarchy like in your mental health center? What does the formal organization chart describe, and how does that diverge from actual practice? Who makes decisions and who carries them out? Is there a power (or powers) behind the throne?

• *Boundaries.* How functional are boundaries between components and personnel within work components? Do they permit adequate separation *and* adequate interaction between components to allow them to work cooperatively, or do components "guard turf"? Are boundaries rigid, with components functioning virtually as separate entities, or are they so diffuse that some people have a hand in everything?

• *Coalitions.* Does decision making actually follow prescribed channels, or are there "cross-generational" coalitions that bypass formal authority and undermine implementation of new ideas? Will a nurse on your staff form a coalition with the medical director to sabotage a non-medical-model approach?

• *Triangles.* Under stress, agencies (or components of agencies) will tend to bring in a third party (triangle) to alleviate the stress. Will your proposal for a new approach create an agency triangle or even "triangle" a family in treatment between you and another component or another "cooperating" agency? (See Chapters Nine and Ten for further uses of the concept of triangles in guiding the therapist's thinking.)

• *Life-cycle issues.* Mental health centers, like people, have life cycles, especially when federal declining grants are involved. Is your mental health center at an early-to-middle phase, flush with funds, or in a declining phase, with attendant belt tightening? How will a systems approach, with its emphasis on cure, affect the flow of state and federal monies? Is head count a critical funding factor?

• *Outside influences.* How will the community react to a new approach? The state umbrella agency? Other allied agencies? Can you frame the systems approach as advantageous to all involved?

From a strictly practical point of view, you need to determine how and where ideas are implemented in your system. It may be well and good to get fired up about a family systems approach, and perhaps you will have some initial success in initial implementation of family systems treatment. But will it stick? What will happen when a pivotal case goes to review or to the medical director? As practitioners we have not usually chosen the paths of implementation wisely in choosing to start clinically and to gather a band of adherents around us. The more advisable approach might have us first persuading the center director or the citizens' advisory council on the advantages *to them* in embracing this approach before actual implementation. (For some strategies used to enlist the support of upper administration, see Chapters Three and Nine.) As emphasized throughout this book, the context in which treatment occurs is at least as important as the treatment occurring within that system. Treatment and context cannot be separated in terms of treatment setting any more than individual behavior can be separated from the context (system) in which it occurs. A great many treatment interventions fail because the context in which they occur will not permit change to take root.

Practical Issues in Implementation

Once you have examined critical issues of organizational structure and function, there are certain practical adjustments that must be made in the mental health setting before embarking on effective interventions with families. The potential instigator of family systems intervention must decide whether these pragmatic changes can be instituted in the particular setting. I have included some implementation suggestions in each area that should be helpful in the assessment process. Keep in mind that at any time these procedures could bump up against traditional procedures and thereby force a "strategic reevaluation."

Intake Procedures. You need to begin at the beginning with incoming clients. If someone comes into the center in crisis, and the intake worker directs that person to the psychiatrist for medication, you have missed an excellent opportunity to intervene systemically. For example, if the presenting problem is acute depression, and the client gets the message that the medication will provide the cornerstone of treatment, you have the makings of a long-term or continual patient. Such a patient may then actively resist involving the rest of the family on the grounds that they are extraneous to the problem. This also sets the stage for the family to resist because the problem clearly *be-*

longs to the patient (see also Chapter Two on the importance of initial contacts and Chapters Three, Five, and Nine for other views on the importance of how a client's problem is initially defined and handled).

The initial contact person may also have quite an impact on the *modality* of treatment that the client desires. I cannot overstress the importance of having systems-oriented persons in key intake positions. Often one must "sell" a family on treatment as a unit rather than treatment for the individual. The client may have in mind compelling reasons that he or she should be seen alone—compelling unless one thinks systemically. An intake worker schooled in systems intervention will continue to press for all family members to accompany the identified patient, even under extreme duress (but in a way that makes it seem beneficial for the family). And the duress will indeed be extreme in many cases. People have been indoctrinated to think "mental illness" for a long time; add the fact that the families of many of our clients have been through long years of "treatment," and they resist further cooperation (even when they are being asked as a family for the first time). As mental health workers become more comfortable with systemic interventions, they may turn to more strategic approaches with partial family groups in order to entice all family members. In all fairness, many family members feel that the only purpose of the family session is to fix blame for the patient's current condition; they may, in fact, have been blamed on other occasions. Recently I saw a family with previous experience in "family therapy." An analytically oriented psychiatrist had conducted these sessions and had left the family with a very clear message: The patient's problems stem from contact with all of you; so it is best for the patient if she has no further contact with the family.

Since community mental health centers are mandated to provide service to anyone in their designated catchment area, an issue especially likely to upset staff embarking on a sytemic program is the question of appearing to refuse treatment—that is, of not just offering the treatment modality requested by the client when he or she first contacts the center. In my experience, a good systems-oriented intake worker can head off most of the trouble with tactful but firm diplomacy. In actuality, a good many of those who refuse to accept a family appointment end up reconsidering and calling back when they are sure the center is firm in its resolve to involve the entire family whenever possible. For this reason, you will have to ensure that the center is firm in its resolve, and the issue must be broached with the powers that be before it reaches a crisis stage.

The refusal of a spouse to cooperate is the most common form of client-dictated treatment. A prospective client may say that a spouse refuses to come in or that he or she does not want the spouse to come in and to be part of treatment because there are things the spouse should not know about. In the former situation, I have found that about half the time the spouse *is* willing to come in—it is just that the prospective client wants the spouse excluded. Whenever I hear that a spouse will not come in, I tell the prospective client to ask again and to tell the spouse that I feel that the spouse will be a genuine help and will be really important in helping to change things for the better. Then I tell the prospective client that I will be happy to call the spouse if his or her efforts fail. Usually I do not have to make the telephone call myself, because both parties get the message that I am firm in my request. All this negotiating takes place either on the telephone or in a setting such as a waiting room, where therapy will not begin "accidentally." When a prospective client absolutely refuses to include a spouse, I may respond by saying that I would not risk threatening the relationship by seeing only one person in treatment. My experience shows that seeing one person only has a high-risk potential for damaging a relationship, while seeing both parties increases chances for mutual satisfaction (see Gurman and Kniskern, 1978).

Sometimes it is children who refuse to come in with the parents. I understand the parents' lack of leverage with grown, independent children. But I flatly reject the idea that a dependent child, living under the parents' roof or from the parents' support, cannot be persuaded to attend at least one family session.

So the intake procedure is the optimum early intervention/education opportunity. You will be pleasantly surprised at how much the initial intake orientation will contribute to later success in treatment. If your center will not take a systems-oriented stand on intake, your chances of success are greatly diminished.

Evening Hours. Recently I began consultation with a local mental health group. As I outlined the pragmatics of systems intervention, one group member said, "Well, it sounds like this family work means more evenings. I guess that leaves me out." What this person said was true. Family systems work requires evening hours and even occasional weekend hours. Private practitioners are used to this kind of scheduling; people in the public sector may not be. The prime middle-of-the-day working hours are usually almost useless for family work. Occasionally you will find a family with no one working, so that the family members may be willing to come in during the day. However, sometimes with such a family your successful intervention may lead to someone's obtaining a job. Your lack of availability for evening appointments may be just the excuse a family member needs for not seeking employment. Those of us who work regularly with some flexibility of hours forget how difficult it may be to ask a new employer for time off during the day, especially for a therapy appointment! In the same vein, do not be too quick to label a husband or wife "resistant" when he or she fails to agree to daytime appointments. Many professionals do not understand the impossibility for assembly line workers, clerks, or other working people to get time off during the day. They may risk their jobs in doing so.

So you need to decide at your center who will work what evening hours or even early mornings. If a staff of five will each agree to work two evenings per week (5:00 to 9:00 P.M.), that is the equivalent of ten evenings of staff time, or forty hours of evening appointment time per week. Forty hours of evening time should easily accommodate twenty to twenty-five families per week or more.

The question is, will your staff agree to work in the evenings? My guess is that child-oriented therapists will agree more readily than adult-oriented practitioners because child-trained people already orient themselves to the reality of school hours.

History Taking, Recordkeeping, and Diagnosis. Standard
social or psychiatric histories do not provide us with the kinds
of information we need to do effective family intervention.
They can even interfere with effective systems work in that
they orient our thinking to past "causal" events and they focus
unnecessarily on a medical orientation. Most states require mental health centers to complete some sort of standardized history
for inclusion in a client's chart or file. Unfortunately, these histories focus on the identified patient, and so the inclination is
to gather the data for such a history by seeing that person
alone. Resist the inclination. You need to do your history taking
in the family session and to use the interaction patterns as yet
another assessment tool. It may surprise you that mother knows
more about the history of the problem than the identified client. Maybe daughter answers questions for mother. Of course,
there will be no opportunity to make such observations unless
your center will allow you to have control of the history-taking
process. Can this be accomplished?

Recordkeeping can become a bit more complicated. Some
centers require a separate file on each family member seen so that
the center gets credit for rightful head count. This means process notes on each family member for each session—an almost
impossible glut of paperwork. Only slightly better is the practice of opening the chart in the name of the identified patient.
This identifies the client all right, as the "sick" one. Sometimes
one can ask who in the family is willing to have the case in his
or her name, but this practice also creates complications. For instance, if you are working in a child/adolescent unit, and the
father agrees to have the case put in his name, then the age does
not fit the unit reporting requirements. Ideally, one file could
be opened for each family in the *family* name. Not many centers can accommodate this practice. None of these recordkeeping problems is insurmountable, but they *will* arise (compare
Chapter Eleven).

Often one can avoid difficulties concerning diagnosis. The
pathologizing latent in individual diagnosis has no place in systems work. However, the description of an individual's difficulties contained in such diagnoses as learning disability and men-

tal retardation is often useful to the clinician. The reality is that most centers require individual diagnoses. The DSM-III adjustment reaction diagnostic series will provide the least pejorative labels. Will your center balk at a rash of adjustment reaction diagnoses?

There seems to be a trend afoot to tie diagnosis to permissible treatment or, at least, the treatment for which Medicaid will pay. In practice such a move would mean that there would be a distinct limit on what would be authorized for treatment of, say, an adjustment reaction. The more severe the diagnosis, the more treatment or the more intensive treatment would be authorized for payment. Such a policy would be detrimental in two ways: It could require the use of a more pejorative diagnostic label in order to concentrate treatment on a family, and it could require that only certain forms of intervention be used in treatment of severe cases. Both options would work counter to a systems approach and would work to further the status quo—that is, medication as the primary treatment for chronic clients.

You need to assess the willingness of your center to accept less emphasis on diagnosis. Does the center have an investment in reporting a higher number of chronic clients in treatment? Sometimes centers with the heaviest concentration of schizophrenics reported stand the best chance of retaining or increasing funding levels.

Cotherapy, Fees, and Components. Two basic considerations about cotherapy warrant examination. One concerns staff harmony and staff support, examined later in this chapter. The other involves administrative issues, specifically costs and fees. As therapists, we may not enjoy looking at costs and fees, but these items may well determine what you are permitted to do on the job (compare Chapters Two and Nine).

When you begin to do family systems work, it will be unfamiliar to you, and you will experience everything from unabashed elation to unsettling anxiety. Most therapists like to share these burdens and rewards by having a colleague in the room with them as cotherapist. Many centers do not feel that they can justify cotherapy from a cost standpoint. Certainly it is not practical to charge the client a fee for the services of both therapists, as happens in private practice. This may seem a minor matter to the therapist, but it proves a major concern to administrators. If the implementation of a systems orientation in your center depends on the staff comfort received from cotherapy, make sure that you know where you stand with your administration on the issue.

One way to justify the cost is to present cotherapy as a training or supervisory procedure. In addition, it is sometimes possible to charge a therapy fee based on family income, rather than the income of an individual, who may be an unemployed or underemployed chronic client. This extra fee may help to justify cotherapy.

The cotherapy arrangement may present a special problem when there are children in the family or drug addicts or a mentally retarded person. If you see a family with a cotherapist who represents one of these specialties, then you need to decide which component or which therapist will receive credit for the service. Many components in a center are mandated to maintain certain levels of service. Alcohol and drug components in Georgia centers must maintain a certain level of patients or lose funding, and they are reviewed quarterly.

In any event, it is important to gain the cooperation of other components in your center, cotherapy or not. Suppose a woman calls in depressed. You succeed in having her come in with her husband and children only to find that the husband is a client in your drug unit. Maybe your drug people do not believe in a systems approach. You are then in trouble. (Chapters Two, Three, Seven, Eight, Nine, and Eleven describe some ways to collaborate usefully with other agencies or with other components within an agency.)

Ideally, in systems terms, a center would not have components. Systems problems would receive attention as a whole, without regard to age or symptom. There would still be room for people to specialize in psychosomatic families or alcoholic families or leaving-home problems, but treatment would not be bound by the limitations of territorial issues. Under current circumstances, however, you will need to assess the flexibility in your center for dealing with various contingencies between components.

Medication. The medication issue remains the most difficult to deal with in the public sector. Medical people have a lot to lose in terms of status and hierarchy should the system change. Many of the people we see and who see the physicians in mental health centers need to be on medication for at least some specified period of time. Too often they are told that the period of time is for the rest of their lives. The serious obstacle with medication for the systems therapist is that only the psychiatrists among us have control over the amount of medication or the duration of the prescription. This brings us to a very realistic consideration for most mental health practitioners: You will not be successful with cases in which the prime consideration when you get the case is medication and in which the physician will not let you manage the case.

Staff Harmony. Haley (1975) has observed that treatment outcome is of little concern to mental health centers and that staff harmony constitutes the primary concern. Whether or not you agree with Haley's observation, it is clear that harmony will be directly affected by a move to a systems orientation. Staff members will be uncomfortable because they do not know how to work with a systems approach. I remember one staff member saying to me shortly after my arrival as her new supervisor: "Dr. Carl, I know what you've been teaching us really works and really makes sense, but I'm not going to do it. I just don't feel comfortable working in a room with all those people!"

You will encounter this posture in various forms and configurations, overt and covert: Downright refusal. Extra individual sessions "on the side." Seeing the family with key members not present. Staff coalitions aimed at your defeat (especially cross-generational ones between staff members and administrators). You must be able to assess just how far the staff is willing to go—and how quickly (compare Chapter Three). Doing effective systems work in a public setting involves much more than simply being a proficient systems therapist. Therapy skill alone is not enough. A great deal of spadework is required before the impact of a significantly different therapy approach can be absorbed by the treatment system. Most of us, as trained therapists, dislike dealing with the problems of organizational structure and management. However, here is where the systemic approach can serve you well, as it offers an overall orientation to change in *systems,* not just in *families.* These initial issues offer you an opportunity to test your skills!

A Typical Multiproblem Family

The following case example was chosen for several reasons. First, it involves a family with three generations of stubbornly chronic mental health problems—the kind of situation that might traditionally be treated with an emphasis on deeply ingrained pathology, individual psychotherapy for one or more family members perhaps being prescribed. Essentially, the family systems orientation allowed the therapist to approach the presenting problem—chronic encopresis—as a normal child problem and to deal with the adults as essentially competent executives rather than as chronic, untreatable patients. The focus on the child problem and the resulting solution then provided access to other dysfunctional aspects of the system. Second, socioeconomically as well as diagnostically this family is exactly the kind of family that typically shows up in MHCs and not in private practice. And third, the multifaceted resources of the MHC are tailor-made for handling the many aspects of this three-generational dilemma.

The author first encountered the Bailey family while acting as a consultant to the child and adolescent component of a mental health center. Joey Bailey, eleven, was encopretic and was being seen for that problem. Joey's mother and grandmother were also mental health center clients of the chronic variety, both involved in some form of treatment in the adult services component of the same mental health center. The mother, forty-four, had also attended day treatment in the past. Currently she saw an individual therapist once a month and attended a monthly medication group. She carried a diagnosis of schizophrenia, chronic undifferentiated type. The grandmother,

Mrs. Clark, seventy-seven, attended a different medication group and had earned a similar diagnosis with a secondary OBS level. The grandmother, mother, and Joey all lived in the grandmother's house. Joey attended fifth grade, but neither the mother or grandmother worked, although Mrs. Bailey had worked intermittently as a waitress. They lived on the grandmother's Social Security and Mrs. Bailey's disability payments. Mrs. Bailey was also involved with vocational rehabilitation through the mental health center, with the goal of helping her return to work. The family genogram looked like Figure 1.

Joey had been seen for about ten sessions, both alone and with his mother, at the time of the initial consultation. A variety of behavioral and strategic plans had been used, which had resulted in the encopresis becoming less frequent. Because the symptom was still persisting, however, I was asked to consult with the therapist and the family: son, mother, and grandmother. In the early part of the session, various family members provided a somewhat rambling description of Joey's problems while the therapist underlined instances of the boy's competence and normality as an eleven-year-old boy.

The therapist then switched to talking about the encopresis, which, he noted, was not a normal problem. In the course of pursuing information about the symptom (when it occurred, what family members had done about it, and so forth), the therapist found out that on a number of occasions the boy had been encopretic but had successfully kept the symptom secret. The therapist used this information to begin a new reframing of the problem.

Therapist: Well, you know, it's normal for eleven- or twelve-year-old boys to have secrets from their mothers and fathers and grandmothers. That's part of growing up. You think you're normal in that way?

Joey: Um-hum.

Ther.: I see the problem a little bit differently than maybe you two do [To adults]. First of all, we talked about there being two problems: one, the normal one, having a little trouble with

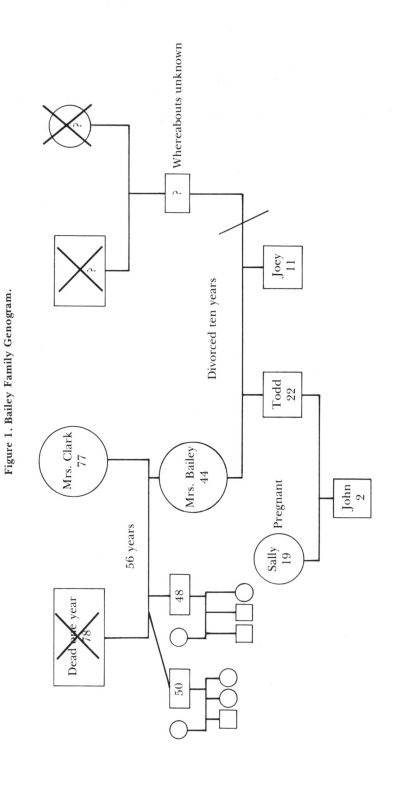

Figure 1. Bailey Family Genogram.

the police and learning not to get in trouble. That's normal. And then there's this other problem you describe, where Joey goes to the bathroom in his pants, and that is not a normal problem for an eleven-year-old. Now one of the things I know about this problem—the fancy name is *encopresis*—that with some kids it happens, no one knows why, and then it just goes away by itself. Sometimes they are eleven, sometimes twelve, sometimes thirteen. But it just goes away. And the problem that I see you're having is that Joey has trouble keeping it secret around you. There's an old saying: If a tree falls in the forest and there's no one around to hear it, does it really make a noise? And with this problem, this isn't a problem for you, Joey, when you're with Charles or Jamie or Dana [Joey's friends]. They don't know that you have the problem, because you're real good with them at keeping a secret. And the problem that I see, Joey, is that you're not very good *yet* at keeping a secret from your mother.

Joey: She doesn't know it any old time!

Ther.: Just when you want her to! One of the things I know about boys around your age is that they start changing from children to adolescents or young men, and I think you are right on the verge of going through that change. Your mother and grandmother know what I mean. And one of the things that happens when people get that age, when they change from kids to young men, is that they learn to keep some secrets. They don't tell everything to their mothers. They're more likely to tell their friends than they would their parents. When kids are younger, then they tell their mothers or fathers or grandmothers. And I think that you're right at that time of your life when you're learning—you said before you keep some secrets—but you haven't learned how to keep a real secret. And when you learn how to keep a real secret, that's going to be the beginning of your really growing up! So what I see as the problem is that you need to learn to keep a secret from your mother, and I don't know whether you can do that yet. What do you think?

Joey: I dunno.

Ther.: We'll see. Do you and your brother talk much?

Joey: Sometimes.

Ther.: I wonder whether you and your brother could talk about keeping a secret from your mother. 'Cause he's twenty-two, and he knows. He doesn't tell your mother everything. You think you're grown up enough to do that?

Joey: Yep!

Ther.: We'll see. We'll see. You'll find this business about messing in your pants will stop. One week and it will be less, then less, and you may not even notice, but suddenly you'll realize— "Hey! I don't do that anymore." So we're not going to worry about that. That's going to happen all by itself. Think about it.

The mother's overinvolvement with the son had been a prominent characteristic in this family from the start. In fact, all three generations were overinvolved and enmeshed with one another. The intervention involved a reframing of the problem as one of a transitional developmental milestone: The boy had difficulty keeping secrets from parental adults, and he needed to develop selective keeping of secrets to begin the path toward adolescence. He would "discover" that older boys had certain secrets from their mothers. (He had already shown an uncanny ability to keep his soiling behavior secret from peers but was all too willing to continue sharing that part of his life at home.) The session also dealt with the mother and grandmother in a normal context as mother and grandmother to the boy.

Six weeks after the session, Joey reported only four accidents, compared with everyday occurrences or greater on previous occasions. Three months later, the encopresis ceased to be a problem. But we expected we had not heard the last of the Clark/Baileys.

In addition to the consultation session, the various therapists and caseworkers were advised to involve the two adults in more peer-related activities. Mrs. Clark began attending senior citizen activities daily. Mrs. Bailey became more actively involved in her vocational rehabilitation activities. As Joey's problem lessened, however, another family member appeared to take his place: son Todd, twenty-two and unemployed, his pregnant wife Sally, and their two-year-old son got grandmother's permission to move into the house about six weeks after the consultation session. Initially the family therapist used the occasion to promote some older-brother/younger-brother activities. But more and more Todd and Sally left the house during the day, with their two-year-old in Mrs. Bailey's charge. This interfered with her vocational rehabilitation training and happened at a time when she was about to go out on a job test.

Shortly thereafter, Mrs. Clark sprained an ankle and took to bed, refusing to leave her bed for weeks and engaging in more and more "crazy" talk. She heard her dead husband's voice and other voices. She began accusing people of trying to poison her. After several weeks she did attend her medication group, where she complained constantly of bad headaches and demanded a prescription for tranquilizers.

Chronically dysfunctional family systems require tight management for changes to stick. In this case it was necessary for someone to coordinate various maneuvers in order to consolidate the gains made. The family therapist and the case manager for the adults (we had transferred Mrs. Clark to Mrs. Bailey's case manager) worked together to prompt the senior citizens' van to come for Mrs. Clark, ready or not, using peer pressure from other attendees to reinforce that move; to send the message to Mrs. Bailey that she had moved too fast with vocational rehabilitation and that maybe she needed to "sacrifice" herself even more for the time being and take on even more care of the two-year-old grandson; and to use the leverage already developed with the family to get Todd and Sally to attend family sessions, so that an appropriate strategy could be developed to accommodate all of them without the unproductive enmeshment.

This case illustrates some of the everyday complications as well as resources available in mental health center cases. It is by no means uncommonly complicated, yet it has the potential to develop numerous and time-consuming triangles among the case manager, the therapist, and the family as well as triangles within the family system itself. The advantages for handling a case such as this in the public sector were discussed earlier in this chapter.

Conclusions

The time has come to look seriously at changing the treatment model in public mental health. Sometimes it seems a monumental job. Yet good systems therapists know that a series of small changes can lead to a major change. The trick is in knowing when and where to plant those small changes. So far we have overlooked some opportunities.

First, we have largely failed to take into account the mental health center as a system and new therapeutic approaches as challenges to the balance of that system. We have not dealt with resistance as an interactional artifact; rather, we have "assigned it" to mental health centers, calling them resistant to change. In reality there is no such thing as a resistant system, only systems impervious to inopportune interventions. This is a fact of life we need to face if we choose to implement change, be it in families or mental health centers. So one thing we need to learn is to assess the systems in which we work, find our opportunities, and *then* come up with the same kind of creative interventions we use to help families change.

Next, there are procedural changes in operation that will naturally fall into place once we have intervened effectively in the system. Staff members who are excited about working systematically will even find themselves volunteering for evening duty when such participation is encouraged throughout the system.

We also must not ignore the community, which can prove to be one of our greatest assets. Untutored or uninitiated in the machinations of professional therapists, community members mostly have no axes to grind regarding the form of treatment if they can be convinced of the ultimate benefit to them and to the community on the whole. Get your citizens' advisory group on your side, and you have a powerful ally.

Finally, there is the issue of treatment. When all the other elements are in place, effective treatment can begin with actual families, individuals, and their satellite systems. Then and only then can the skill of the therapist begin to show results. As therapists, we are tempted to do treatment first, but we also need to learn patience.

5

Martha A. Foster

Schools

Typically, children spend at least six to eight hours a day in school and additional time on the bus or in car pools, in after-school activities, and doing homework. Thus, the school is a major context for children and for their families and deserves attention and understanding from therapists working with child-focused problems. Family therapists need to take school problems and the school context seriously because academic and behavioral problems at school are a major reason for referral to therapy. Common presenting problems include behavior problems, peer conflicts, academic underachievement or failure, school avoidance, and symptoms of social immaturity at school.

Because school problems have obvious immediate effects on both the child and the family, successfully treating a school problem is helpful to both. Siblings of referred children may also benefit when parents are helped to negotiate positive school/family relationships and thus become better prepared to handle later school difficulties with other children. In addition, there is growing evidence that adjustment problems in adults are often preceded by school maladjustment (Bower, Shellhamer, and Dailey, 1960; Cowen and others, 1973; Robins, 1969). Ac-

Many of the ideas in this chapter evolved from my collaboration with Michael Berger, Carrell Dammann, and Gregory Jurkovic over the past years. I am indebted to them for their input and particularly to Michael Berger for his unflagging conviction of the importance of social systems beyond the nuclear family.

110

cordingly, remediation of school adjustment problems in children may serve a preventive function in adult mental health. Because of the potential for both short- and long-range benefits, then, the school is a critical context for intervention with children.

Schools are "self-contained cultures" (Lightfoot, 1978). They have a particular language, organizational structure, and set of functions that must be understand if the school context is to be effectively and appropriately used in treatment. The goals of this chapter are to provide the reader with an understanding of the school as a system, to evaluate how this system interacts with the family system and with the therapy system, and to offer guidelines and techniques for working with school personnel and families in the solution of child and family problems. Although I have worked for several years within a school system, this chapter is written from the perspective of an "outsider" to the schools, a role I have taken during the past few years as a family therapist in private practice treating many families who have a child with a school problem. I recognize that the school counselor or school psychologist who does systems therapy may, as an insider, need to operate somewhat differently. Potential constraints, as well as advantages, of working systemically from a position within the school system will be addressed later in this chapter.

Culture of the School

In America there is no one "school," only diverse modes of schooling. Schools vary in their size, source of funding (public or private), pedagogical orientation, and organizational structure. The differences between a small alternative school that emphasizes free expression, individuality, and socialization experiences and a larger, more traditional public school can be considerable. Each talks a somewhat different language, holds different expectations for child behavior, and seems to appeal to and work best with different types of families and children. Even among apparently comparable schools or among classrooms within the same school, there can be considerable diversity in such things as curriculum, standards for child behavior, amount of contact with families, or flexibility in schedule. Therefore, although schools have many functional and structural features in common, there remains sufficient diversity among schools to warrant caution in generalizing from one school environment to another.

In all schools, though, there is an underlying assumption that they are in existence for children—to educate, socialize, monitor, and protect children. The way these functions are carried out may vary, but the orientation of educators is toward viewing the child as an individual agent, apart from family and social context. This view is shaped during teachers' own professional education, with its emphasis on methods of instruction and on child development, and is continually reinforced by the structural features of schools that segregate children from families and thus limit teachers' opportunities to see children contextually. For example, it is becoming less and less common for teachers to make home visits or to interact with parents and children in other than formal parent/teacher conferences. Their training and the ongoing structure and purpose of schooling act to maintain educators in intraindividual explanations of behavior and result in school treatments and interventions primarily at the level of the individual child—for example, psychoeducational assessment, special education classrooms, and individual counseling.

I think this individualistic viewpoint of educators is shaped and maintained by yet another phenomenon that is best understood by looking at the school as a major institution. As an institution, the American school is charged by society with a very broad array of functions, including education, health maintenance, values training, child caretaking, and evaluation. No other institution, except the family, is given so much responsibility by society, or maintains its influence for such a long period, or is required to interface with the total spectrum of citizens. Furthermore, because children legally must be educated, the school is not a voluntary institution. Therefore, in comparison with institutions with a delimited purpose, a nonmandated membership, or time-limited contact, such as the health system,

Schools 113

religious organizations, or even the judicial system, the school is more at risk of direct competition with the American family. In order to avoid competition and allow the family its traditionally central role with the child, the institutional policy of schools is to focus on the child as an individual. Consequently, the systems therapist who attempts to alter the belief system of educators toward more systemic thinking should bear in mind the likelihood of institutional as well as individual sources of resistance. I have found that a more effective stance is usually to work strategically, accepting the individual frame and tailoring interventions to fit it.

Functions of Schools. Schools have at least four major functions: education, evaluation, socialization, and childcare. Although individual schools and school systems define these functions differently and give them different priorities, these functions are common to all schools.

All schools teach basic academic skills such as reading and arithmetic; however, methods and theories of instruction vary, and schools are quite diverse in their definitions of a curriculum. For example, in some schools the educational curriculum is designed to promote awareness of cultural diversity, values differences, and sex-role stereotyping. In other schools such issues are explicitly defined as not the school's responsibility.

All schools also play an evaluative function (Henry, 1963). Report cards and achievement tests provide teachers, parents, and children with feedback about the child's performance relative to age peers and normative standards. However, schools differ in the manner and frequency of feedback and in how broadly they define their evaluative function. Some emphasize the traditional academic areas, while others include more detailed assessment of social and emotional functioning. Clinicians must keep in mind that although evaluation may be routine from the perspective of school personnel, for families it is seldom routine. The school evaluation, particularly the more formal tests and procedures, arouses considerable anxiety in many parents as well as in their children.

This evaluative function also legitimizes the school's role as a labeler of deviance for society. However, diversity in educational orientation among schools results in variation in the kinds of behavior in children labeled as atypical and resulting in referral. For example, shy behavior in an academically achieving student might be coded as problematic in a school that places a high priority on social development, while the same behavior in a child in a school that emphasizes academics might be ignored. Thus the values and educational focus of a school influence its evaluative function. Although families may not view such judgments as relative to a school's pedagogical agenda, therapists are advised to evaluate assessments of children in context.

The third function of schools, the socialization function, may be directly or indirectly acknowledged. All schools provide an organizing framework for peer relationships. Children are at school with age peers for a large portion of their waking hours, and it is here that friendships develop and the child's relative status in the peer group is defined. The elementary school peer group is unique, for unlike the child's set of siblings, the school peer group is often tightly age- and sex-segregated. However, with the onset of adolescence and usually by high school, the composition of the school peer group usually changes to include children of both sexes and a broader age range. These changes can be disconcerting to parents who are unused to seeing their child socializing with older friends. Schools thus serve a critical function as a laboratory for peer socialization. This is an area that is generally not widely open to adult scrutiny and yet is presumed to be critical for child development (Minuchin and others, 1969).

Schools differ in how much influence they attempt to have on peer relations. Some schools take into consideration friendship patterns and the "climate of the group" when assigning children to classes; others do not. For the clinician, the school offers a setting for intervention when peer relationships are poor, a common presenting problem in referred children. In addition, the school provides an alternative setting and source of stability for children when family stress is high, a setting where they can interact positively with both other children and adults.

A fourth, often unrecognized function of schools is their

child caretaking functions for parents and society (Goodman, 1960). Mandatory education laws removed children from the labor force during an era when child employment was becoming increasingly unacceptable socially and economically. Schooling provided a benevolent rationale for removing children from competition in the labor market and corralled them during the day in a highly structured environment. Today, issues of child labor seem archaic, but the concern for where children are to go during the day remains. Schools offer a safe, supervised, and ideally stimulating care situation. Moreover, for dual-worker families and single working parents, the presence of schools is essential for the family's economic stability (Bane, 1976). Although most schools still operate on a schedule geared to an agrarian economy, some schools are beginning to alter their programs to accommodate working parents by offering after-school daycare, full-day kindergarten, and summer programs. The importance of this childcare function of the school was brought home to me recently when a divorced working mother confided that she was doing her daughter's homework for her because she was anxious that her daughter be perceived by the school personnel as doing well. The youngster's school was the only one convenient and affordable to the mother that provided after-school care, and the mother felt she could not risk the possibility of a recommendation to another school because of poor performance by the child.

Structure of Schools. Like other systems, schools are hierarchally organized. Principals are over teachers, and teachers are over students. However, this simplistic assessment grossly underestimates the complexity of the school's structure. Several factors that express themselves in idiosyncratic ways in different schools must be assessed before the hierarchy in a school becomes clear.

First is the administrative style of the principal (Sarason, 1971). Principals generally set the tone for the school. They may assume a position that is central, involve themselves in educational and disciplinary issues, and promote high contact and information sharing between themselves and the teaching staff. Such a principal will be more likely to pursue contacts with families and be aware early of problems in children. Alternatively, principals may take a more distant stance, choosing to leave most educational and child management concerns to teachers while they focus more on administrative issues. With the latter style, the boundaries between the teacher and the principal are clearly delineated and the roles differentiated by function as well as status, while with the former, the boundaries are more permeable, as the functions and roles of teacher and principal overlap. In bypassing a central principal, the therapist may be overlooking an important participant in the sequence around the problem. Triangles that include principals as well as teachers, parents, and children are not uncommon. It is therefore wise to contact the principal first when making a school visit; this respects the hierarchy, and it often reveals an important actor in the problem sequence.

Principals vary, too, in how broadly or narrowly they interpret school system guidelines and rules as applicable to their own school. Sarason (1971) links this variation in principals to their degree of locus of control. Principals who themselves feel that they determine the destiny of their school are willing to bend rules and experiment with unorthodox procedures when needed. However, when dealing with a principal who adheres closely to procedure and tradition or invokes the "system" as his or her guide, it may be necessary to obtain the support of the principal's superiors in the hierarchy for an unusual request. Moreover, the therapist should demonstrate sensitivity to such differences among principals in choice of language and frame for the problem.

A second factor to remember when assessing the structure is that schools contain many more actors than the principal, teachers, and students. There are counselors, speech or special education teachers, and support personnel such as secretaries and bus drivers. School counselors often have considerable influence because their position, by definition, marks them in the school context as an expert in dealing with emotional or behavioral problems. Moreover, their role allows them greater access to confidential information. Less obvious is the secretary. Access to the principal or to teaching personnel is often controlled by the secretary. Moreover, in many schools, the office personnel have a great deal of contact with children and families.

In addition to staff members who work at only one school, there are a myriad of professionals such as school psychologists, special education consultants, "itinerant" teachers, supervisors, and area coordinators who travel among several schools, entering and leaving the system. These consultants complicate the hierarchy when their role or authority is unclear. Some, such as school psychologists, wield considerable power at decision points, such as placement staffings, but may have little or no authority in the day-to-day operation of the school. In general, the more serious or entrenched a child's problem, the more specialists there will be from the greater school system. Not unlike working with a large extended family system (Dammann and Berger, 1983), determining the hierarchy when a youngster's school problems have mobilized the school system's network of special education personnel can be challenging. Typically, during formal meetings such as staffings, ascribed or achieved status determines the hierarchy. Thus the school psychologist or educational supervisor has more influence than a teacher in a placement decision. However, implementation of a treatment plan depends squarely for success on the consent and cooperation of the teaching staff and the principal.

A third factor that influences the hierarchy of the school is the fact that most schools are embedded in a complex structure, the "school system," with its own agenda and rules. Furthermore, all schools are under scrutiny from parent and consumer groups and from society as a whole. The impact of these forces from the broader context of schools can be seen in how schools define and assign priorities to their functions. Principals and teachers may change their positions suddenly under pressure from superiors in the school system or from parent or consumer groups. The way a therapeutic plan for a child at school can be jeopardized when school personnel change their stand under such pressure is demonstrated in the following example: A young girl with learning and behavioral problems was enrolled in a private school. Although she was showing some behavior problems, problems not typical in this particular school, the principal and teachers had repeatedly reassured the parents she was appropriately placed and doing well. Suddenly, one day, when the child acted out in school in a manner not unlike previous transgressions, she was summarily expelled. Only several weeks later did the therapist inadvertently learn the reason for the expulsion. Some parents of other pupils in the school, pupils who showed learning difficulties but not severe behavioral difficulties, had complained to the principal that this child was a bad influence on their children. Although the teachers were well trained and equipped to deal with behavioral problems, because of the principal's response to parent pressure, the educational component of the therapeutic plan for this child had to be precipitously revamped.

School/Family Relationships

As an institution, the school has a set of functions that overlap considerably with those of the family. Yet, in important ways, these functions are and must remain different. Lightfoot (1978) examined the differences between the teacher/child and the parent/child relationship. First, the parent/child bond is an enduring, lifelong relationship, while a teacher's relationship is time-limited. Second, a parent has a more exclusive relationship with a child; the teacher must divide his or her time among a much larger number of children at approximately the same developmental level. Even a parent with several children does not have more than one child with exactly the same needs (except possibly in the case of twins), so that a more individualized response to the idiosyncratic needs of the child is possible. The availability of many age peers in the classroom also seems to pull the child toward peer relationships and away from developing a relationship with a teacher that is as exclusive as that with a parent. Third, whereas children know teachers in only one context, their relationship with their parents exists across many contexts. Last, and most important, there are differences in the scope and emphasis of the socializing and nurturing roles that both teachers and parents provide for children. In families, the socialization function (values training, limit setting, education) and the nurturing function (protection from harm and provision for emotional and physical security) are of paramount and equal importance. In fact, parents of children with behavioral or emotional problems often present to the therapist with these functions out of balance (too "hard" or too "soft"). Teachers, too, have both socialization and nurturing roles vis-à-vis children, but the scope of these roles is different. The socialization role entails more imparting of "universal truths" in a context that is less emotionally charged than a family, while, generally, the nurturing function is secondary to the socialization function.

These divisions in function between the family and school permit the child, ideally, to evolve two very different types of relationships with parents and with teachers. When the functions of the two settings are respected and the boundaries clear and supported by both parents and teachers, children are free to use the school and the family as alternative environments for growth (Erikson, 1950). Schools provide a setting in which children can begin to move away from the emotional and dependent constraints of family and experience greater autonomy and connection with social systems beyond the family. Simultaneously, the family provides the security of ongoing relationships and the protection and guidance appropriate to a child's still dependent status.

Parents and educators must achieve a degree of "institutional symmetry" (Lightfoot, 1978), that is, coequal status, for there to be true dialogue and mutual support and for the child to avoid being triangulated between the two settings. Problems arise when the boundaries between home and school are blurred or too distinct or the divisions in function are not clear.

Entry into the School System. Educators share a common language that demarcates their profession from others. The systems therapist who talks this language will find it easier to enter the educational system. At the very least, the local terms for disability categories and their abbreviations (BD, SLD, SED), for special education services (resource rooms, Project Re-Ed), for evaluation instruments and nomenclature (stanines,

PIAT), and for the steps in referral into special services (screening, staffing, IEP meeting) are important. Although it is sometimes a useful joining step to support the expertise of the educator by asking for an explanation of such terms, usually ignorance will handicap the therapist's ability to assess the situation or communicate with the educator. Moreover, familiarity with educational jargon and terminology allows one to serve as a translator for families and to equip them to interact more competently with specialists.

In addition to acquiring a new language system for working with educators, the therapist is advised to avoid psychiatric terms and nomenclature and find other ways to demonstrate expertise. Diagnostic labels carry extra meaning and may not be well understood. In fact, even the term *therapy* is best avoided in the school context. *Counseling* and *meeting with the family* are preferred alternatives because they raise less anxiety among staff and are generally more acceptable to families as well.

There is no one point in the course of treatment when the therapist predictably makes contact with the school system. Contact can be initiated before seeing the family, after the initial family interview, or at some point during the course of treatment; the decision about timing depends on who initiates referral, the nature of the school problem, and the degree of agreement between the parents about the problem.

When the school identifies the problem and either makes the referral directly or indicates to the family that therapy for a school problem is needed, contact with the school is necessary early in treatment to obtain a clear problem definition and to map a course for intervention. Early school contact is particularly important when a problem is occurring within the school setting but not at home. Aponte (1976a) suggests conducting the initial interview in such cases with the school personnel and the family, so that the school staff can present their view of the problem to the family and to the therapist directly. This procedure eliminates the need for the family to interpret to the therapist the school's view of the problem, a difficult task for many families when they do not experience themselves as having trouble with a child. An initial school/family interview frames the problem from the beginning as a school-defined concern and can reveal resources in the school setting for resolution of the problem that might be overlooked if only the family were seen. The intent of the initial family/school interview is to avoid prematurely identifying the child as a patient and to promote joint problem solving between the family and the school personnel. Usually, because of schedules and the number of school personnel involved, the interview is held at the school; the use of a cotherapist may be helpful if the number of persons involved is large. Aponte advises staying focused on solutions rather than searching for causes of the problem, a stance that serves to protect the privacy of both the parents and the teachers and discourages the mistake of dealing with school personnel as clients.

In my own experience of beginning therapy with a family/school interview, I have found that when school personnel were able and willing to commit sufficient time for the interview, and when anxiety in both the school personnel and the family was not overly high, the method worked well. It is less successful when the participants are pressed for time or highly anxious about dealing with each other. The latter seems to be more likely when the problem has been a long-standing one for which many solutions have been attempted or when the family has a history of conflicts with school personnel. In such cases, separate initial meetings with the family and with school personnel are preferable because they allow the therapist to establish firmly a working relationship with each and to reduce anxiety before bringing them together.

More commonly, families enter therapy well aware of and concerned about their child's school problems. The decision on when to contact the school depends on the nature of the school problem and the therapist's assessment of the degree of discord between the parents about the school difficulties. School phobia warrants immediate evaluation of the school situation to determine whether there are legitimate reasons for the child to be avoiding school. If the school environment is not safe for the child, this must be remedied or another school found before a treatment plan to return the child to school is implemented (Haley, 1980). In addition, for children who present with symptoms of school failure or underachievement, the appropriateness of the school program for the child must be evaluated early in treatment.

However, in many families where a child has a school problem, considerable discord exists between the parents about either the definition or the handling of the problem. Unless the problem requires immediate intervention in the school setting, it is best to resolve the disagreement between the parents before recommending a school/family conference that would expose the disagreement or result in an impasse because of the conflict at home. Even merely calling the teacher to get information about the situation may be construed as entering into a coalition with one parent against the other if their disagreement concerns whether a problem at school really exists. For example, a family came into therapy because their eleven-year-old son was receiving poor conduct and academic grades at school and showing aggressive and impudent behavior at home. During the first interview, it became clear that although both parents were upset by the child's behavior at home, the mother was much more distressed than the father by his transgressions and underachievement at school. The child attended an achievement-oriented private school that the mother had selected. The father, who had considerably less formal education than the mother, opposed the mother by his passive, unconcerned stance about the child's school performance. Despite the mother's vigorous suggestions during the first session that the therapist meet with them and the school staff about the child's problems, the therapist wisely elected to refrain from doing so until the parents had come to some agreement about the child's school behavior. When this had been achieved, the parents were able to meet with the child's teachers to jointly implement an intervention directed toward problems they both wanted remediated. Had the therapist sanctioned a school conference before resolution of the conflict between mother and father, the therapist would have entered into a coalition with the mother against the father and increased the distance between them on this issue.

In other situations, the parents may be in clear agreement

that a problem in school exists but may lack expertise in discussing the problem or comfort in dealing with school officials. It may then be wise to postpone a meeting with the school until the parents have sufficient information about school procedures or an understanding of the requisite language to communicate effectively with school personnel about the problem. Even though the therapist may be well trained to serve as the family's spokesperson at the school staffing or parent/teacher conference, it makes more sense in the long run if the parents are helped to learn how to negotiate such routine school contacts themselves (Milan and others, 1982). The therapist who initiates contact with the school as soon as the parents bring up a school-related concern may be missing an opportunity to assist the parents in learning to deal with the school directly. Empowering parents to be effective in dealing with educators is often an important goal of treatment.

Assessment of the Family/School Relationship. The family/school relationship goes through predictable stages that change as a child shows increasingly problematic behavior at school (Haley, 1976; DiCocco and Lott, 1982). In the absence of serious problems in the child, the two authority systems, the parents and the educators, each retain primary responsibility for the child's behavior in their respective settings. The boundaries between home and school are clear, and the teacher/student relationship is clearly distinguishable from the parent/child relationship. The parents and the teachers each are relatively certain about the extent and limit of their responsibility toward the child.

When a child's school problems escalate to the point that school personnel find themselves unable to solve them, responsibility for the child's school behavior is returned to the parents. DiCocco and Lott (1982) term this "Phase II." Essentially, the parents are brought in at this point with the expectation on the part of the school staff that they should get the child to behave or perform at school. Thus the parent/child relationship is expanded to a parent/child-student relationship. This phase may be marked by notes and calls to the parent about the problems at school, increased homework supervision and tutoring by the parent, behavioral contracts about school behaviors with the parents dispensing rewards and punishments, or suspension to the home. When problems are not entrenched and the parent/ teacher relationship is positive, it is productive for parents to step in temporarily to help teachers solve school problems. This procedure works when the child perceives the parents as backing the teacher's position about school behaviors and both authorities agree about the plan of action—in short, when the hierarchy and the expectations for change are clear. A large number of school problems are handled in this manner without involving mental health professionals.

Referral to a therapist often occurs at the point when the youngster's school problems have not been corrected after considerable effort by the parents to solve the problem at home. The parents and the educators at this point are confused about who is responsible for the problem and how to solve it. Blame and lack of confidence prevail on both sides. The problems escalate and become chronic as the child is caught in this confused hierarchy between home and school. DiCocco and Lott (1982) term this "Phase III." Several factors may contribute to the development of this state of affairs, including conflicts between the parents, logistical limitations or skills deficits that prevent parents from following through on treatment plans, or failure of parents and teachers to agree on treatment strategies. Moreover, parents who at first readily step in to deal with a child's school problems often find that as they are unsuccessful in changing the school problems, other new difficulties also begin to appear at home. As problems escalate and spread to the home situation, parents often turn back to the school for solutions. By the time the therapist enters, the home/school relationship is tangled, emotionally negative, and sometimes adversarial. A recursive sequence, marked by transmittal of negative information about the child between parents and teacher, serves to escalate the feeling of blame and incompetence on both sides. The parents and the teacher are allied only in the sense that they share a sense of frustration and anger with the child.

Interventions. Breaking a negative sequence and restructuring the hierarchy so that the parents are the authorities at home and the educators are in charge at school are the long-term goals for the systemic therapist. Different tactics may be used to reach these goals, tactics that often involve creating an initial "abnormal structure" (Haley, 1976) as an intermediate stage in the therapy.

One tactic involves restructuring the hierarchy so that, temporarily, the parents are above the teachers and are responsible for developing a plan for handling the child's behavioral problems *at school* (DiCocco and Lott, 1982). In this approach the parents are directly involved in setting up, and sometimes implementing, consequences in the classroom situation for the problem behaviors. The approach requires that the school staff have exhausted all resources within the school for managing the child and are sufficiently desperate that they are willing to relinquish control of the problem to the parents. Because the parents can use the child's full school day as a source of consequences for school problems, their range of possible management techniques is increased over what was available when there were consequences in the home situation only for school misbehavior—for example, the withholding of television privileges. This can be a boost to the parent who is feeling that the number of home consequences has been exhausted; moreover, even though the parent is directing the plan, because school behavior is being handled at school, the amount of punishment at home for school behavior can be reduced, resulting in a clearer separation between home and school problems and sometimes an immediate and positive change in the parent/child relationship. DiCocco and Lott (1982, p. 101) stress that "the therapist's primary maneuver must be to create and orchestrate a scenario in which the child's parents assume a hierarchical position superior to that of the teacher *while the child observes* [italics mine]. The parents must openly direct the teacher in how to manage the classroom behavior of their child. Once this scenario has taken place, in front of the child, new behavioral sequences can begin to transpire between child and teacher, between child and parents, and between the two sets of adults."

From my own experience in reordering confused hierarchies by temporarily giving parents greater authority for school problems than teachers, several comments about the tactic are in order. As DiCocco and Lott stress, it is critical that the child observe the parents directing the teacher to implement the plan, thus underscoring the change in order of command. For the technique to work, disagreements between the parents about the school problems must be resolved first or set aside so that the child or the teacher is not caught in a triangle with them. If a covert disagreement becomes overt during the process, as often happens, it needs to be settled. This may entail a recess to meet with parents separately to help them resolve their differences before continuing the negotiations with the teacher. The therapist must also be particularly sensitive to reluctance of any of the adults to implement the plan. Failure leads only to further confusion in the hierarchy. Finally, the therapist must shift to a more normal hierarchy once the abnormal structure has been effective in getting the child to behave. Often the process of putting the teacher back in charge at school while distancing the parents requires as much attention from the therapist as did setting up the intermediate structure in the first place.

For example, in one case the parents had been helped to develop and endorse a method for the teacher to use when their child was verbally abusive at school, a long-term problem over which the parents and teacher had repeatedly clashed. The consequences set up by the parents entailed restriction from favored classroom activities and chores distasteful to the child in the school cafeteria. Conflicts between the parents and teacher lessened as they joined together around this agreed-on strategy, and the verbal abuse subsided in frequency. The parents experienced considerable relief when their negative interactions with their son about his school behavior were reduced, freeing them to focus on difficulties with him at home. However, the teacher required consultation with the therapist to reassume her rightful authority in the classroom. Because the tactic of placing the parents in charge of the verbal abuse problem had proved so effective, she turned to them for help with other, less entrenched problems that the child showed. The procedure had been effective in clarifying the hierarchy and changing the presenting problem, but it had temporarily robbed the teacher of her sense of competence as a manager of routine classroom difficulties. With some brief consultation and support by the therapist, she was able to discover her own solutions for new problems with this child. Therefore, continued contact with the teacher is recommended beyond the abatement of the presenting complaint, to ensure that parity between the home and the school is fully reestablished.

An alternative approach to breaking a negative sequence between parents and teachers and reordering a confused hierarchy around school problems is to arrange a temporary severance of contact between home and school. Such a move may be appropriate when tension in all parties is being increasingly fueled by the child's escalating problems in both home and school. Neither the parents nor the teachers are successful in handling the child's behavior, and mutual blaming and a history of negative interaction between them preclude the kind of cooperation required in the former procedure. In this case, the therapist positions herself between the parents and the school staff and secures a time-limited commitment from each that they will not communicate with the other. Further, the teacher must agree not to discuss home problems with the child, and the parents agree to refrain from dealing with the child's school behavior problems at home. The therapist works separately with the two systems to help each resolve the problems in its respective setting. This procedure forms an extremely rigid boundary between the home and the school as a temporary measure to reduce the tension and allow each authority an opportunity to begin to bring the child's behavior under control. Lusterman (1982) terms this type of intervention "interdiction" because it interrupts the negative recursive cycle between parents and teachers. He argues that therapists should secure the parents' written approval for the tactic and their support for using any method at school that the therapist and teachers deem appropriate to change the child's behavior. Clearly, for parents to give such latitude to the therapist requires that they have joined well with the therapist and trust his or her judgment. The therapist must be prepared to assume an active role in working with the teachers to resolve the school problems, including being readily available to them for emergency consultation. Again, this is an intermediate stage in the therapy and creates an abnormal structure, much like the abnormal structure a therapist creates by putting one parent totally in charge of a child's behavior for a time while the other parent "takes a vacation" from dealing with the problem (Haley, 1976). In both cases, therapy must continue to the final stage, in which the boundary between the two authorities is less rigid, with appropriate degrees of communication and collaboration. As the adults are helped to handle the child's behavior problems, and the child improves, tension diminishes. The therapist then needs to orchestrate the exchange of positive communications between parents and teachers and highlight places of agreement to counter the history of negative interactions. As the therapist moves them back toward more direct interaction with each other, he gradually loosens the boundary and removes himself from the "go-between" position.

I have used various types of "interdiction" tactics in my own practice as intermediate strategies to block dysfunctional sequences between parents and teachers as well as between parents and children about educational concerns. For example, in one family where a girl had a history of underachievement in school, the solution initially recommended by the school involved the mother, a single parent, tutoring the child in extra homework in the evening. However, the mother was temperamentally a poor teacher for the child and was very anxious about her daughter's academic success. Mother and child engaged in heated battles around homework that further increased the child's anxieties about academic work. By the time I became involved with them, the tension between mother and daughter had spread to encompass their interactions around non-school-related concerns, such as chores and house rules. The child was disobedient and belligerent toward the mother and the teacher, and both were distressed by her poor grades and problem behavior. The mother asked for more homework and the teacher kept giving it. However, "the solution had become the problem" (Watzlawick, Weakland, and Fisch, 1974).

Blocking the mother as supervisor of homework was the first step in changing the problem. Since the child went to a neighbor's home after school, a plan was worked out that for a month the child would do her homework at the sitter's home, and the teacher would check the homework before school started. The mother was responsible for bringing the child to school early so the teacher could review the homework. The plan entailed securing the cooperation of mother, teacher, sitter, and child and was framed as necessary for the mother to allow her to focus on the home problems. The child was challenged to demonstrate her maturity, a bet she readily accepted to prove her mother wrong. Although this was but an initial step in the therapy with this family, it blocked the negative sequence around homework and created a clearer boundary between home and school.

In another situation, a girl was enrolled in a private school after not succeeding in an academically oriented public school. Her father, the custodial parent, had had tense, sometimes conflictual contacts with the previous school's staff and for that reason was suspicious of the new school. His anxiety was legitimate in that some problems had been mishandled in the previous setting; however, his frequent calls and unannounced visits to the new school were distressing to the teacher and the child and were beginning to re-create some of the tensions the father had felt in the prior school. I discovered that a major problem was that he needed a large amount of information to feel comfortable about the child's school experience, while the teacher was not used to sharing detailed information about her students with parents except during scheduled parent/teacher conferences. Armed with these observations, I persuaded the father to let me provide him with the information he needed, arguing that the information would be more accurate and less likely to be slanted to make him feel comfortable. Since the father was already suspicious that he was not hearing "the real story," he accepted my offer and agreed to suspend contacting the teacher. I established regular contact with the teacher, who was relieved to talk with someone other than the father. After a semester of using this procedure, the teacher had much positive information to share with the father, information that he could readily accept because the girl was succeeding in school. Following the creation of a firm boundary between home and school through positioning myself as a "go-between," the anxiety between the father and the teacher lessened sufficiently to allow them to begin to connect in a more appropriate manner.

Thus, the therapist can block dysfunctional sequences centering on educational concerns by arranging a rigid boundary for a period of time between home and school. This may entail blocking *all* communication between the adults in the two settings for a while (Lusterman, 1982). In this case the procedure must be viewed as an intermediate stage in the therapy, a therapy that will continue until appropriate communication between parents and teachers is reestablished. In other cases a clear but less rigid boundary may need to be drawn to help parents, teachers, and children reestablish school and home as separate environments for the child.

Predictable Triangles. Certain triangular relationships among children, parents, and educators deserve highlighting. Though not inclusive of all possible relationship configurations, three types of triangles are common.

Parent/Teacher/Child. When conflicts between parents and teachers are handled by involving a child in the dispute, a classic triangle is formed. Whether the struggles between the adults are overt or covert, the child is caught in a loyalty conflict between the two authority figures. One such triangle involves a parent and teacher who are competing with each other over the child. The parent may be a mother who is having difficulty allowing the child to form strong attachments to other adults. When the child's teacher moves in too quickly to establish a close, warm relationship with the child, the mother is threatened. This sequence often seems to involve a single-parent mother and a young teacher whose uncertainty and lack of experience with teaching make her need a close relationship with the child to affirm her teaching abilities. Essentially, mother and teacher are competing over the nurturing function. In other cases, parents may seek to protect children from their teachers, thus entering into a coalition with the child against the teacher around issues of classroom discipline.

Such conflicts between parents or teachers, whether about the nurturance or discipline of the child, must be resolved before the child can be removed from the middle position. The teacher, who is often better trained to deal with children than with adults, and the parent, who may be anxious about talking with the teacher because of his or her own educational experiences, need a third party to help them resolve their differences. A conference at the school, often in the classroom, can be used to help the adults establish points of agreement. Including the child in the session(s) depends on the degree and nature of the conflict between parent and teacher; in any case, the child should be included at least to the extent that he or she can observe the new united front. Carl and Jurkovic (1983) offer additional examples of this type of triangle.

Mother/Father/Teacher. Usually when parents, in extreme disagreement about a child, pull a teacher into their dispute, the therapist is advised to work with the parents to help them resolve their differences before holding a meeting with the teacher and the family. However, in many cases work with the teacher is also indicated, particularly when the teacher's strong relationship with one of the parents is contributing to the maintenance of the triangle. Many educators operate as though "parent" meant "mother" (Foster, Berger, and McLean, 1981). Conferences and meetings are often scheduled with mothers because, historically, mothers have tended to be more accessible during the schoolday and perhaps because teachers (who most often are women) are more comfortable dealing with mothers. The therapist can assist fathers and teachers in establishing a direct relationship with each other in a number of ways. For example, until the problem is resolved, the parents can be directed to talk together with the teacher, even to the point of using extension phones. Separate conferences with the father and the teacher may be needed to unbalance a tight alliance between mother and teacher. When a parent and a teacher have established a coalition against the other parent, informational meetings between the teacher and "outside" parent can help the teacher see this parent in a new light. For example, when one mother and father disagreed about the seriousness of their son's learning disability, the therapist discovered that although the child had been in a special school for three years, the father had been to the school only twice. The mother drove the child to school daily and had an intense and intimate relationship with the child's school counselor. The mother and the counselor agreed that a major problem was the father's "uninvolvement" and lack of support for the child's many learning problems. The school counselor had accepted the mother's view of the father as reality without getting to know him or trying to understand his assessment of his child. The first stage of the therapy was directed toward helping the father establish a separate relationship with the child's teacher to counter the strong coalition between mother and counselor. With his own ally in the school, an ally with much direct information about the child, the therapist then helped the father establish a working relationship with the counselor as well.

Teacher/Teacher/Child. Triangles that include teachers or other members of a school's staff and a child are also common. Such triangles may involve a regular education and a special education teacher, a teacher and a counselor, or perhaps a principal and a teacher. The adults may differ in their view of the child's needs, often with one advocating for "stricter controls," the other for more "understanding." In addition to triangles in which the adults disagree along a "tough/soft" continuum, I occasionally see children who become caught between two teachers who are struggling over who should be in charge of the child or who understands the child more. The latter situation is similar to the loyalty conflicts that children experience when two parents compete for a child's affections. For example, in one school the counselor and one teacher had a poor working relationship to which the therapist was alerted by the principal's offhand comment that "those two *never* saw eye-to-eye." When a boy who had been working with the school counselor for the previous year and a half because of home problems was promoted into the teacher's classroom, the ingredients for an intense triangle were in place. When the counselor began to inform the teacher about the boy's home situation and need for special handling, old antipathies were triggered in each of them. The teacher felt the counselor was siding with the boy against her classroom rules, and the counselor felt the teacher was unsympathetic to the boy's needs. The stricter the teacher became with the boy, the more ways the counselor found to rescue him. A series of interventions that established firmer boundaries between the teacher and the counselor and between the boy and the executive subsystem at school were needed to break this sequence and disrupt the triangle. For example, the counselor repeatedly interceded on the boy's behalf when a problem in the classroom emerged. The therapist convinced the counselor that the boy needed to learn "negotiation skills" to use with his parents and that she could help him develop these by coaching him in how to negotiate directly both with his parents and with his teacher. This blocked the counselor from interceding with the teacher herself, drawing a boundary between the boy's relationship with the teacher and that with the counselor. The therapist chose to work initially only on the adult/child relationships, never directly addressing the teacher/counselor relationship until the boundaries were clearer. This tactic avoided exposing the intensity of the negative feelings between the teacher and the counselor and thereby avoided the risk of the therapist's getting involved in directly working with the teacher and counselor as clients. (Additional tactics in handling staff differences are described in Chapter Nine.)

Using the Peer Network. When I work with families experiencing a major stressor such as divorce, death, unemployment, or marital conflict, I inquire about the degree of involvement of the children with peers in school. When children, particularly adolescents, have had well-developed peer relationships prior to the family stress, they can often retreat temporarily to the peer group for the support that is unavailable at home. For children who are isolated from peers, teachers can be excellent resources for helping parents orchestrate a peer network for the child. The teacher can usually identify an appropriate potential playmate from the class, introduce the two families to each other, and suggest to the parent of the isolated child appropriate play activities to encourage in the home. And after being alerted to a child's difficulties with peers and asked to help the parents with this problem, many teachers "spontaneously" also begin to intervene in the classroom setting to support peer relationships for the isolated child.

Using Routine School Events and Processes. Regularly scheduled parent/teacher conferences and staffings, routine events from the school's viewpoint, offer opportunities for the systems therapist to alter family/school relationships. Whenever possible, I try to use such routine meetings in the conduct of therapy because they are naturally occurring events that both school personnel and parents attend. Parent/teacher conferences are opportunities to implement strategic moves aimed at changing teacher, parent, and child relationships in a context that is defined as educational and not therapeutic, an advantage in many situations. Because parent/teacher conferences traditionally do not include other professionals, I often coach the parents and/or the teacher rather than attending myself, although clearly in many situations the presence of a therapist to orchestrate the interactions is essential. However, after accurate assessment of the system and planning, I have found I can often effect change quite well from a distance. For example, to unbalance a tight coalition between a mother and a teacher, I might join with the father by supporting his expertise, encouraging him in ways to take a more active role during the parent/teacher conference. I also work through teachers, coaching them in particular tactics to produce change. This might involve only asking them to avoid or minimize some topics. For example, parents who experience themselves as incompetent because they cannot get their child to complete his homework will only be further demoralized if the teacher makes the homework problem the focus of the conference. The therapist should anticipate the potential impact of a parent/teacher meeting and plan ahead with the participants so that the conference serves the direction of treatment.

Staffings are formal meetings attended by parents, teachers, and specialists from the school system at which special education placement decisions are made or reevaluated. Public Law 94-142, the Education of All Handicapped Children Act, which legislated a greater degree of parental participation in educational decisions as well as other assurances for children with handicaps, stipulates that parents must be included in placement staffings and involved in the decision-making process. I fully support the importance of involvement of parents in educational decisions, particularly those on labeling or a segregated placement; however, placement staffings as sometimes structured serve more to rob parents of their sense of competence. The typical staffing includes one parent, the mother, and generally three to eight teachers and specialists, including a school psychologist, an "area coordinator," and the principal. Many parents are unaware of the purpose of the meeting, the fact that they can request a postponement, and the fact that they do not have to agree to the plan recommended at the time. While staffings are probably stressful for all parents, for families with a history of a conflict with the school, an initial placement staffing is often a disaster, with both sides bringing to the meeting accumulated tensions and frustrations. Some orchestrating ahead of time can significantly reduce tension, leaving parents and educators better able to communicate and make decisions. For example, I strongly recommend that parents attend staffings together and that they postpone staffings until they have a relatively united position themselves; this often entails my working with the couple, helping them sort out their individual reactions to particular educational choices. I also strongly urge parents to find out before going into the staffing the agenda and the nature of decisions to be made. In addition, if new evaluation information is to be shared, particularly information that may be complicated or painful, I encourage parents to request a separate feedback session with the school psychologist before the staffing in order to have ample time to assimilate the new information before having to make a decision based on it.

Rather than coaching the parents, the therapist might work with the teachers to alter their transactions with the family during a staffing. This is generally easier when the therapist has an ongoing relationship with the teachers, either because of being employed in the educational setting or because of having been on the case for some time.

A good example of a strategic intervention with teachers

at a staffing comes from one of my students employed in a special education program as a consultant. A staffing was planned to discuss the continued enrollment of a four-year-old girl, identified as possibly retarded. The child had made considerable progress but was seen as troublesome by the teachers, who were used to children less verbal and independent than she. The teachers had given the mother many suggestions about how to help the child, which the mother had not followed. Moreover, the mother and teachers had had some conflicts, and at the time of the reevaluation, the mother, a single parent, was threatening to remove the child from school precipitously. The teachers saw the mother as odd, difficult, and aloof. The mother confided to the consultant that she too found the child very difficult to handle at home but that she was fed up with people giving her advice that she could not carry out. She was depressed, overwhelmed with life stresses, and feeling incompetent as a parent. The consultant immediately recognized that intervention was needed before the staffing to block the teachers from giving more advice to the mother and probably precipitating the child's removal from school. Before the staffing, the consultant met with the teachers to describe his view of the home situation. At that time he described the mother's severe depression, evoking sympathy to counter their prior anger at her. The teaching staff began to argue that, for the present, the child was better off in this school than at home and expressed concern that the mother might withdraw her. This was a radical shift from their previous position about this family. With the consultant, they evolved a plan for conducting the staffing in a way that would lower anxiety and make the mother feel more competent. They decided to offer *no* suggestions for her to carry out at home and, whenever possible, to support her perspective on the child. What seemed critical was that the consultant did not tell the teachers how to conduct the staffing but, rather, focused on changing their belief system about the mother, a change that permitted a new range of behavior during the staffing. (Still other uses of the staffing will be found in Chapter Six, as will examples of the therapeutic use of other common school procedures, such as psychological testing.)

Special Considerations. Parents who are educators themselves deserve special attention by the therapist. To be both a teacher and a parent is difficult, and particularly so when a child is showing problems at school, the work domain of the parent. The child's difficulties take on extra significance in that they call into question the parent's expert status in the community. A comparable situation may exist when the parent is a therapist, child psychologist, or minister. Often the parent is intensely upset by the school problems and may be fueling them by his or her own concern. When outrage or embarrassment in the parent is extreme, it may be more related to the parent's own work insecurities and probably is best dealt with at that level. Many of these professional parents deal with school problems in their children by functioning more as teachers than as parents at home. They may be adding their own extra homework, grilling the child about school behavior, and generally monitoring in a teacherlike fashion. Moreover, because of their job, they may have access to information that other parents would not have, making it difficult for the child to feel there is a boundary between home and school. Generally, in such cases I enforce a rigid boundary between home and school, arguing that the parent needs a change of role after three o'clock as much as the child does.

The therapist also needs to attend to developmental differences in children when selecting treatment tactics and formulating goals. For example, I always have the parents of a young child who is failing in school meet with the youngster's teacher to determine the cause of the problem; however, I often send adolescents initially by themselves to talk to teachers about school problems. This tactic both supports and tests their maturity and draws a boundary between home and school. For adolescents who have depended on their parents to rescue them when they experience difficulties at school, this type of task is both a restructuring move in the family and an opportunity for the adolescent to learn an age-appropriate skill.

Therapists working with schools and families have a responsibility to be very clear themselves about their own role vis-à-vis the family and the school personnel. As noted earlier, when employed by a family, they must be wary of stepping into a therapeutic role with the school staff. Although some of the tactics presented in this chapter are focused toward teachers, they are framed as dealing only with educational issues.

In addition, in most cases the therapist will need to maintain a position of neutrality with both the family and the school. By avoiding taking sides when controversy emerges, the therapist remains "meta" to the system and available to both teachers and parents in the negotiation of differences. Whether the therapist is "outside" the school system, in public or private mental health, or "inside" the system, as a school psychologist or counselor, a position of relative neutrality allows the therapist the greatest latitude for effecting change. Occasionally, the therapist may choose to shift from this role of consultant to the role of advocate for a family if injustice is occurring or if the family needs the weight of an expert to effect a change in the school system. I have acted as an advocate for families primarily around issues of child testing and special education placement when appropriate procedures were not being followed or testing data were not being interpreted accurately to parents. But as quickly as possible, I prefer to move back to a more neutral stance. To step in and act as an advocate for parents reduces their own sense of power and competence and creates a coalition with the parents that restricts the range of therapy and limits the therapist's role with the school personnel. (For an example of the therapist's advocate role, see Berger, in press.)

Operating from "Inside" the School System

Although this chapter has been written from the perspective of the systems therapist who is not employed by the school system, the thinking and many of the tactics are appropriate for school psychologists, school counselors, or other school personnel working with children and families. In fact, the therapist who is "inside" the system has the advantage of being familiar with the language and policies of the school as a system and of being able to intervene into a problem sequence early in its evolution, perhaps even before it is identified as a problem (see

Chapter Nine). In fact, for many families, a meeting with an outside practitioner is much more threatening than a more routine meeting at school with the counselor or school psychologist. In this sense, the counselor or school psychologist can play a preventive role in child and family problems. Several recent publications have argued the relevance of family systems thinking for school personnel and suggest that this conceptual framework is gaining in support in training institutions and among practitioners in the schools (for example, Johnston and Fields, 1981; Perosa and Perosa, 1981; Worden, 1981; Green and Fine, 1980; Smith, 1978).

From my own experience working with school system personnel on clinical cases and through training seminars, I think professionals in the system experience a number of constraints on their work with families. First are the constraints on the professionals' time and responsibilities by the school system. For example, many school psychologists are so overwhelmed with assessment and staffings that little time remains for other activities. Moreover, many report that they are limited to having very few sessions with a family. This limitation is not necessarily incompatible with a brief model of treatment, such as structural or strategic therapy, but it does hamper the therapist when more contact is needed. Second, professionals working within the system must work harder to secure a position of neutrality about school-related concerns. Parents may perceive them as representing the school system's viewpoint and even siding with the school against the family. Rapport may thus be threatened, and concern about such issues as confidentiality or professional bias may emerge. Lastly, because of the pervasive child focus of the educational system and the small number of counselors and psychologists working with families, they often must work in isolation, without a peer or support group. To the extent that the broad context of the work system organizes our thinking in particular ways, these professionals inside the school are in particular need of a like-minded peer support group with which to discuss cases and plan interventions. (A similar point is made by Dammann in Chapter Two with regard to systemic therapists in private practice and by Greiner in Chapter Nine with regard to nurses practicing in medical settings.) Because of the work load and the often rigid schedules of schools, freedom to seek such support is often more restricted for the school counselor or psychologist. Although none of these constraints need prevent a therapist within the system from working systemically, they make such work more difficult.

Besides being in a position to work personally with child and family problems, the school psychologist or counselor is often in the important position of being the person in the school system who determines when referral to a practitioner outside the system is warranted. How the referral is framed and presented can have a major impact on the therapy to follow, and hence the process of making a referral deserves attention. Making a good referral, a referral that will be acted on, often entails the same systemic thinking and strategic planning entailed in therapy. In fact, I see it as the beginning of therapy and as one of the ways in which therapists working inside the school play a critical role in the treatment process. For example, referring persons who respect the family's view of the problem, using their language, and understanding notions of family structure and hierarchy will be more successful in getting families to follow through on their referrals. The wise referring person does not highlight a marital issue when suggesting a referral if the parents are more worried about a child's acting-out behavior. And the school counselor, wary of triangles and coalitions and therefore careful to get both parents' views of the problem before making a referral, avoids setting up resistance in a father because he was not consulted about a proposed referral.

Just as important as understanding how to present a referral to a family is knowing to whom to refer. Being a family or systems therapist does not guarantee interest or expertise in dealing with school-related problems. I think it is important to find out whether the therapist is willing to work with the school, is willing to make school visits, and is informed about educational policies, issues, and practices.

Despite the impact of television and other media, schools and families are still the major settings in which children are personally educated and nurtured in our culture. For the sake of children and the future of our culture, it is crucial that these two institutions support and complement each other. Therapists can help make this possible by understanding and respecting both systems and by practicing in such a way that the resources of both settings are employed to further the development of children and families.

6 Michael Berger

Special Education
Programs

Special education settings appeared in the
United States during the latter part of the nineteenth century,
following closely on the nearly simultaneous passage of state
mandatory education and child labor laws. The functions of
special education settings, functions not consistent with each
other, are described in a 1913 definition of the special class:
"any form of class provided for a group of children who are in
some way exceptional and who cannot, therefore, be instructed
to advantage in the regular classes of the school system, either
because they fail to receive the instruction suited to their special
needs or because they receive such instruction at the expense of
the remainder of the class" (Whipple, quoted in Sarason and
Doris, 1979, p. 275). Special education settings deal with individuals who are exceptional either in their needs or in the demands they place on regular education settings, demands these
settings are not prepared to meet.

Reflecting the low regard in which handicapped people
are generally held in our society, special education settings have
been stigmatized and segregated from regular education settings

Both in my thinking about families with handicapped children and
in my clinical work with such families I am heavily indebted to the work
of Martha A. Foster. I am also grateful to Stephen Berger, Mary McLean,
Debby Guthrie, Lisbeth Vincent, and Beatrice Lampiris for their comments on drafts of this chapter.

even when the two kinds of settings are housed in the same building. This segregation extends not only to the students in special education classes but to their teachers as well. Special education teachers are trained in separate academic programs from regular education teachers. Often this segregation extends as far as the theories of development that teachers are taught, theories that take for granted implacable internal differences between handicapped and nonhandicapped persons (Sarason and Doris, 1979).

Special educators are trained to focus on the needs of individual handicapped persons who are thought to possess some sort of deficit that requires remediation in the form of outside intervention. Most special educators think of their client as the individual handicapped person, viewing him or her in isolation from any social context, including the family and peer group. The theories of development, the theories of problem formation and solution, the intervention techniques that are taught to special educators define the isolated handicapped individual as the unit of concern.

Most special educators consequently have, at best, a vague view of families, family development, and the needs of family members other than the handicapped individual (Foster, Berger, and McLean, 1981; Sarason and Doris, 1979). In general, when special educators think of families, it is in terms of their relationship to the handicapped individual. This means, for example, thinking of parents or siblings as possible teachers for the handicapped individual, persons available to supplement the efforts of special educators by carrying out additional programming with the handicapped individual. Family members are also noticed when their needs conflict with what special educators think are the needs of the handicapped person. Hence, in the special education literature, therapy is most often discussed in terms of helping parents "adjust" to the fact of the handicapping condition and to the needs of the handicapped person. The aim is that parents will either help remediate the handicapped person's deficits or not interfere with the efforts of professionals to do so (Berger and Foster, 1976; Wolfensberger, 1967).

The most common triangle in special education settings is therefore one in which professionals are in coalition with the handicapped person against his or her parents (see also Chapter Five). A major goal for therapy in such settings is to prevent this triangle from forming or break it up once it has occurred. Strategies for doing this will be discussed later.

Predictable Issues in Therapy

Although much of family therapy with families with a handicapped child follows similar lines to therapy with any family with a child problem, there are some special issues and circumstances to be considered when working with such families. First, families with a handicapped child generally spend large amounts of time and energy finding the services needed to support the child's development. Because services for handicapped individuals are usually organized and funded on a categorical basis (that is, a given agency provides services only for individuals having a particular label or disability), and because service settings tend to specialize and to provide only one kind of service (for example, medical services or educational services), families with a handicapped child face the task of locating appropriate services, qualifying for them, obtaining them, and combining them in as satisfactory manner as possible. When a child has several handicapping conditions or requires a variety of services, this can be a huge task (Gorham and others, 1975; Schwartz, 1970). This task is made more difficult by the habit of professionals who work with handicapped children of demanding strict attention to their prescribed treatment at all costs. This practice cues family members to believe that the needs of the handicapped child must be given priority over the needs of other family members.

Because the task of arranging for the youngster's treatment falls mostly on mothers, a predictable structure for families with a handicapped child is one in which there is a very close mother/child dyad. The closeness of this dyad is reinforced by the fact that when agencies that serve handicapped children seek "parent involvement," they tend to mean mother involvement and will ask mothers to work with their children in the treatment setting or to carry out tasks with the children at home. Such agency requests for maternal involvement place mothers in a double bind: If a mother complies with the request, the result is to intensify an already close relationship; if she refuses to comply or comments on the double bind, she runs the risk of being viewed by agency personnel and by herself as being "uninterested" in her child (Foster, Berger, and McLean, 1981).

Another common structural characteristic of families with a handicapped child is that these families often organize around the handicapping condition as if it were the central fact about the family. This occurs for several reasons. First is the amount of effort required to obtain services for the child once the handicapping condition has been diagnosed, an effort so large as to make it often necessary to put aside or sacrifice the needs and wishes of other family members. Second is the stigmatizing character of handicapping conditions (Goffman, 1963). Families with a handicapped child live in a society in which it is better not to be handicapped. Living in this society, family members are likely to share this view, becoming ashamed of themselves as well. Often, parents of a newly diagnosed handicapped child cut off contact with their social network, becoming increasingly isolated. This isolation, in turn, increases the family's focus on the handicapped child, making it more likely that the child will become a target for parental anxiety and concern. Cutting off contact with the social network of extended family, friends, and neighbors also has the effect of establishing a feedback loop in which initial isolation leads to additional isolation as family members find it more and more difficult to explain the handicapping condition to network members and to explain why the family has withdrawn from the network. By this point, parents often identify themselves first as parents of a handicapped child rather than simply as parents. They then join groups that reinforce this identification and out of these groups create new social networks that define the presence of the handicapped child as the central fact about the family. In the extreme case, the family ceases to deal with persons who are not connected with the handicapped child, limiting its contact to service providers and other parents of handicapped children.

Defining itself as a family with a handicapped child often has the additional consequence of freezing the family and its organizational structure at the point in time when the presence of the handicapping condition is acknowledged. Such a rigidified structure, of course, limits the future growth and development of family members, since both individual development and family development are likely to require change in family organization (Haley, 1973; Minuchin, 1974). For example, it may be appropriate for one or both parents to be extremely involved with a handicapped child while the child is still an infant. But when the child begins to function as a toddler and contact with peers becomes more important, family structure needs to change so that the previously intensely involved parent pulls back and behaves more distantly with the child, permitting the child to be more involved with peers. If, however, family structure rigidifies around dealing with the needs of an infant, it may be difficult for the more involved parent to pull back from his or her intense relationship with the handicapped child. Not only does such rigidity increase the chances of the child's missing out on peer contact and the resulting social and cognitive development, but the overly involved parent is likely to be denied the opportunity to develop parts of his or her life that are separate from the needs of the handicapped child.

An additional consequence of self-definition as a family with a handicapped child is that family members tend to focus on deficits and failures rather than on strengths and successes. It is therefore even more important than usual, with such families, for the therapist to highlight competencies and accomplishments in order to alter the atmosphere of disappointment and failure so that the talents of family members can be employed and supported.

Conduct of Therapy in Special Education Settings

I have worked with special education settings in three contexts: as the director of a special education agency, as a consultant to special education agencies, and as a private practitioner to whom families with a handicapped member are referred. I will begin by describing in detail the special education setting I directed (the Family Intervention Project), because the procedures developed there are the basis for my work in the two other settings.

The project was funded by a grant from the Office of Special Education* whose regulations specified that the ticket of admission to the project would be the presence in the family of a pre-school-aged handicapped child. Families were referred to the project by family members, by physicians who worked with young handicapped children, or by social workers at agencies for young handicapped children. The median age of children at the time of referral was twelve months (this was generally several months after the handicapping condition had been diagnosed). Half the families seen were single-parent families (these households were generally headed by teenaged mothers), and the median income of the families served was $7,200, which was well within the range defined by the federal government as poverty-level.

The project was defined by the funding agency as an educational program that happened to have a strong interest in families. The local service agencies that worked with handicapped children held a similar definition of it. Their view of the project made sense because all previous early intervention programs for handicapped children in the city in which we were located had been directed either by physicians or by special educators and had therefore been defined as either medical or educational in orientation. Since our project was located at a university, it was thought of as educational.

Given these circumstances, it seemed futile to explicitly define the project in other than educational terms. We therefore deliberately structured the project in many ways as a typical early childhood special educational program, though as one that provided only parent-implemented services. (Our staff did not

*Direct service funding for the project was provided for three years by the federal Office of Special Education and, for a fourth year, by the City of Atlanta and Fulton County. The project was administered through the Department of Psychology, Georgia State University, Atlanta.

work directly with handicapped children; rather, we served as consultants and trainers of family members who themselves worked directly with the handicapped child.) For example, when a parent called to ask for our services, he or she was told that we offered a variety of child-focused services, such as educational programming, speech and language therapy, behavior modification, and physical therapy. If the family wished to use our services, they then completed an intake form that asked for detailed information about the child's medical history and development, his or her previous and current involvement with other service providers, and parents' concerns for their child.

Staff then arranged for an initial interview to be held at the family's home. Two staff members were present at this interview. One met with the adults in the family to discuss their concerns about the child and to obtain a history of the family's involvement with the child's disability. The second staff member observed the child in a semistructured situation to obtain a rough initial idea of his or her skills and deficits. At the end of this interview, an appointment was made with both parents to bring the child into the project's offices for a formal assessment, and dates for a meeting with the family social network were discussed. Network meetings were usually attended by nuclear and extended family members, although at times they also included neighbors, members of the clergy, babysitters, and friends of the family.

Following the formal assessment and the network meeting, project staff shared their findings with one another and mapped out the areas in which they thought it useful to work with the child (for example, training to develop language skills or to help the child walk). These recommendations were then reviewed with the adults in the family. After this review, a tentative treatment plan was devised. This consisted of our objectives for the child, the activities designed to lead to the accomplishment of the objectives, and the person(s) who would be asked to carry out the different activities with the child.

Next, a staffing was held with the family and project staff, to which all other agencies and service providers involved with the child were also invited. At this meeting, the involvement of all the agencies was reviewed and, if necessary, plans for their coordination devised. Then the findings and recommendations of our staff were presented to the family for their comments.

Following the staffing, family members indicated whether they wished to work with the project. If they did, a treatment plan was written and discussed with the family and a contract drawn up formally acknowledging the obligations of family members and of staff as embodied in the treatment plan. Once this contract was signed, formal work with the family began.

The description of the project thus far has stressed its similarities to most special educational programs—for example, its emphasis on working with the handicapped child and on devising activities to remediate the child's deficits. However, our interests went beyond this to a concern for the welfare and development of the families we served. Accordingly, we deliberately set up the procedures of the project so that they would support the aims of a systemic therapy. Let me carefully review how this was done.

Initially, when a parent called to ask about our services, in addition to being informed about the child-focused services we offered, the parent was told that our staff's major concern would be to help the parents and the other members of the family deal with the problems *they* thought were important. This was done both to indicate that we thought of the family, rather than only the child, as a legitimate focus of our concern and as a way of supporting parental competence (a key concept in the systemic treatment of child problems) by indicating that we would place great emphasis on the issues parents thought important. Further, the parent was told that we were interested in meeting with the family social network, the relatives, friends, and neighbors who were important to family members or were involved with the handicapped child, to help the network members and the family, if necessary, in dealing with their concerns.

To maintain our focus on the family and on supporting parental competence, the initial interview was held in the family's home rather than at our offices. We did this because we thought that family members would be more comfortable in their own home. The interview was deliberately scheduled at a time when all the adults in the family could be present; this usually meant evenings or weekends. Our ability to do this rested, as did other aspects of our program, on hiring staff members who were willing to work nights and weekends and on the director's ability to compensate staff for this work (Chapters Four and Eleven also stress the importance of this). We sent two staff members to this meeting and had one of them meet only with the adults in the family to stress that our concern was as much with the other family members as with the handicapped child. This staff member reviewed with the family members the history of the family's involvement with the child's disability so that we would understand how family members viewed the child's problems and what solutions they had already tried. This initial interview also served as a means of obtaining information that guided our initial hypotheses about family structure.

In addition to serving its manifest purpose, the formal assessment provided a context in which enactments were set up that let staff see how each parent interacted with the handicapped child and with the other parent about the child. For example, while testing the child, the examiner would ask the parents whether the child could successfully complete a given test item. If the parents said the child could do the item and the examiner failed to get the child to do the item, it then seemed natural for the examiner to ask one or both parents to get the child to complete the item successfully. The assessment also provided a context in which the examiner could underline and call to parents' attention previously unnoticed competencies in the child. In addition, the assessment could be used as a situation for teaching parents methods of observing child behavior, how to understand test scores, and medical and educational terminology. Further, the tester would discuss with parents how they wanted the information obtained in the assessment used in the writing of the child's treatment plan (for example, which skills did they wish to focus on teaching?). Lastly, the assessment was a situation in which parents were able to ask questions about various aspects of child development or about particular child behaviors without having to define these concerns as "problems." In order to use the assessment in these ways, we routinely pressed to have both parents present (we succeeded over 90 percent of the time). This not only permitted our staff to observe how each parent dealt with the child and allowed each parent to voice his or her concerns but kept mothers from once again having to carry the burden of interpreting the remarks of professionals to the rest of the family.

Most commonly, the network meetings served both a problem-solving and a ritual function. Usually, network members would discuss their concerns about the handicapped child and, often, about how the disability was affecting other network members; when parents agreed with these concerns, network members would then focus on which members of the network could best help family members deal with shared concerns. In addition, the experience that network members had in meeting together and talking about the handicapped child and the effects of the child's handicap on different network members served as a ritual affirming both the relatedness of network members to one another and the family's ability to prevail over the handicapping condition (Dammann and Berger, 1983). Finally, network meetings also served a diagnostic function for the therapist, permitting him or her to observe the sequences between network members and family members that were influencing how family members dealt with the problem of the handicapped child and giving the therapist information about family functioning and the sharing of responsibilities.

As noted earlier, after the assessment and the network meeting, staff members shared their findings with one another and mapped out the areas in which we thought treatment would be helpful. Then the staff member with primary responsibility for the case met with the adults in the family to review our findings and recommendations and to ask family members their views on the issues on which treatment should focus. Strong and repeated efforts were made to reinforce parents' sense of their own competence: Copies of all test reports were given to parents and reviewed with them so that their questions could be answered and their concerns heard; staff recommendations were presented tentatively; family members were encouraged to tell staff members their priorities for treatment; and staff members were directed to incorporate the family's suggestions into the treatment plan whenever feasible.

We worked this way for two reasons. First, by attending so closely to family members' concerns about the child, we laid the groundwork for family members' accepting of our often intrusive demands for change in family organization. Second, with families who have experienced a great deal of failure, it is crucial to begin working on a task at which success is possible within a short time and which is important to family members. Succeeding with such a task quickly renews family members' sense of competence with the child. Thus, an important part of this first meeting was a negotiation between the staff member and family members about where intervention would begin. If family members' objectives were too far off target to permit successful intervention, staff members would reframe these concerns so that they could successfully be met.

We used the activities necessary to reach agreed-on goals for the child, established in the treatment plan, as the tasks through which we would influence family structure (Haley, 1976). For example, in a family in which we thought the mother was overinvolved with the handicapped child while the father was too peripheral, we would set up educational and therapeutic tasks that required the father to interact more with the child in a context in which he would be successful with the child. (For some reason, physical therapy tasks, perhaps because they relate to motor development and to physical activities stereotypically thought of as masculine, were particularly effective for this situation. Fathers were willing to do these tasks, and mothers were willing to let fathers do them.) In such cases, it was crucial either to give the mother something else useful to do (either another task or a consultant role vis-à-vis the father), rather than merely asking her to pull back from her child, or to give her a reasonable explanation for pulling back (for example, "You've had to do this so long by yourself that you've become exhausted and need to take a little rest so you can gather your forces to be even more helpful"). Asking people to give up something for nothing does not work.

Or if we thought one parent was overwhelmed by his or her involvement with the child, we would search the family network for other individuals who could and would pick up some of the responsibility for the child. We would then devise ways of framing the situation so that the parent would permit these other persons to help. And if we thought a parent was greatly overestimating or underestimating a child's capabilities in particular areas, we would invent tasks that would lead the parent to notice the child's actual abilities.

The next step was to hold a staffing between the family and project staff to which all other agencies involved with the family were also invited. Throughout the handicapped individual's life, important decisions about the handicapped person will be made at staffings involving the person, his or her family, and service agencies. We thought it important, therefore, to train families to be effective advocates for their child and themselves. Toward this end, a staff member was assigned to provide any assistance the family members wished in order to make themselves heard by our staff at the staffing. This staff member was the one who had met with the family previously to explain our staff's findings and suggestions and to help family members formulate their goals for the child. This person sat with the family at the staffing, and his or her job there was to ensure that project staff were responsive to the ideas of family members. (Other ways in which we trained parents as advocates can be found in Muir and others, 1982.)

At the staffing, each member of the project who had been involved with the family reported his or her observations and recommendations. Representatives from other agencies were also asked to report their contacts with the family and their findings and recommendations. Then family members were given time to ask any questions they had or to put forth recommendations for our staff or the staff of other agencies to consider. Often these questions and recommendations showed a need for closer coordination between the different agencies involved; when this occurred, the staffing was used to begin to achieve that coordination. Staffings were also used as a ritual through which staff and family members would share, agree on, and thus make real their new (reframed) understanding of the problem. In addition, staffings were used as a context in which parental disagreements about child issues could be enacted, intensified, and at times resolved.

The staffing was the end of our formal assessment procedure. After the staffing, family members were asked to take some time and decide whether they wished to work with the project. If they decided to work with us, a treatment plan was drawn up and agreed on with the family, and then formal work began with the family.

In the project's "assessment" procedures, as in all systemic therapy, what we were formally terming assessment was also intervention. An excerpt from the transcript of one initial interview may help make this clear.

The Harris family was referred to the project by Dr. Martha Foster, who had tested the thirteen-month-old daughter (Caroline). After a large number of diagnostic medical tests and many consultations from different specialists, Caroline had been diagnosed as having an infectious disease that varies widely in its severity. In this particular case, the girl showed no signs of retardation and appeared to have lost only peripheral vision. In addition to Caroline, the family consisted of Sarah (aged five) and two parents. There had been another daughter (who would have been three at the time of the interview) who had died suddenly two years before.

Therapy Session	*Commentary*
Ther.: Hi, I'm Dr. Berger, and this is Debbie Gunther, our coordinator. I guess the two of you have spoken on the phone.	
Mrs. H.: Yes.	
Ther.: Okay. We've gotten the report from Dr. Foster, and we saw that she tested Caroline only five months ago, when she was eight months old. Now,	The therapist is trying to associate himself and the project with Dr. Foster, whom he knows the parents like and respect. He is also trying to un-

Therapy Session

Commentary

normally, we would test her now ourselves, but I'm not sure it's necessary, since Dr. Foster has done it so recently.

derscore her findings, which were that Caroline was of at least normal and quite possibly of superior intelligence.

Mrs. H.: We'd like to have it done.

Ther.: Fine. But—I'm curious —how come?

Mrs. H.: [Looks at husband, who looks away from her] We just want to be sure—to be sure that she's going to do anywhere as well as Dr. Foster said she would.

Ther.: You have doubts?

Mrs. H.: Yes.

Ther.: Any particular reason?

Mrs. H.: You tell him, Marshall.

Mr. H.: We just don't—our experiences have led us to think that doctors tend to be overly optimistic. They don't want to give families bad news. [Therapist looks confused, so Mr. H continues] We lost a child two years ago. She was a little under a year old.

The therapist takes Mr. Harris's statement about doctors tending to be "overly optimistic" as an indication that Mr. Harris has been hurt by physicians' optimism and therefore as a cue to the therapist that he should not speak optimistically.

Mrs. H.: Ten months.

Mr. H.: And she was doing just fine, and then she got sick, and the doctor put her in the hospital and said she was going to

Therapy Session   *Commentary*

be fine, and then suddenly they said she had a heart condition, and then she was dead.

Ther.: I'm sorry.

Mr. H.: And it's been the same doctors this time, and now they're telling us she'll be all right. And I can't believe them.

Mrs. H.: I was lying there in the hospital, and she was only a few hours old, and they took Caroline away from me, and they called Marshall and told him they had rushed her to the Children's Hospital because she needed special treatment. And then it took weeks to find out what was wrong with her and they couldn't be sure, and they were calling in all these specialists to tell them, and finally they decided what it was and that she would be all right, that she would have some eye problems, but that she would have a normal brain. And it was all so sudden.

Ther.: So you couldn't be sure whether to believe them?

Mrs. H.: [Fiercely] Would you?

Ther.: I don't know. I do know that the two of you have made sure that Caroline's had excellent treatment. But you're

The therapist agrees with the parents that they should be cautious (and thus does not himself proceed optimistically)

Therapy Session	Commentary
right—you should be cautious. So let's test her again. We'd like you both to be there when Debbie does the testing so she can explain what she's looking for and so you'll be sure you know what we're doing. Okay?	and with their request to have Caroline tested again. Rather than fighting the parents' pessimism about Caroline's future or their anger at the experts, he asks them both to be present at the testing so they can monitor what the staff is doing during the assessment. This is also the beginning of a set of probes to find out how much each parent knows about Caroline's ability, whether they agree about her condition, and how comfortable each of them is about dealing with her.
Mrs. H.: Sure. I was there when Dr. Foster tested her.	
Ther.: [To Mr. H] But you weren't?	
Mr. H.: No.	
Ther.: I think it's important that you both be here for this one. I know your wife is a strong person—the two of you wouldn't have survived if she wasn't—but I think she could use your help here. Okay?	Guessing that the father has distanced himself from Caroline, the therapist goes out of his way to ensure that Mr. Harris will involve himself in the assessment. The therapist does this first by framing participation in the assessment as a way of helping his wife (focusing Mr. Harris's attention on the wife rather than Caroline), then by joining with Mr. Harris by discussing his new business ven-

Therapy Session   *Commentary*

ture, then by stressing the importance of Mr. Harris's presence by indicating the therapist's willingness to schedule the assessment at Mr. Harris's convenience.

Mr. H.: Okay. But it may be hard for me to arrange. I've just started my own business and—

Ther.: What kind of business?

Mr. H.: Accounting. I used to be in a large firm, but I decided to go out on my own.

Ther.: Quite a change? If it's like private practice in my business, it would be pretty scary.

Mr. H.: Well . . .

Ther.: Anyway, I think it's real important that both of you be there, so we'll schedule the testing at your convenience. Will you give Debbie some times when you can make it, and then the rest of us will schedule around you?

Mr. H.: Okay.

Ther.: By the way, what have the two of you told your other daughter about Caroline? She's five, right?

The therapist continues to probe how the parents think about Caroline's condition.

Mrs. H.: Nothing.

Therapy Session   *Commentary*

Ther.: Does she ask about her?

Mrs. H.: Sometimes. And sometimes she calls her Karen.

Ther.: That's the name of the daughter who died?

Mrs. H.: Yes.

Ther.: Okay. Well, down the line I'd like to have somebody on our staff talk with Sarah to see how she's doing. And I think it will be helpful for the two of you to make clear to her that Caroline is not Karen.

Mrs. H.: I don't think this is the time for that.

Mr. H.: I don't want Sarah involved with Caroline now.

Ther.: Okay, I must be off base. You know how clinicians are—always looking for trouble even when there isn't any. Let's just go ahead and have Debbie test Caroline and have the physical therapist look at her, and then we'll know a lot more about where we are and what we need to do. By the way, when we set up the staffing, which of the other doctors would you like us to have there?

Mrs. H.: Dr. Alfred, the neurologist. He worked with both Caroline and Karen.

The parents' responses cue the therapist that their anxiety over Caroline's condition and its resemblance to Karen's fate is so high that he needs to back off at this point.

The therapist is looking for allies, other professionals involved with the family whose opinions carry weight with Mr. and Mrs. Harris. His use of Dr. Alfred will be discussed below.

Therapy Session   *Commentary*

Ther.: Okay. I'll make sure to
call him and schedule the staffing so he can be there.

From this interview, the therapist thought it likely that
both parents were demoralized by the death of their child two
years earlier, that they often confused Karen's fate with Caroline's, and that the experience of having had Karen's doctors
prove to be overoptimistic had led them to doubt anything positive said to them about Caroline. The therapist also wondered
whether Mrs. Harris felt that her husband was too distant from
both children or from Caroline. Confirmatory evidence for the
latter hunch was obtained during the assessment procedure
when the examiner noted that Mr. Harris interacted frequently
and well with Sarah but would not have anything to do with
Caroline.

At the network meeting, which included Mr. and Mrs.
Harris and Mrs. Harris's parents, it became even more clear that
Caroline and Karen were blurred in the adults' minds and that
family members expected something terrible to happen to Caroline but were trying to be stoic about it. Noting that of all the
physicians involved with the family, Mrs. Harris had most trust
in the neurologist (the one physician she wanted to invite to
the staffing), the therapist called him and asked for his help.
The neurologist said he would be glad to help. The therapist
indicated that what he expected to happen at the staffing would
be that after the staff members had presented their reports and
indicated that their findings were consistent with Dr. Foster's
testing (namely, that Caroline had lost peripheral vision but was
functioning at a normal or superior level cognitively), Mrs. Harris would question these findings. The therapist asked the
neurologist to be prepared to intervene firmly at this point and
to reiterate to Mrs. Harris what he had told the therapist, that
all damage that would occur to Caroline had already occurred.
The neurologist agreed to do this.

The staffing was one of those fortunate times when a
therapist's predictions prove precisely accurate. Staff members

presented their reports; Mrs. Harris thanked them for their time and then turned to the neurologist and asked him whether what the staff was saying was true. The neurologist, who is very tall, looked down at her, banged his fist on the table, and said: "All the damage that will be done has been done. She will get no worse." Mrs. Harris looked both stunned and relieved, and the therapist commented that he hoped she would not grasp this fact too quickly, "because it is always stressful to change, even when a change in views or perceptions seems obviously positive." Mrs. Harris agreed not to change her views too quickly.

From this point on, therapy proceeded quite easily and quickly. Tasks were set up for the father to observe the way Caroline carried out certain visual-motor tasks (he was quite concerned about her visual-motor coordination). In the process of doing this task, he noticed some things that caused him to comment that "Caroline was looking more and more normal to me." The therapist met with Mrs. Harris and her parents to discuss how to talk about Caroline's condition with Sarah and how to help Sarah distinguish between Caroline and Karen. Helping Sarah accomplish this discrimination task helped the adults to do it as well. Much later, when both parents were convinced that Caroline was a basically normal child, behavior modification procedures were taught to the parents so that they could help her control her temper tantrums; earlier, they had refused to use such procedures, since they had thought of her tantrums as emotional manifestations of her abnormal condition. As a final note, by the end of the project, the parents asked the staff to help them locate a private school for Caroline that had a gifted program she could enter.

This example clarifies some of the ways in which project procedures were used to accomplish therapeutic aims. Our use of the initial interview and of the formal assessment in this case was quite characteristic.

As noted earlier, network meetings served both ritual and problem-solving functions. The following excerpt from a network meeting illustrates some of the uses made of the meeting. The Hugheses had two children, a five-year-old boy who was doing very well and Eric, then eighteen months old. At six months Eric had been identified by the mother as a slow learner. He had been seen by a number of physicians, who had prescribed cognitive activities for the mother to carry out with him. However, his rate of cognitive development had not improved during the ensuing twelve months. At the initial interview, it became clear to the therapist that family members disagreed about the nature of Eric's condition, with his mother being most firm that he was in fact mentally retarded, but with a number of other family members—most important, Mrs. Hughes's mother—believing that he was just a slow learner. It was the consensus of all the professionals who had been involved with Eric that he was moderately to severely retarded. The parents also hinted at long-standing clashes between the two extended families. The therapist felt that Mrs. Hughes was almost wholly exhausted, both mentally and physically, but was unlikely to ask for help with Eric. The parents and therapist agreed that the specific agenda of the network meeting would be for the therapist to tell the network that Eric was retarded. Neither parent wanted to be the one to deliver this piece of "bad news." The therapist also obtained the mother's consent to his pushing her to let other people help her with Eric.

The therapist began the meeting by having various members of the staff describe their work with Eric and their findings. After the results of the physical therapy and cognitive assessment had been presented, the therapist moved to his agreed-on agenda.

Therapy Session	*Comments*
Ther.: Let me put the testing in perspective. Eric has been tested three times during the past twelve months. He was tested by Dr. R___ when he was six months old. [Various adults indicate they had not known this] And then Debbie tested him recently, when he was twelve months old. [Vari-	Forewarned by Mr. and Mrs. Hughes, the therapist assumes that members of the network will have difficulty with the diagnosis of mental retardation. He therefore proceeds slowly and factually, underlining the amount of information and thinking that has led to this conclusion.

| *Therapy Session* | *Comments* |

ous adults indicate they had not known this] And then Debbie tested him recently, when he was eighteen months old. So he's been tested three times. Okay, what Debbie is holding up is a graph of the three testings. You'll see two numbers for each testing. One is the score for the testing; the other thing is this fancy number we call developmental rate, which is really the age equivalent of the child's score, divided by the child's age. For instance, if a six-month-old scored an age-equivalent score of six months, his developmental rate would be 1. Now, what the graph shows is that while Eric's absolute score has not changed much over the twelve months of testing, his developmental rate has dropped. And that, considering all the work Polly and Dr. R____ have been doing with him this past year, is discouraging. It means that even with excellent care, his rate of development is not improving— in fact, it's getting a little worse. I'm sorry, I'm so used to lecturing I go on and on. Are there any questions? [Mr. Hughes's father asks to have developmental rate explained.

Therapy Session   *Commentary*

Debbie does so. One of Mrs.
Hughes's sisters says, "It doesn't
look good, does it, doctor?"]

Ther.: I wish I could tell you
differently, but, in all honesty,
I can't. My job tonight is to
give you bad news. What this
means is that Eric is retarded
and that, even given the best
possible help, like the kind of
help his mother has been doing
with him, he'll remain retarded. He won't grow out of
this. [Murmurs of "How can
you be sure?"] What makes
me think this is the decrease in
developmental rate over time.
If he had only been tested
once, I wouldn't flat out say
that he was retarded or anything. I wouldn't be sure. But
if after a year of people working with him intensively he has
not improved, then I think I
owe you our best judgment.
Besides, I think some of you
have known this in your hearts
already [Some nods], and you
probably haven't known what
to say about it because it's so
upsetting and you didn't want
to hurt Polly or George. [More
nods] I'll tell you the truth,
I'm less worried, just now, for
Eric than for Polly. Eric has
been getting superb care, and

Therapy Session   *Commentary*

knowing his mother, and seeing you all, I know he'll continue to receive superb care.
I'm more concerned about
Polly now, because I think that
not only has she been doing
most of the care for Eric, but
that she's been carrying a lot
of the burden of knowing that
he wouldn't grow out of it. And
she's a proud woman and
doesn't like to burden other
people, even her family, by
asking for help. [Comments of
"What can we do to be helpful?"; small groups in conversation of "Did you know?"
"Yes, I thought so," and so on]

Mr. H's father: All right, doctor. You've laid it out for us.
Now, give us our marching
orders. What do we do?

Ther.: A couple of things.   Focus is kept both on what
First, in terms of Eric, Debbie   needs to be done for Eric and
and our staff will be working   on how to help Polly help Eric.
up a plan of activities that will   Network members are chal-
help him learn certain skills or   lenged to show that they will
strengthen certain muscles.   help Polly help Eric if she is
What we'd like to do is to have   hesitant to ask for help.
various family members work
with Eric on different activities
—otherwise, I'm afraid that
Polly will rush in and insist on
doing everything herself. Now
I need help. How can we arrange things so that Polly,

Therapy Session   *Commentary*

who's going to murder me soon
if I don't stop talking about
her, won't do everything?

Mrs. H's sister: I would just
come over and tell her, "Polly,
today I'm working with Eric."

Ther.: Great! Could you do
that on a regular basis, like
schedule it so every Tuesday
you would do it and Polly
would know you were com-
ing? I'm nervous that if you
did it only once in a while, Polly might pooh-pooh your efforts and tell you that you
weren't doing it just right.

Mrs. H's sister: Sure. In fact, a
bunch of us could arrange to
do that, on different days.

Ther.: Wonderful. In fact, I
think what we'll try to do is,
every time we start programming on a new activity, we'll
schedule it at someone else's
house so that it will be real
clear which of you is in charge
of that activity. Okay?

Mr. H's mother: What can *we*
do to help? We don't see Polly and George all that much;
we're busy and we don't like
to meddle in their affairs.

Ther.: Ask Polly and George.   Therapist supports Polly and
They'd know better than I.   George vis-à-vis others in the

Therapy Session   *Commentary*

network, thus supporting their competence. Note the delicate line the therapist has been walking between asking that network members help Polly and George whether they ask for it or not (a move that may threaten their competence) and supporting their competence. However, the fact that Polly does not challenge the therapist's attempts to get others to help her serves as a tacit cue that she approves of these efforts and will let the therapist act for her.

Mr. H.: Well, mother, you could invite both Eric and Tommy over to play instead of just Tommy.

Mr. H's mother: Do I do that?

Mrs. H.: Yes.

Ther.: Mrs. Hughes? Have you been unsure of what to do with Eric when you're with him? [She nods] Polly's real good with Eric—could she, maybe, show you a couple of things? [She nods] Would you do that, Polly? [She nods]

Mr. H's father: Doctor, it's still important that we love the child, isn't it?

Mrs. H.: Of course it is, daddy,

Therapy Session	*Commentary*
he's just like any other little boy.	
Ther.: Of course, Eric is fortunate to have such a large and such a concerned family. And he will need your help. And Polly and George will need your help. They've been going through this alone for too long now. And it's going to be hard to help them, because Polly will say she doesn't need it, and George—[To George's brother] Do you know when George is down about Eric?	Therapist both strokes the network members (telling them how important they are) and challenges them to be helpful to Polly and George.
Brother: I know when he's down but not what he's down about.	
Ther.: I don't know. I'm leery about sounding like a therapist and saying people ought to talk to each other more. You're his brother, you've known him so much better than I do. Could you help him when he's down?	
Brother: Yes.	
Ther.: Polly—would that be all right with you?	
Mrs. H.: Sure.	
Mr. H's mother: And you know that Big Daddy and I will always be glad to help you.	

Therapy Session   *Commentary*

[George doesn't respond; Polly looks a little irritated]

Ther.: Okay, unless there are more questions . . .

Many of the suggestions put forth at the network meeting were adopted in the treatment plan. Initially, Mrs. Hughes was put in charge of all the activities with Eric. Once he had mastered a given activity, Mrs. Hughes was then asked to teach that activity to another network member, who then continued to work with Eric on the activity. Over time, we moved to a procedure of asking Mrs. Hughes to begin work on some new activities while assigning other new activities to different members of the network. The staff's job was to monitor the program to see that network members followed through on their commitments and to mobilize the network if there was a breakdown in the plan.

Particular attention was paid to involving Mr. Hughes in the programming for Eric in ways that were comfortable both for him and for his wife. Much effort was also devoted to working with the couple on how they wanted to deal with the long-standing conflicts between their two families, conflicts that were also expressed in disagreements about the nature of Eric's condition and its prognosis. Basically, the couple decided not to deal with these issues by avoiding them in general, while, in specific, not assigning responsibilities for Eric in such a way that the two families would compete or collide.

The preceding case examples overemphasize the front-stage role of the family therapist in the project. The project was a collaborative enterprise, involving family therapists, special educators, physical therapists, speech therapists, and behavior therapists. All the knowledge and skill of these different disciplines were needed and used (see Berger and Fowlkes, 1980, for a more comprehensive description of the project). I know of no family therapist who has the skills in physical therapy, in language and speech therapy, and in special education to do all the work necessary with these families alone. Rather, professionals in these other areas have much to offer therapists, and we should welcome them as colleagues rather than treating them as mere adjuncts to what the family therapist thinks of as the "real" treatment (see, for example, Chapter Eight). In fact, in the main, the family therapist's role in the project was that of an orchestrator, diagnosing family structure, helping to plan activities that would restructure the family, and helping the professional who was directly working with family members to propose activities in such a way that they would be accepted. It was also the family therapist's job to train the rest of the staff in the basic therapeutic skills (for example, reflective listening, giving directives) needed to work well with families.

Project Failures. Like all programs, the project was not always successful. We had our greatest difficulty with families whose belief system strongly contradicted ours—that is, families whose belief was that someone from outside the family should work with the handicapped child, while family members would not be involved with treatment. With some families holding these beliefs, the discrepancy between their view and ours was so great that once the project and its procedures were described, the family member indicated that he or she would prefer to work with an agency where a professional would work with the child and that would be all. In these cases, referral to an appropriate agency or practitioner was made. With other families holding these beliefs, the assessment procedure served as a process through which an acceptable compromise between the family and staff positions was negotiated (one, for example, in which our staff would, atypically, directly work with the child in a particular area for a short time in exchange for family members' agreeing to be involved in other activities with the child). In still other cases, family members apparently bought our point of view, either because it came to seem reasonable to them or because they did not think they could obtain equivalent child services elsewhere.

Other failures included families in which chronic marital problems were intermingled with child problems, and we were not successful in untangling the two sufficiently to solve either set of problems. Still other failures included families that, by the time they came to the project, had cut off so definitively from their network that we could neither restore it nor help the family create a new one that was workable. Finally, in a small number of families, adults did not carry out assigned tasks. These tended to be families who had been referred to the project because of a referring person's concern about the handicapped child, a concern that family members did not at that time share.

Applicability to Other Settings. Although the population served by the Family Intervention Project was mainly low-income and heavily single-parent, my experience in private practice and consultation leads me to believe that many of the project procedures are appropriate for therapists in private practice or those employed by special education settings. Therapists in both settings can use child assessments as situations in which parental interaction with the child can be evaluated, parents taught about testing and observation, and parents' concerns about child development explored. Therapists in both settings can use staffings or Individualized Educational Plan meetings as chances to inform parents and to create truly collaborative efforts between families and special education agencies. Therapists in both settings can probably use network meetings as we did so long as they are careful to define these meetings as being necessary in order to help meet the needs of the handicapped child. An alternative to network meetings that has also proved effective is to coach each parent, using a Bowenian framework, to work with his or her own extended family around the issues raised by the handicapping condition.

Therapists in both settings should be aware of the requirements of both state and federal law with regard to the education of handicapped students. In particular, Public Law 94-142, the Education of All Handicapped Children Act, specifies not only assessment procedures and the development of a written Individualized Educational Plan (IEP) for each child but also the rights of parents to be involved in the development of their child's educational program and to due process if they object to the program offered by the schools. To work effectively with educational programs, therapists should be familiar with the procedures for referral, assessment, and placement of exceptional students followed by the schools and with the rights and opportunities for involvement that are provided to the family.

Interventions in these two settings must be phrased as being in the service of the handicapped individual. Although it is impossible to predict the discipline of the director of special education settings, it is likely that the director and most (if not all) of the staff will have a client-focused orientation and will tend to think of the client in isolation from other social systems and contexts. To be successful, therefore, family interventions need to be described to, and seen by, special education staff members as resulting either in the provision of additional help for the handicapped individual or in the cessation of family efforts to block staff members' work with the handicapped individual.

For very good reasons, professionals working with handicapped persons and families of such persons often have different priorities and goals. Professionals are paid to devote their efforts almost solely to the welfare of the handicapped individual. Moreover, they are trained to believe that this is in the client's best interest; and given the low esteem granted handicapped people and the lack of adequate services for them, this belief is often correct. Parents, however, must attend not only to the needs of the handicapped individual but to their own and other family members' needs.

In an earlier paper on parent involvement in early intervention programs (Foster, Berger, and McLean, 1981), we noted that the difference in roles between parents and professionals often leads to conflict.

From the perspective of the professional, more services for the child or more effort expended on the child is better. For the parent, more services provided to the child may be better for the child, and for other family members as well, for example, when the family of a newly diagnosed handicapped child receives help in understanding and managing the child's condition. On the other hand, the provision of more services to the child may harm family members, as when a parent devotes so much time to the handicapped child that he or she becomes exhausted or depressed, and the needs of other family members are neglected. Indeed, at times the provision of more services to the child may even be harmful to the child, such as when an overly intense mother/child dyad is encouraged toward even more extensive involvement under the guise of parent-mediated intervention [pp. 58-59].

These role conflicts cannot be wholly avoided, but in my experience they can usually be managed successfully. A useful role for the therapist here is to serve as a negotiator between the family and the special education setting, representing each group to the other. While working to accomplish this, it is often useful for the therapist to use himself or herself as a go-between or boundary between the two groups, restricting their direct contact when tension is high by having each group communicate with the other only through the therapist. (This tactic, called "interdiction," is discussed more fully in Chapter Five.)

The negotiator role is probably more easily taken by a private practitioner than by a therapist working for the special education agency, since the therapist in the latter case is likely to be under more pressure to side with the agency's view. However, the negotiator role can be employed by an agency therapist if he or she has the support of the agency director. This support is most likely to be obtained if the therapist can persuade the director that the therapist's taking the negotiator role will be helpful to the handicapped individual. Sometimes, however, it is preferable for the agency therapist to refer the family to a private practitioner who will have more leeway to negotiate. What is most crucial, however, is that the therapist help the family and agency staff collaborate, since each has much to offer the handicapped individual. It will be easiest for the therapist to do this if he or she respects both the competence of the family and the skills and interests of special educators. A competent family therapist is more likely to have such respect for the family than for special educators. If the therapist does not respect the skills and interests of special educators but wishes to practice successfully in such settings, it would be salutary for the therapist to do some direct interventive work with handicapped individuals, because that kind of clinical experience teaches that the different skills of the various professionals involved in special education settings are all very necessary. (Reamy-Stephenson, in Chapter Three, provides nice examples of how to demonstrate that the therapist values other staff members' expertise.)

There are times when the agency therapist (or family members) will think that the role conflicts cannot be successfully negotiated, at least without more effort than seems reasonable. In such cases, it is useful for the agency therapist to know how to refer the family to an appropriate private therapist. In my judgment, an appropriate therapist will be competent to deal with the family's issues, will have a detailed understanding of the special education system, its procedures, and its values, and will be willing and able to move between the two systems of family and special education settings. When talking to a potential therapist, I would look for cues that the therapist is willing to go out to the special education setting, seems comfortable dealing both with that setting and with the family (see also Chapter Five), and has no rigidly prescribed notion of the "grief process" to which he or she believes the family must adhere.

This last characteristic is important because, too often, families with a handicapped child encounter professionals who believe that all family members must "accept" the fact that they have a handicapped child and must grieve for their lost hopes of a "normal" child. For these professionals, "acceptance" is manifested by parents' examining their feelings in the presence of professionals and moving through a prescribed series of stages that presumably characterize the "grief process" (for example, denial, anger, and bargaining), ending with a final and total "acceptance" of the handicapped child.

Let me be clear—this process does capture the experience of *some* families. In these families, parents may need to articulate their feelings before they can treat their child differently and can move beyond the stage in which the fact of having a handicapped child is the central characteristic of the family. However, I think it is disrespectful of families for therapists to act as if there were only one way in which family members can or should come to terms with the handicapping condition. It is also simplistic to assume that family members do come to terms with the handicapping condition once and for all. Rather, their views on the matter alter with changes in the child's capabilities and in family circumstances.

Some parents deal with these issues by first talking about them and then treating the child differently. Other parents do not appear to talk directly about these issues. Rather, they interact with their child in ways that enhance the child's development, notice his or her competencies and characteristics, and then, because of their new transactions with the child, change their views and feelings about the child.

A separate but important issue is to whom parents should talk about these issues. Rather than encouraging parents to discuss these issues primarily with therapists, my own strategy has been to encourage parents to talk to members of their social networks, to people who have a shared history with them and who care for them as people rather than as "parents of a handicapped child." What is crucial, however, is that therapists not impose a monolithic solution on families. Our job is to respect and facilitate the diverse ways in which families organize to deal with the issues raised by having a handicapped child.

Existential Issues and the Therapist. Like certain other clinical populations (for example, families in which someone is dying), families with handicapped individuals are often dealing with truly existential issues, issues which may plague the therapist as well and for which his or her professional training affords no real wisdom. Yet, it is necessary for the therapist to be helpful to family members as they confront these issues, rather than either being overwhelmed by his or her own helplessness or denying the issues and forcing them into a form that is apparently amenable to a purely professional solution.

Families with a handicapped person are constantly facing a difficult dilemma. On the one hand, the handicapping condition is chronic, and family members are constantly reminded that the handicapped person is not wholly "normal." On the other hand, the extent to which the disability will interfere with the handicapped person's life can never be totally predicted and depends, in large measure, on the kind and intensity of intervention efforts afforded the handicapped person and his or her family. Ironically, one effect of such intervention is to cause family members to hope and to overestimate the degree to which these services will enable the handicapped person to lead a wholly "normal" life. Family members are thus often disappointed and depressed when, after massive intervention efforts that often result in great improvements in the handicapped person's behavior, they notice that the handicapped person is still not behaving in a totally "normal" fashion (Berger and Foster, 1976).

Many special educators place more emphasis on one or the other side of this family dilemma. Characteristically, special educators primarily involved with assessment and diagnosis tend to put great weight on the family's need to "accept" the fact that the handicapped person is not normal. Interventionists, by contrast, tend to be optimistic, stressing that we do not know what the handicapped person will be capable of, given optimal support.

It is family members who, over the course of their lives, must make their own sense of this dilemma. How can therapists help families do this? First, I think, by being clear with themselves and with families that their professional training gives them no special wisdom in dealing with this particular situation. Second, by helping the family to be as flexible as possible in creating their idiosyncratic solution to the problem.

Several examples may help to clarify this point. I recently saw a couple who had a young child with Down's syndrome. This was their second child (they had a boy several years older), and the wife had been in her midthirties when pregnant. She had asked her gynecologist to do an amniocentesis, but he had dissuaded her from this. When she and her husband came to see me, she wanted to give the child up for adoption. Her husband refused to consider this and indicated that he had already become attached to the child. He spoke in an extremely optimistic manner about the child's future. During the course of the interview, the wife commented on the pictures of my son in the office, asking whether he was my first child. I said he was. The following dialogue ensued:

Wife: How old was your wife when she was pregnant?

Ther.: About your age.

Wife: Did you have an amnio?

Ther.: Yes.

Wife: If it had been [positive], what would you have done?

Ther.: I'm not sure. I would have wanted an abortion, and I think my wife would have, too—but she would have had more trouble than I doing that. [At this point the wife started crying, so I continued] But it's too late for that now. Your husband has already become attached to your child, and for all I know, you may have, too. Besides, what we did isn't relevant. The two of you need to work out your own answer.

The couple were silent for a while, and I asked the husband whether he always talked as optimistically about the child as he was doing during that interview. He said he did. I then asked whether he always felt as optimistic as he told his wife he was. He said he didn't, but he thought it was always important to "look on the bright side of things." I commented that I thought this style made it even harder for his wife, since she thought not only that she was the only one of the two of them who did not want the child but that she was the only one who had any negative feelings. I then suggested that he spend some time just listening to her talk about her view of the matter without trying to change her mind or to suggest that she be more optimistic.

The husband followed this suggestion and allowed his wife to share her feelings with him. As part of this effort, he agreed to take her to look at a possible place for adoption, although he was still clear with her that he was doing this for her and that adoption was not an alternative he would consider. After about two weeks, the wife felt less depressed, noticed she liked the child "a little," became more involved with the child's training center, and agreed to keep the child.

In another example, two colleagues and I were asked to evaluate a sixteen-year-old youth who suffered from a genetic condition that leads to obesity, blindness, and mental retardation. The young man lived with his mother (his parents were divorced) but spent weekends with his father, who was responsible for the son's medical bills. Two years previously, the young man had "become violent" (he had verbally abused and threatened to hit his mother) and had been hospitalized in a psychiatric facility for several months. His condition had been diagnosed early in life. The intensity of the parents' efforts to obtain appropriate treatment for him could be indexed by the stack of files and letters about him, several inches thick, which the mother gave me before the first session and which my colleagues and I read prior to that meeting.

About thirty minutes into the interview, my colleague observing behind the one-way mirror (Douglas Carl) phoned in and asked me to ask the young man whether he wanted to be thought of as "a crazy boy," as "a retarded boy," or "as his own age." Quite angrily, he replied that he wished to be considered a boy of his own age. I then told the parents that, on the basis both of the records we had all read and of the young man's behavior in the session, we did not think he had a psychiatric problem. "If I could believe that, I would be the happiest woman in the world," the mother replied. "Don't be so sure," I said. "If he is not crazy, then you and your husband are the people who are in charge of his treatment—not us. Because while we don't think he's crazy, we do think he is very, very lazy."

Both examples show the therapist seeking to permit more flexibility in the family system. In the first example, I worked to get the husband to acknowledge his own divided feelings, thus permitting his wife to express the previously ignored part of her feelings. I also directed the husband to modify his style in the service of his wife's needs, so that she could know that he cared for her and her opinions even if he would not change his position about adoption. In the second example, we used a common reframing, changing "mad" behavior to "bad" behavior. Here, because of the long years of involvement with experts, the parents were used to being told, first, that there was nothing they could do to help the young man and, second, that he would not improve. They had, understandably, come to feel helpless to help their son. This feeling had been intensified by the psychiatric hospitalization—for if their son was crazy, it made sense to walk on eggshells so as not to upset him. By saying he was not crazy, we told the parents that there was a lot they could do to help him—in fact, that they were the primary people who could help him—but stressed how hard a job that would be, implying that they would prefer to feel helpless rather than to take on that job.

In both cases, I hope it is clear that although we paid attention to both aspects of the parents' dilemma, we placed particular stress on aspects of the situation that would permit new behavior, or a wider range of behavior, in the family. In the first example, I think it is evident also that I felt it important to stress that my professional training and expertise did not give me a solution to the couple's dilemma that was better than one they would jointly devise.

Working with families with a handicapped individual is likely, at times, to test the therapist's faith in himself or herself, in families, and in the justice of the therapist's society. This experience is useful because it places the therapist in an analogous position to that of handicapped individuals and their families, who live in a society that does not value handicapped persons and who have to make sense of their situation, which is socially created but which confronts families with a handicapped individual as implacably and as fearfully as if it were Fate itself.

7

Helen Coale Lewis

Child Welfare
Agencies

A discussion of family therapy and child wel-
fare requires some orientation to the history and structure of
child welfare services in this country. According to *Webster's
Third New International Dictionary*, welfare, in its most general
sense, has to do with "the state of faring or doing well: thriving
or successful progress in life." Definitions of what constitutes
"the state of faring or doing well" vary according to country,
region, class, and ethnic affiliation.

The Child Abuse Prevention Act of 1973 reflects hopes in
the United States for adequate welfare for children:

> Every child, despite his individual differences and unique-
> ness is to be considered of equal intrinsic worth, and hence
> should be entitled to equal social, economic, civil, and political
> rights, so that he may fully realize his inherent potential and
> share equally in life, liberty, and happiness. Obviously, these
> value premises are rooted in the humanistic philosophy of our
> Declaration of Independence.
>
> In accordance with these value premises, then, any act of
> commission or omission by individuals, institutions, or society
> as a whole, and any conditions resulting from such acts or inac-
> tion, which deprive children of equal rights and liberties, and/or
> interfere with their optimal development, constitute, by defini-
> tion, abusive or neglectful acts or conditions [U.S. Senate, 1973,
> p. 14].

180

The clear implication is that every institution of which children are a part and by which they are affected has a stake in determining their welfare.

Until this century, child welfare was intricately connected to the welfare of entire communities. Children were integral parts of each community's work and play, age segregation was minimal, and the entire community's needs came first. When the fields needed working, school was closed. Technological and industrial changes during the last century contributed to increased segregation of children from the mainstream of society. Child labor legislation and compulsory school attendance enhanced their unique status, and specialized institutions were established to serve and protect them.

The Social Security Act of 1935 was the first major source of public funding for welfare services to children. Unlike education, child welfare services were established not for all children but only for those in need of protection because of familial abandonment, abuse, or neglect. Unintentionally, segregating such children and their families into a specialized service track amplified their deviance, restricted their access to mainstream services, exempted the larger community from responsibility for their plight, and reinforced the child welfare bureaucracy's cry for additional resources with which to cure the problem. As a result, child welfare services have evolved into a large conglomeration of public and private agencies that claims ownership to the following: protective services (abbreviated to PS throughout this chapter) abused and neglected children and their families, crisis pregnancy (often termed "unmarried mother") services, foster care, and adoption. Powerful organizations such as the United States Children's Bureau and the Child Welfare League of America and professions such as social work have solidified the child welfare bureaucracy's ownership of these services. Other institutions, organizations, and professions have been only too glad to yield to this monopoly on such difficult services.

Since the late 1960s, involvement in child welfare services of professionals from other fields has diluted the child welfare monopoly. It is a major contention of this chapter, however, that the child welfare monopoly, even as it has been diluted by the addition of such professionals, is a significant contextual factor in any intervention with "child welfare families" (similar points are made in Chapters Five and Eight). In those child welfare services in which the monopoly has been diluted the most, such as protective services, the dilution itself creates hierarchical problems among the professionals involved as they struggle to determine who is in charge of what. With adoption and foster care services, in which child welfare still has preeminent control and in which other professionals are only minimally involved, difficulties stem from the absence of meaningful dilution of the monopoly.

In the following sections, primary attention is devoted to the family therapist's work with abused children and their families. It is with these families that the family therapist is most likely to intersect with the child welfare system. Brief discussions of foster care and adoption services follow.

Protective Services

Working with abused children and their families requires special attention to hierarchical issues and other professionals, hierarchical issues and the family, solutions that compound problems, and the lethal possibilities of the abuse problem.

Hierarchical Issues and Other Professionals. PS staff are experienced in both collateral and hierarchical teamwork, more so than many other professionals and often to a fault. Consensual validation rather than evidence often justifies decisions, and the practice of unending close supervision that limits professional autonomy frequently replaces factual information and competence. The fact that staff generally operate without sufficient training or skills reinforces the need for group decisions and extensive supervision.

Nevertheless, PS staff are used to negotiating on a collateral basis for a wide range of services for their clients from community agencies and are routinely involved with other professionals in delivering such services. The expectation is that, regardless of whether PS receives a family first and then refers for supportive services or receives the family after many other services are already involved, there will be more than one professional or agency working with the family.

As for the issue of hierarchy, PS workers are used to a clear chain of command within their own agency and do not generally struggle for total control in the way that more autonomous professionals often do. If anything, they are likely to abdicate what control they have rather than push for more.

The PS worker's experience with collateral and hierarchical teamwork can facilitate interdisciplinary treatment. Predictable problems occur, however, when the hierarchy among the various professionals is not clear. The greater the perceived overlap in function, the more confused the hierarchical structure can become. The overlap between the PS worker and the therapist, for example, is greater than that between the PS worker and the physician, especially when the PS worker and therapist have the same academic training but view their jobs as markedly different in status. Social workers are especially susceptible to this problem, because they frequently staff both child welfare and community health services. The built-in status differential for social workers in the two settings created by discrepant salaries, mental health's identification with the psychiatric profession, and the community's perception of "crazy" families as less deviant than abusive ones can escalate competition problems between the PS social worker and the mental health social worker.

Moreover, since the child welfare system as a whole has had some fairly grandiose notions about what it should be able to do for children and families separate and apart from the assistance of the rest of society, PS staff often feel grateful for help from the outside with their overwhelming caseloads but also deficient in their capacity to do an adequate job (even if the job is impossible) and, hence, guilty or uneasy about their perceived deficiency. This guilt or uneasiness often surfaces immediately after a conference with the PS worker's supervisor and manifests itself through attempts to outdo the rest of the professionals on the team in helping the family. The therapist who thinks PS work is low-status work compounds the problem, inviting the PS worker to compete.

Families are experts in utilizing hierarchical struggles to their own detriment. They may triangulate the PS worker into their relationship with the therapist by suggesting to the worker that he is far better at understanding the family's problem than the therapist is, the therapist into their relationship with the physician by complaining that the physician is cold and uncaring, and the physician into their relationship with the PS worker by alluding to the PS worker's negligence in visiting them once in six months and then only for fifteen minutes. Pretty soon the family is running the show by defining who is in the dominant position that all the professionals are struggling to attain.

The appropriate hierarchical structure, as I perceive it, is as follows. The PS worker should function at the top of the hierarchy with respect to all decisions about severity of abuse, court action, foster home placement, and obtaining auxiliary services from community agencies. This position is congruent with the legal mandate given to the PS worker for the treatment of abusive families. Professionals outside the child welfare system are required to *report* suspected cases of abuse and have professional, ethical, and programmatic expectations to *treat* such cases, but only child welfare staff have the authority, backed by court and legislative sanction, to *require* treatment. Over the PS worker is the supervisory structure of the agency and, in cases requiring court involvement, the judge. All other professionals should function at a collateral level under the PS worker, with differential authority according to their particular areas of expertise. Hence, the physician is obviously the top expert on medical issues, the police officer on law enforcement issues, the therapist on family treatment issues, and so forth. These experts operate autonomously in their own areas of expertise but only make recommendations to the PS worker on severity of abuse, court action, foster home placement, and required auxiliary services. Decisions about such recommendations are deferred to the PS worker and the courts.

With this view of the hierarchical structure, problems can arise in three main ways (for other examples, see Chapter Eight). First, professionals at the collateral level may attempt to usurp the PS worker's authority by telling her, for example, to place a child in foster care rather than recommending such a placement. The PS worker will reestablish her authority by forgetting to submit the purchase order for the professional's services or by talking her supervisor into disagreeing with the foster care recommendation. Even when the PS worker seemingly offers the dominant position to another professional, it is a trap for the other professional to accept it, because he or she is powerless to control decisions that only the PS agency and the court can make. To accept responsibility for a decision over which one has no control reduces credibility with the family and invites both the family and other professionals to compete for the power created by the PS worker's abdication.

Second, a professional at the collateral level of the hierarchy may try to outdo another professional at the same level by functioning within the latter's domain of expertise. If a physician tells Mrs. Smith to supervise her child's bedtime routine after a therapist has put Mr. Smith in charge, for example, the therapist may start talking about an excellent new pediatric service that just opened two blocks from the Smith home.

Third, the PS worker may cross hierarchical lines and usurp the functioning of someone at a lower level of the hierarchy. This occurs frequently with the PS worker and the therapist because of the overlap in perceived job functioning described above. As the therapist works with Mr. Smith to help him become more involved in parenting, the PS worker weakens Mr. Smith's attempts to do so by rescuing Mrs. Smith every time there is a crisis with the children.

The professional hierarchical structure must be clarified continually throughout the treatment with the family. This means viewing the entire system as the unit of treatment and, through joint staffings, telephone contacts, and written correspondence, assuring opportunities for interventions with the entire unit. Some of the following suggestions can be facilitative.

First, although the majority of PS workers are not professionally trained social workers, the theoretical orientations and rationales for action that guide them are determined mainly by the social work profession, a profession that routinely trains its members in "macrosystem" as well as "microsystem" theories and whose original roots are in the charity organization societies and settlement houses of the late nineteenth century. The social work approach to systems does not typically examine the social worker's contributions to, as well as solutions for, problems (except in broad institutional terms), but it offers at least some background in analyzing human beings within their social context.

The therapist should defer to the PS worker's expertise on environmental and institutional contributions to family problems and develop some credible knowledge himself about such issues. The traditional focus of all the mental health professions on individual and family pathology has, until recently, given them tunnel vision with respect to environmental pathology and its effects on families. The PS worker is part of a larger welfare system whose function has been to cope with the impact of environmental problems on families, often to the detriment of individual families. The therapist can provide a bridge between these two points of view and thereby reduce the risk that the PS worker will try to rescue the family from him because he does not understand them. It is useful to know, for example, that Aid to Dependent Children monies, first issued in 1935, exacerbated family problems by the fatherless-home eligibility requirement or that most states did not enact child-abuse reporting laws until the 1960s.

Second, praise without condescension for a job well done reinforces the PS worker's status in the hierarchy—for example, "Your periodic checking on the child's safety makes it easier for me to treat the family." Even for jobs not well done, the therapist can reframe the reality to produce the desired effect: "Your lack of checking on the child's safety demonstrates great confidence in my ability as a therapist; but since you have had more experience than I in working with abusive families, I wonder whether you would mind checking on this child more regularly and giving me your opinion." Another tactic for reinforcing the PS worker's status is to ask someone who is clearly lower or clearly higher in professional status to approach the PS worker with the request. A police officer's request, for example, does not jeopardize the PS worker's status, and a pediatrician's request may enhance it.

Third, because of the schism between the child welfare and family therapy literatures, most family therapists have little credibility with PS workers concerning their specialized knowledge of child abuse. Family therapy journals and texts contain almost nothing about child abuse, foster care, or adoption. Similarly, there is very little about family therapy in child welfare journals and texts, and what there is often misinterprets family therapy as dependent on the number of bodies in the room rather than as a way of thinking about families (see for example, Sgroi, 1982, pp. 241, 264; Meiselman, 1978, p. 342). In a setting in which getting an entire family together is often logistically impossible, it is no wonder that family therapy has been relegated to a backseat in child welfare services in favor of behavioral and educational models of treatment. It helps if the family therapist subscribes to *Child Welfare* as well as *Family Process* and at least knows who Helfer and Kempe (1968), Gil (1971), and Justice and Justice (1976, 1979) are. (For other ways of showing service providers that the therapist takes other professionals seriously, see Chapter Three.) It is also important to make clear in the beginning the therapist's views about family treatment so that the PS worker does not think that it is applicable only to families whose members can/will all get to the therapist's office.

Fourth, the family therapist should be both multitheoretical and multilingual. I once made the mistake of explaining on cross-examination in court how families operate systemically as a rationale for involving the nonabusive as well as the abusive parent in treatment. A judge generally listens more receptively to statements derived from theories of individual pathology: "Mr. Jones is so out of control with his children that I shall need all the help I can get in treating him; therefore, I would like Mrs. Jones to assist me." Other therapists may respond best to psychoanalytic, ego psychological, or Gestalt rationales. PS workers like an eclectic approach. Physicians respond best to theories of individual pathology but will accept other orientations as long as the communication is qualified by an attitude of deference.

It is useful to speak jargon-free language in court; this requires sufficient knowledge of the theoretical model being used to explain it in plain English. In other settings, it is often imperative to use just enough jargon to convince the other professional that one has professional (as opposed to common) knowledge of a particular theoretical framework and/or to create empathy by matching the other professional's language. The proper amount of jargon often depends on hierarchical considerations: Less jargon can be deferential to another professional; more jargon can maintain or increase one's status in the hierarchy.

Hierarchical Issues and Families. The family, along with the professionals, has a clear place in the hierarchy, and it should be at the top. Although the family members have lost control of some aspects of their lives, they are still the experts on themselves and must be respected as such.

The family's expertise is often relegated to no-man's-land in current interdisciplinary efforts to treat child abuse. All parties are so busy trying to rescue the child from the family and the family from itself that they often undermine the family functioning they are trying to improve. The family's dilemma is similar to the dilemma of the inpatient; to be discharged, the patient must demonstrate his capacity to function autonomously and responsibly as an adult in a setting that treats him like an irresponsible child, creating a "power struggle that can end with the patient's demeaning or destroying himself as a person" (Haley, 1973, p. 287).

There are three responses that families can make to this kind of dilemma. First, the "cooperative" (and hence "treatable") abusive family allow various professionals to take charge of many aspects of their lives. No one can understand why this family, which is trying so hard (to please), does not get better.

Second, there is the family who passively allow the professionals to take charge of just about anything and, in so doing, defeat everyone. Initially, their helplessness is viewed as cooperation; later on, it is labeled "resistance." The helplessness is generally explained by professionals as the result of emotional problems stemming from generations of deprivation and/or abuse (for example, Steele and Pollock, 1974). Although generations of abuse can certainly contribute to helplessness, so does a helping system that does not respect a family's power. Helpless families act the way they think the system expects them to act; their helplessness evokes more help from the system, which evokes more helplessness, which evokes more help, and so forth. Somewhere in this escalating cycle they are then labeled "multiproblem" families.

Third, there is the "nonvoluntary" family. *Nonvoluntary* means that the family will not volunteer to do what the professionals want them to do and generally make this clear in an aggressive style. Little attention is paid to the helping system's contributions to a family's nonvoluntary stance—the anonymity of reporting laws, for example, which contributes to a family's mistrust of community agencies, or the constant stream of professionals asking personal questions. Instead, the nonvoluntary stance is perceived primarily as a defense against internal feelings of inadequacy and helplessness.

The family's competence in the hierarchy is also affected adversely by the nature of the protective services system as an agent of social control whose function includes protecting the larger society from facing the many ways in which children are abused by institutions and by society as well as by their parents. Treating abuse as mainly a problem of individual and familial pathology exempts the larger society from responsibility and thus puts additional pressure on individual families. The therapist who, for example, directs some parental rage toward a society that provided the parents themselves with no protection from being battered as children (since reporting laws were nonexistent until the 1960s) may relieve some of the rage the parents feel toward their children, while the therapist who focuses only on the parent/child system may escalate that rage, rather than reduce its intensity. The parents know they have failed to meet societal standards (and are therefore in a one-down position with respect to other parents) and yet, at some level, are also aware that society has failed them. When the helping system focuses primarily on the family's failure, it compounds the problem. Moreover, perceptions of abusive families as categorically different from nonabusive families (though inaccurate,

since rageful feelings toward children are universal) are powerful general public attitudes that exacerbate the abusive family's
feelings of failure. The therapist who acknowledges the normality of rageful *feelings* (as differentiated from rageful *behavior*)
can help decrease the family's sense of isolation and deviance
from the rest of the community.

Working within a system that does not generally recognize the family's expertise means that special attention must be
given in the therapeutic process to helping families feel more
powerful. The following suggestions are offered.

The family should always be included in contacts with
other professionals. Telephone calls can be conference calls or,
at the very least, can occur in the family's presence; copies of
letters should be previewed by the family before mailing; and
meetings should include them. Their involvement is a clear message from the therapist that she expects them to take control of
their lives. Furthermore, in a system that encourages distrust because of anonymous reporting and free exchange of information
among professionals, the family can at least be sure that the
therapist keeps no secrets from them. They may not *like* everything she says, but at least they will *know* what she says. An
additional fringe benefit to the family's involvement can be the
dilution of turf struggles among professionals, who are less likely to vie for power in front of a family than behind closed
doors. If they do struggle in spite of the family's presence, the
therapist gains additional information about hierarchical problems in the system and an opportunity to intervene. The family,
in observing the struggle, can be forced to take more control of
their lives, since it is clear that the squabbling professionals are
out of control.

Hierarchical problems within the larger system must be
kept in mind throughout all treatment sessions with the family
as well as in interdisciplinary meetings. Often, for example,
once a family are in the PS system, they are frightened of as-
serting themselves with anyone for fear of jeopardizing their
situation even further. Professionals compound the problem by
violating the family's boundaries with unnecessary as well as
necessary intrusions, rendering the family even more helpless. A

family, therefore, may need coaching in how not to tell their private business to everyone who asks about it, a symbolic ritual with which to express their rage at the daycare center operator who reported them anonymously rather than facing them with his or her concerns, or assistance in simply saying no to the Parents Anonymous chapter's request for volunteer time.

The therapist, as part of the system, must include himself in efforts to increase the family's power. Maneuvers designed to produce resistance to the therapist's suggestions, for example, can be useful. "Perhaps you should continue to punish yourself for being a bad child to your mother and a bad mother to your child by depriving yourself of all pleasure in life" or "Perhaps you should continue to rescue your husband from all frustration with the children by taking total responsibility for them yourself and then taking the rap for what happens when you carry his frustrations as well as your own." Such maneuvers must be used cautiously and only when the therapist is sure the family will resist them.

Other ways to increase the family's power include taking a one-down position ("I don't know; they're your children, so what do you think?"), telling anecdotes that reveal the therapist's normal human feelings, reframing events in the family's life to emphasize how they *are* powerful ("The way you fought with your wife instead of your child demonstrates much strength"), staging enactments in which the parents are encouraged to take control, assigning nonparental tasks that enhance both power and pleasure, and designing rituals to celebrate increased control in the family's lives. Defusing parents' rage at themselves and their children by framing their problem in a broader context is also important: "Our society is hard on parents and does not do much to help with the things that parents need in order to be successful."

Lastly, a nonrescue stance toward abused children is essential, as rescuing undermines parental power. This is tricky because parents cannot be allowed to batter their children, but efforts to stop the battering must be framed in ways other than simply "for the sake of the children." If they could have stopped "for the sake of the children," they would not be in the PS system. For families who deny the abuse or deny that the abuse is problematic, the therapist must find some reason that will motivate the family to stop, such as getting the PS agency off their backs, staying out of trouble with the courts, or doing a better job with their children than their parents did with them. It is a trap to insist that the family acknowledge the abuse, as only the family will control that kind of power struggle. Families do not *have* to acknowledge the abuse to define staying out of trouble with the courts as a goal they can work on with the therapist, and the therapist is more likely to obtain later acknowledgment if she does not push for it initially. For families who do admit the abuse and want it to stop, reasons other than "for the sake of the children" must also be found (even if the family itself state this as a reason), as no one changes only for the sake of someone else: "You were deprived of pleasure as a child; you deserve pleasure as an adult with your own children" or "Abusing your child plays right into your mother's predictions that you would be 'no good'; don't you want to prove her wrong?"

Even when the child's safety must be assured by taking action out of the family's hands, the family can maintain some control: "Would you like me to call PS and request a foster home placement, or would you like to make the call yourself from my office?"

In situations in which the therapist finds herself chronically anxious about the child's welfare, it will be especially difficult to avoid trying to rescue the child. A second therapist to work with the children can relieve the first therapist of the total responsibility for this worry and thus reduce the risk that the first therapist, out of her anxiety, will undermine the parents' decision-making power, however circumscribed that power may be. The second therapist should be at the same location as the first, work with the children from a systemic perspective, and acknowledge the parents' therapist as the primary therapist for the family. (For still other maneuvers to empower families, see Chapter Six.)

Solutions That Compound Problems. Child protective services are organized to protect children. Staff members, therefore, emphasize fairly direct ways of reaching that goal, such as teaching communication and parenting skills. Even with the recognition that parents have their own needs and problems that interface with parenting (the literature is replete with psychological profiles of the typical abuser) and therefore may need individual or marital therapy to address such problems and needs, everyone's agenda is to provide help for the sake of the child (Berger in Chapter Six notes that this is also the case in special education). This agenda is not enough to motivate people to change, as discussed above, and it can also exacerbate the problems that contribute to the abuse. For example, referring a couple for marital therapy in order to help them become better parents can add fuel to the fires of their resentments toward a child who had already "caused" them much difficulty by being hard to manage and getting them into trouble with the community. Referring them for therapy to help with the stress their child has "caused," in contrast, gives them the opportunity to defend the child from the helper's accusations that the child is troublesome. Or requiring an abusive mother to work in her child's daycare center as a way of learning new parenting skills may be pushing her toward the very situation in which she feels the most inadequate and helpless rather than toward a situation, such as employment, that would develop her competence in a less toxic area and enhance her power and status in the family. Building in daycare services for overwhelmed parents may provide necessary relief in a volatile situation but may also facilitate further abdication of parenting responsibilities by the nonabusive parent. The therapist must critically examine every "solution" offered the family by helpers in the system for its potential for creating more problems than it solves.

Another difficulty with the emphasis on direct attempts to improve parenting is that many of the skills that are perceived as desirable are based on middle-class standards. Although there are certainly many problems associated with middle-class standards, one of the most powerful ones derives from dichotomous thinking about parenting. One either is or is not a parent, has custody or does not have custody, can or cannot provide what is necessary to one's child. There is little room for parents who can function five days out of every seven, share custody with the state, or meet only some of their child's requirements. Nor is there room for parents whose method of childcare depends on extended family support systems, as is the tradition in many ethnic groups (Chambers, 1980).

Because of this all-or-nothing mind set, professionals feel pressure to *make* parents perform, because if they cannot perform, they lose parenting rights and privileges, and the professionals have failed. Ironically, this not only keeps the system from supporting flexible ways of parenting but also interferes with realistic identification of those parents who genuinely cannot function as parents even in the most minimal ways with maximal supports. The huge numbers of children stranded in "temporary" foster care reflect our discomfort in giving up on the hope that parents will eventually be able to "perform."

As stepfamilies and single-parent and dual-career families work out more flexible models for parenting, families in the child welfare system and the professionals who work with them have an opportunity to broaden their definitions of "successful" parenting. At the individual case level, this means asking what the family really need in order to function. Do they need better parenting skills or relief from some of the pressures to "perform"? Would a cooperative living arrangement with extended family or foster care placement one day a week help? Limiting ideas to what is actually available within the system just puts more pressure on the family to fit the mold, a mold that is unrealistic for many families but particularly so for abusive families, whose perfectionistic expectations of themselves are often a contributing factor in the abuse in the first place.

A colleague related the story of a family in which the father lost his arm in an industrial accident and, as a result, also lost his job. The son asked the father to build a doghouse. When the father bought a doghouse instead, the son complained that it was not as good as the doghouse that the man next door had built. So the father bought lumber and struggled with hammer and nails. As his frustration with the one-armed carpentry work mounted, the son criticized his clumsiness. The father abused the son. Often what professionals do with abusive families is to push one-armed men into building doghouses that can be acquired in other ways—if they are even necessary.

Lethal Possibilities of Abuse Problems. The family therapist dealing with abusive families is in a life-and-death arena that requires absolute clarity about the therapist's power and responsibility, caution in the use of strategic maneuvers, expertise in court, and humility.

With abusive families, *the therapist has more power over and more responsibility for what occurs in treatment* than with other kinds of families; the fact that a child's life may be at stake ups the ante. The therapist's power derives from the legal mandate, either through PS or through the court, that the family be in treatment. Even if the family starts with the therapist and is then referred to PS, rather than the other way around, the referral itself triggers the mandate. This means that the therapist, from the start, must be clear with herself, and with the family about the parameters of her power. She does, for example, have both the power and the responsibility to alert the PS worker and/or the court if the child sustains an injury while in treatment, if the family drop out of treatment prematurely, or if the family undergo changes that increase the potential lethality of the abusive situation (as when an abusive father loses his job and is now home with the children every afternoon after school). She does not, however, have the power to make the family talk in treatment sessions or agree to improve their lives; only they have that power. Nor does she have the responsibility to report intimate details of the family's life that have no direct bearing on the abuse. The therapist may have the responsibility in many cases to make recommendations to the court about custody, foster care, severance of parental rights, and so forth, but only the court has the power to make the final decision. The parents, however, can share in decisions about the therapist's recommendations, whenever possible prior to the court process. They may, for example, choose voluntary rather than court-ordered foster care or request that their weekly visits with their child occur immediately after therapy sessions rather than at the PS worker's office.

Clarity about power and responsibility not only minimizes the risks of treatment in possibly lethal situations; it also is good role modeling for the family. The clearer the therapist is about her own power, the clearer she can be with the family about their rights.

The lethal possibilities of work with abusive families requires *caution with paradoxical and other strategic maneuvers,* particularly those that prescribe the family system and restrain change. Because the treatment system is complex and unwieldy, the effects of such maneuvers can be unpredictable and therefore potentially dangerous. Other professionals can misunderstand them, and they are hard to explain in court.

Since child abuse is against the law, work with abusive families often requires *expertise in court.* Most therapists do not like to go to court. Its adversarial format is alien to their training and professional comfort. They often put their energy into thinking up creative ways of getting out of going to court rather than creative ways of being involved in the court process. It is essential to have basic information about rules of evidence, how to qualify as an expert witness, how to avoid irritating the judge with hearsay testimony, jargon, or inaudible answers, what to do when an attorney interrupts, discredits, or badgers, and so forth. In addition to possessing basic information, it is a plus if the therapist enjoys the challenge of court involvement. For example, presenting recommendations in a public courtroom can sharpen therapists' skills, can heighten their awareness of how a family feels with the court in control, and can teach them how to hold their own in an adversarial format. The minimum information is available in courses, texts, and journals. The enjoyment comes with experience.

Lastly, the lethal potentialities inherent in work with abusive families require *humility and a knowledge of one's own limitations as a therapist.* Consultative and or supervisory supports are essential, as is a clear limit on the number of abusive families worked with at any single time. Legal consultation and, in some cases, safeguards for one's physical protection may also be required. No one can do good work while frightened.

Case Example

The following case example illustrates some aspects of working with the entire system as the unit of treatment.

Virginia and Doug Knapp, a professional couple in their early thirties, had two children, Sam, age five, and Sandra, age three. Doug was one of five children whose father had functioned marginally owing to chronic alcoholism and whose mother had overfunctioned with respect to instrumental tasks but had been emotionally detached and distant. Doug, the eldest son, was identified early in his life as the family rescuer. His professional legal training as an adult perpetuated his rescue functioning as one sibling after another got into trouble with the law. His worst fear was that he would end up like his father, a "bum." Overwork was his way of ensuring that this would never happen. Consequently, he worked seventy to eighty hours a week.

Virginia was the youngest of three girls born to a mother who had grown up in orphanages and had been sexually and physically abused at the hands of her caretakers. By all descriptions, her mother had been psychotic most of the time and had subjected Virginia to bizarre and sadistic forms of sexual and physical abuse. Virginia's father, a traveling salesman, "did not know" of the mother's maltreatment. The two times that anyone tried to intervene, the abuse got worse as "punishment" for the interference.

In the Knapp family, the first incident of abuse occurred when Sam pushed his new baby sister in a typical two-year-old's maneuver to get rid of the competition for parental attention. Virginia gave Sam a concussion in her attempts to protect her daughter (herself) from injury. This kind of incident was repeated over the years until, by the time the family was identified, Sam, then age four, was routinely injuring Sandra in desperate attempts to feel more powerful in the context of his mother's abuse. This triggered Virginia's "protection" of Sandra (herself), and the cycle escalated.

The abuse was also the only thing that got Doug to give attention to and be involved with the children. With the couple, it gave Doug an opportunity to use his skill in connecting through rescue attempts and Virginia an opportunity to be rescued. The only other avenue for connection between the two of them was over the same rescuer/rescuee theme, when Virginia developed serious medical problems that often required as many as ten hospitalizations in any one year. The couple never fought, rarely played, and almost never had sexual relations. Nor did they have friends or outside activities.

The Knapps' connections via abusive incidents and illness exacerbated the abuse problem. Doug, exhausted from his lifelong rescue missions and his workaholism, would retreat further behind his desk after an abusive incident, and Virginia, feeling both deficient because she should have been able to rescue herself (a belief she carried from childhood) and abandoned (because the rescue attempts did not work), would try harder with the children, becoming even more frustrated when her efforts did not produce the unrealistically happy children she needed as proof of her good mothering.

At the point of referral to this therapist, the family were involved with a pediatrician, a neurologist, a PS worker, volunteers from a special outreach program for abusive families, the local Parents Anonymous chapter, a daycare center, and a lawyer. They had already been in treatment for over a year with a therapist affiliated with a specialized early childhood program in which Sam had been enrolled and where the abuse had first been identified and reported. Sam was no longer eligible for the program—hence the referral. In spite of admirable efforts by the former therapist to manage the inevitable hierarchical problems in the larger system, there was still much jockeying for position as each helper tried to rescue the family better than the others. The fact that Virginia was a pleasant, intelligent woman who expressed much gratitude to everyone for his or her attempts to help and who tried hard to follow everyone's recommendations contributed to the competition. Well-meaning efforts to help Virginia when she lost control of herself with the children had interfered with the function the abuse served in the family. Doug knew no other way to be involved with his children, and the couple had no other avenue for connection. The abuse and Virginia's illnesses had thus escalated while busy volunteers and professionals increasingly usurped Doug's involvement and then became angry with him for his withdrawal from his wife and children.

One of the first treatment interventions, therefore, was to put Doug back in charge as "chief rescuer" until there was time to work out other ways of connecting with his wife and children. Virginia was instructed to call him whenever she needed help with the children, and he was either to carry a beeper or to be sure his secretary would know how he could be reached at all times. This intervention had interesting reverberations throughout the rest of the system. The PS worker and the volunteers from the outreach center, who had been receiving several crisis calls a week from Virginia, did not know how to disentangle themselves without appearing rejecting and unhelpful, even though they were in agreement with the plan. That problem was solved when the PS worker left for another job and a new PS worker, without any history of helpfulness to Virginia, took her place, and when the outreach agency decided that their volunteers were needed elsewhere with families less skillful than the Knapps in lining up resources for themselves. At this point the daycare social worker joined Virginia in an alliance against the therapist, agreeing with her that there were some things she could not discuss with her husband. This social worker called the therapist to suggest individual therapy for Virginia because of the intensity of her problems, which the therapist obviously did not fully understand. She wondered whether the therapist was informed about the extent of the abuse in Virginia's background. In a subsequent meeting involving the new PS worker, the daycare social worker, the family, and the therapist, the daycare social worker again presented her concerns that Virginia was not receiving intensive individual work. The therapist deferred to her expertise in early childhood traumas and, utilizing the social worker's model of individual pathology, gave a brief dissertation on the potential curative powers of intimate relationships such as marriage for healing old childhood hurts. The therapist also used the social worker's concerns about Virginia's abusive background as well as her obvious status needs to enlist her assistance in stopping Sam's teacher from asking Virginia personal questions and "trying to be Virginia's therapist." The Parents Anonymous meetings were framed as a place where Virginia could discuss things she could not discuss in front of her husband.

Later, in a session with the couple, the therapist described the social worker's assistance as a violation of the family's privacy, taking her cue from Doug's complaint that "everyone knows our business." Once Virginia received permission not to be cooperative with everyone who asked her personal questions and encouragement for keeping some things to herself, she stopped encouraging the daycare social worker's efforts to help her. The social worker, frustrated in her attempts to outdo the therapist in treating Virginia, then called the therapist several times, usually beginning the conversation with "I don't mean to be critical, but . . ." Initially, the therapist listened politely to the social worker's assessment of the situation, thanking her for her interest and taking a one-down position designed to deescalate the social worker's power struggles with the therapist. After the fifth call, when the therapist was sure that Virginia was strong enough to resist the social worker's intrusiveness, the therapist suggested to the social worker that perhaps the Knapps should terminate therapy and be referred to the daycare center for all further treatment. The calls stopped, as did the social worker's daily efforts to help Virginia.

Encouraging Virginia to obtain employment as a way of enhancing competence in areas of her life other than parenting was also difficult within the larger system. With the goal of improving parenting skills, she had been encouraged by the first PS worker and the daycare center to do volunteer work with the children at the center. At the time of referral to this therapist, she was putting in about three days a week. The daycare staff, finding her to be a very cooperative and talented volunteer, was also giving her free daycare for one of the children in return for the volunteer work, thus saving the family tuition money. Although the arrangement was helping the family financially, it was not helping Virginia do any better with her own children and, in fact, seemed to have made things worse. Both children behaved well when around other people and deteriorated only at home as they helped their parents connect by means of temper tantrums and other abuse-provoking behavior. This reinforced Virginia's feelings that only other people could handle her children and made her feel increasingly deficient and powerless.

Initial efforts to redirect Virginia toward employment failed under the pressure from the daycare center director to keep a good volunteer who owed the center tuition money and Virginia's concern that she had failed at a task that was supposed to make her a better parent. At this point, the PS worker found a daycare center free to children on PS caseloads; this eliminated the tuition issue. A student intern supervised by the therapist was rounded up to provide bimonthly therapy sessions for Sam, with both Virginia and the therapist observing behind a one-way mirror and coming into the session to work on specific tasks with Sam and the intern. This not only provided the therapist with additional diagnostic information about how Sam and mother triggered each other with their behavior; it also took care of Virginia's need to have an avenue for working specifically on parenting skills. Since the therapy sessions were presented to her as higher-level work than what she had been doing at the daycare center, she accepted this substitute. In addition, the husband was encouraged to discuss in treatment sessions the exhaustion he was feeling with his job and his need for assistance in supporting the family. It became clear that he needed Virginia's help, and she later accepted a part-time job doing legal assistance work in a neighboring law office. The fact that she rejected four or five job suggestions from the therapist before finally deciding on one her husband offered was a good sign.

A few months later, Virginia and Doug filed a lawsuit against a manufacturer for a product whose defective structure had contributed to Virginia's health problems. The therapist, after receiving a release-of-information request from the attorney, asked the couple about the relevance of their treatment to the lawsuit and discovered that Doug and the lawyer planned to allege in the suit that the defective product had caused the emotional stress that caused the abuse. Since the product had supposedly caused permanent damage to Virginia, the abuse would have to continue for the couple to win their suit—and it would have to continue as Virginia's problem alone. In a meeting shortly thereafter with the couple and the attorney, the therapist outlined all the factors in the Knapp family that contributed to the abuse: Virginia's predisposition to abuse; Doug's detachment from the family; Virginia's projections onto Sam, which, combined with his exceptional intelligence, made the family perceive him as a difficult child; and the initial crisis that had precipitated the abuse when Sam was two. The family was described, in other words, as fitting the typical profile of an abusive family as discussed in the literature (for example, Steele and Pollock, 1974). Since the therapist's intent was not only to discourage the attorney from his stance on causation but also to provide Doug and Virginia with some respectable way to vindicate themselves other than the lawsuit, the profile was described in normalized, soluble terms. No attempt was made to describe family life cycles or systemic patterns, because the attorney lacked awareness of family therapy as a valid form of treatment; to speak from this point of view would therefore have jeopardized the therapist's credibility with the attorney (and later in court). The attorney was skillful and continued to try to convince the therapist that the defective product should be blamed for the abuse. Hypothesizing that the attorney was working on a contingency basis and was expecting a larger settlement if emotional as well as physical damage could be proved, the therapist appealed to his pocket, telling him that he could probably find some independent expert who would agree with him but that once the abuse issue was brought into court, the Knapps would be waiving their rights to maintain therapy records as confidential, and the lawyer representing the manufacturer of the product would undoubtedly subpoena this therapist to testify. Knowing what the therapist's testimony would be, the lawyer knew that the only way not to jeopardize the lawsuit was to exclude the issue of abuse from it, and he did.

The example of the Knapp family describes only a few of

the many interventions used and how each intervention involved the entire system as the unit of treatment.

Foster Care

The child welfare system is in control of about 400,000 children in this country (Silverman and Feigelman, 1977, p. 554). Even with legal mandates for periodic reviews to protect children from becoming permanent foster children, most of them do not return home to biological parents; nor are they placed for adoption. A Massachusetts study, for example, found that 67 percent of all foster children had been in the system for two or more years and, of that 67 percent, 83 percent were never returned to their parents (Silverman and Feigelman, 1977, p. 554).

Foster children live in a power vacuum. Foster parents, the nonprofessional employees of the foster care system, are charged with the impossible expectation of providing care in a normal family setting without sufficient authority to do so. Often the caseworker aligns with the child or with a supervisor or an agency policy to remind the foster parent that the agency, not the parent, is really in charge of the child. The foster parent may then forget to comply with an agency policy, bend the teacher's or therapist's ear about the caseworker's ignorance, or, as often happens, remind the caseworker who is in charge by returning the child to the agency for placement elsewhere. An unpublished study (Henry, 1976) describing highly discrepant opinions between foster care workers and foster parents about the same child's needs demonstrates a problem that both emanates from and contributes to hierarchal struggles within the system.

Therapists may be turned to as a solution to the power vacuum. They are often asked, for example, to evaluate a particularly troublesome foster child for purposes of planning. In the process, they may unintentionally seal a child's doom by reinforcing, through their diagnosis of the child, the belief that the child is unadoptable or requires institutional care. Often such evaluations occur without access to all significant parties in the total system and with biased information derived from foster care records compiled by a succession of caseworkers trained to think in terms of individual pathology (Goffman, 1961). A child's behavior is then misinterpreted as "disturbed" rather than as an understandable response in a specific context. A child, for example, may refuse to cooperate with foster parents because cooperation would mean siding with them against the caseworker. Even young children know that it is the caseworker who has the ultimate authority over their destiny. The extent of their efforts not to cooperate may appear quite pathological, as in the case of a ten-year-old boy referred to me because he refused to talk and had convinced the caseworker and foster parents that he was totally mute.

Assessing and treating foster children requires assessing and treating the entire system. Clarifying who has control of what is often an important first step. The "mute" boy, for example, was told that only he had control of his mouth and vocal cords. The police officers could not force him to talk when they rescued him from his abusive father; the caseworker could not force him to talk when he picked him up at the police station; the foster parents could not do any better than the officers or the caseworker; and the therapist not only could not force him to talk but did not want him to talk until he was sure that he alone had control of his words. The foster parent who initially kept the boy was relieved of all responsibility for curing him (and hence competing with the caseworker for his job) by reframing the mutism as a healthy, self-healing response to the traumas the boy had experienced and, as such, evidence that the foster parent was doing an excellent job in making the boy feel comfortable in her home. The caseworker was relieved of expectations to cure the boy by framing the mutism as an expectable response to trauma, which would diminish in the excellent foster home the caseworker had obviously taken great care in selecting for the child. Slowly, the boy began talking.

Once the current contextual problems have been addressed, the therapist then has some responsibility for tackling the issue of long-term planning for the foster child. The overriding question must be "How can a normal environment be worked out for this child so that he or she no longer needs treatment simply to help him or her adjust to the pathological conditions of foster care?" The high turnover of casework staff, frequent changes in foster homes, and the limbolike legal status of foster children are all deterrents to long-term planning, reinforcing the day-to-day kinds of power struggles within the system and the abdication of responsibility for the larger decisions. The foster parents cannot shop the sales for next year's winter coat; the caseworker dreads the call advising her to move a child into another foster home; and the child remembers the long list of caseworkers who have been in charge of his life and wonders who will be next. It is no wonder that the system often asks, "Which home will take him now and for how long?," rather than, "How can we get this child out of foster care?" The former question "occurs within a given system which itself remains unchanged" (Watzlawick, Weakland, and Fisch, 1974, p. 10) and makes possible only first-order change. The latter question changes the system itself and makes possible second-order change, or "change of change" (Watzlawick, Weakland, and Fisch, 1974, p. 11).

The therapist must think in terms of second-order change for the foster child. Adoption is one example of second-order change. Thus, in the case of the mute boy, adoption was identified as the long-range goal early in treatment. Not only had the biological mother died, but the father was chronically alcoholic, was a frequent guest in the state psychiatric hospital, and had lost four older children to permanent foster care. The boy, while maintaining some loyalty to his father, responded to foster care with an eagerness to be "just like" other children and with rage when anything reminded him that he was not. The rage was often misinterpreted by both the caseworker and, initially, the foster parent as pathological; much reframing was required to convince both that it was a good indicator of the child's comfort in the foster home and of his efforts to catch up with his peers developmentally. The foster parent, a sensitive, caring single woman, developed a strong attachment to the boy and he to her. It rapidly became evident that the temporariness of the arrangement was creating far more problems for their family unit than anything else that they had to handle together. When the caseworker was convinced of this, she then utilized the therapist's support for negotiating with her supervisor an agreement for filing a petition for severance of parental rights and approval of a subsidized adoption application. The therapist's willingness to testify in court was essential, as the general expectation in foster care units about severance-of-parental-rights petitions is that they are almost impossible to obtain. In addition, the biological father was abusive and angry in the face of such an action. It was important that the caseworker not have to face him alone in court. Severance was ordered, subsidized adoption approved, and a normal environment thus established for the boy.

Treatment continued into the first year of the adoption, mainly to help the adoptive mother work out problems with the school system in obtaining special education services and to provide her with support as the boy, now that he had a permanent home, could begin to talk about some of his experiences before placement and express his rage about them. In spite of the total legal control that adoption confers, the adoptive mother, rather than close off all contacts with the boy's biological family, assisted him in making contacts with his siblings, a move supported by the therapist because of its congruence with the boy's needs rather than with the arbitrariness of legalized cutoffs in the typical adoptive family. Follow-up one year later found the family doing well and facing normal problems associated with adolescence.

When removal from the foster care system is not an option, then the second-order change may be to reframe the foster family as the child's "permanent" family, solidify their power, reduce the caseworker's control, and help the child understand why he lives with a foster family. When foster care is not faced honestly as the permanent solution that it is for many children, the system compounds the child's problems by treating as temporary what in reality is permanent. Everyone's power is dimin-

ished while waiting for a "permanent" solution other than foster care; meanwhile, the child grows up.

Adoption

Adoption services has traditionally been regarded as the
highest-status work in child welfare and, as such, has been
guarded more zealously against intrusion by other professionals
than any other child welfare service. Unlike other services, it has
catered primarily to middle-class clients, sanctioned the exclusive use of psychoanalytic theories in assessing and treating clients, and insulated itself more fully from its mistakes through
the myth of unique competence, the legal strength of sealed records (Kirk, 1981), and the absence of adequate follow-up studies
of agency-placed children. Adoption-agency control of childless
couples' access to the children society has traditionally required
as evidence of "success" has given such agencies immense power. Even though some five million adopted children in this country are intimately involved with some forty million family members through their adoptive ties (Kirk, 1981), adoption is still
considered a specialized child welfare service. When adoption is
discussed outside the child welfare arena, as it is, for example,
in psychiatric journals, adoptive family issues are frequently defined in terms of individual and familial pathology. Little attention has been given to the societal and institutional contributors
to the problems faced by adoptive families. Societal values that
place a premium on biological parenthood, for example, have
created unnecessary problems for adoptive parents, who, by virtue of their family structure alone, have been defined as "second best." Adoption-agency efforts to match the "perfect
child" with the "perfect couple" in a placement procedure that
often simulates biological parenthood (even in the context of
required preplacement discussions about infertility, managing
children's questions about adoption, and other issues not faced
by biological parents) give conflicting messages to adoptive families about their similarities to and differences from other kinds
of families. Sealed records designed to protect the adoptive and

biological parents at the expense of the adopted person have simultaneously reinforced biological simulation in the adoption process and dramatically highlighted the differentness of adoption as a legislated family form. So have laws that differentiate between adoptive and biological children for purposes of insurance, inheritance, and incest. Society and its institutions have given the mixed message that the adoptive family is just like any other family—only it really is not.

Many therapists see adoptive families in their offices long after the adoption has taken place and compound the family's problems by not understanding that the crux of their underlying uneasiness is often the original set of mixed messages itself. Helping them accept their difference from other families as a viable (as opposed to pathogenic) difference can reframe the problem in such a way that other problems stemming from the initial ambivalence and confusion then become more solvable. Increased numbers of stepfamilies and other nontraditional family structures, combined with the volume of interracial and older-child adoptions, in which biological simulation is impossible, have paved the way for advertising rather than concealing (Haley, 1973) the adoptive family's differences from other families.

Since therapists generally become involved with adoptive families after the adoption has taken place, they, like the rest of society, are cut off from knowledge of the adoption experience itself. Including professionals not employed by adoption agencies in the aspects of the adoption process over which these agencies have traditionally had total and exclusive control might be a healthy way of addressing societal and institutional contributors to the adoptive family's problems. A family, for example, can perhaps talk more easily with a therapist about their ambivalence in applying for adoption than with the adoption worker who will be judging their potential adequacy as parents. A family in the postplacement stage of their adoption may feel more comfortable discussing their problems with someone other than the adoption worker, who tends to think in terms of the child's rather than the family's adjustment and who has a vested interest in validating her own competence by not seeing problems that may jeopardize the "rightness" of her placement decision. Especially in older-child placements, the worker's feelings of ownership toward the child can interfere with the family's sense of entitlement (Katz, 1977) and thus compound the family's problems. Adult adoptees, confused about the decision to search out biological roots, may receive more objective help in making this decision anywhere but in the agency that controls access to that information and is most likely biased against giving it to them. A recent Child Welfare League of America study (Research Center, Child Welfare League of America, 1976) showed, for example, that even though 70 percent of all agencies surveyed considered the adult adoptee's efforts "a natural search for identity," and even though 87 percent of the reunions effected were judged successful, most agencies still did not favor helping the adult adoptee obtain complete information.

The increase in independent adoption placements, managed primarily by physicians and lawyers, is a reflection of families' discomfort with total agency control. The Child Welfare League of America, however, views the increase in independent placements mainly as a response to the decreased supply of normal, healthy, white infants rather than as any real indicator that families are rejecting adoption-agency services for reasons having to do with the adoption agencies themselves (Meezan, Katz, and Russo, 1978). The fact that physicians and lawyers report less time discussing "psychologically significant factors" (Meezan, Katz, and Russo, 1978) may be a clue, for example, that families could do with less intrusive discussions in agency home studies, particularly now, when the greater societal permission given to families *not* to have children means that self-selection will increase in families who apply for adoption. Because of only nominal recognition that agencies themselves may contribute to a family's decision to adopt independently, the Child Welfare League's stance on independent placements is to call for increased legal sanctions and greater agency control in the independent placement process. The rationale is the presumption that independent placements do not measure up to the standards set by the Child Welfare League, not on any hard data provided by follow-up studies. In fact, almost all independent placements in the study were rated as good as or better than agency homes in physical and emotional care of the child (Meezan, Katz, and Russo, 1978). Nowhere in the report is the suggestion made to contract some services, such as preadoptive counseling, home study assessments, or follow-up counseling, to qualified mental health professionals or clinics outside the adoption agency itself. These functions are clearly reserved for adoption agencies.

The preceding discussion is not meant to be a polemic recommending a clear course of action for inclusion of therapists in the adoption process. It is meant to illustrate how societal attitudes and agency monopolies segregate adoptive families and to suggest that there may be some advantage to broadening the adoption turf.

The Child Welfare System in Society

Treatment within the child welfare system has much to teach the family therapist. As she deals with the complex network of helpers, she fine-tunes her sensitivity to how societal and institutional contextual factors affect all families. The problems that demand attention in child welfare are problems that all families experience to some degree: how to manage anger, fears of abandonment, loss of control, felt differences from other families, failure, and so forth. Child welfare families are just more symptomatic and, because of a segregated service track, more isolated. Systemic thinking in the family therapy field can inject hope into the "child welfare problem" in the same way that reframing a symptomatic child's behavior as benevolent generosity to the rest of the family can make a family's problems more hopeful—for, in a real sense, child welfare families and the agencies and institutions that serve them are like the symptomatic child offering benevolent protection to the larger society.

8 Gregory J. Jurkovic

Juvenile
Justice System

The family systems therapist is the "new kid on the block" in juvenile justice. Like his or her predecessors, the systemic clinician is hopeful of introducing a new approach to understanding and treating delinquency. Help from the therapeutic community has long been welcomed by court officials. Indeed, shortly after its inception in 1899, the first juvenile court called on William Healy to develop a court clinic. Today mental health services available through the court or other community settings (child guidance and mental health centers, private clinics, university departments) play a vital role in virtually every juvenile court system in the United States (Pabon, 1980).

Unfortunately, despite their long association, the juvenile court and the mental health profession have yet to achieve a satisfactory entente. Like travelers in a foreign country, clinicians in juvenile justice share neither a terminology nor a world view with court personnel. Moreover, they often find their goals subordinated to legal needs and controls. Not surprisingly, many quickly withdraw from the juvenile court, attributing their therapeutic failures and frustrations with court-involved youths to the youths themselves or to the court system (see Lewis and others, 1973; Prentice and Kelly, 1966).

Whether family therapists will fare better than others in their collaborative ventures with the juvenile court remains to be seen. Certainly, it behooves them to do so in light of the judicial system's increasing involvement in the lives of American families. As the authors of the 1976 *Task Force Report on Juvenile Justice and Delinquency Prevention* noted: "More children now have not only a stepparent, but also a judge, probation officer, or a protective services agency social worker" (p. 272). Family systems theory can help therapists understand the part of both the court and the clinician in the larger context of delinquency and service delivery. The challenge, however, is to translate that understanding into effective treatment strategies that are sensitive to the multiple interests involved (families, children, court personnel, community members, and so forth).

For the past several years my staff and I have attempted to develop such strategies in our work on a privately funded project* serving probationers at a large, metropolitan juvenile court. The project is one of many community agencies to which the court refers youngsters for counseling. Working out of an inner-city health clinic located near the court complex, we have served a diverse group. The majority of juveniles, however, have lived in poor, multiproblem families similar to those described by Minuchin and others (1967) in *Families of the Slums*. Although I have worked with numerous court-involved youths in my private practice, it has been in the design and direction of this project that my appreciation for the interrelatedness of court personnel, therapists, and families has grown.

In this chapter I will present what we have learned about the court/family relationship: how to enter, assess, and change its transactional field. Special emphasis will be placed on ways of working cooperatively with the juvenile court and of using seemingly countertherapeutic legal processes as levers for change.

*The Central Presbyterian–Georgia State Delinquency Project, which has received support from the Pollard Fund, Central Presbyterian Church, Atlanta; the Higher Education Challenge Fund, Presbyterian Church, U.S.; the Women's Opportunity Giving Fund, United Presbyterian Church; and Georgia State University. I am indebted to Marsha Weiss, Michael O'Shea, Debbie Daniels-Mohring, David Kearns, Cinda Caiella, Michael Chiglinsky, and Joel Rosenthal for their creative and dedicated work on the project, receptivity to my supervision of their therapeutic activities, and stimulation of many of the ideas presented here.

Because effective work along these lines requires an understanding not only of family process but also of judicial process, it will be important, before discussing particular strategies, to provide a brief overview of the juvenile court.

Juvenile Court: Theory and Practice

Backed by the principle of *parens patriae*, government officials in Illinois were the first to claim the right and the responsibility to act through the juvenile court to meet the needs of youthful offenders (Cox and Conrad, 1978). By 1945 every state had enacted a juvenile court act or juvenile proceedings code. In addition to creating separate courts for juveniles, these codes typically specify the purpose, scope, and procedures of delinquency proceedings (Cox and Conrad, 1978).

Purpose and Scope. Although the juvenile court movement has pursued various and oftentimes competing goals, its founders were concerned mainly with rehabilitating, rather than litigating and punitively disposing of, wayward and troubled children. To achieve this aim, they not only dispensed with procedural formalities but also expanded the jurisdiction of the juvenile court to include youngsters guilty of status offenses, such as truancy, runaway, or incorrigibility, as well as youngsters variously labeled over the years "dependent and neglected," "deprived," or "in need of supervision." These changes enabled juvenile court officials—like "good parents"—to attend more closely to the child's psychosocial condition than to his or her guilt or innocence (Stapleton and Teitelbaum, 1972).

Whether youngsters should exchange their basic legal rights for understanding and treatment, however, has been questioned in recent years, especially in light of little convincing evidence of the state's effectiveness in its parental role (Hazard, 1976). In a landmark decision in 1967, *In re Gault,* the Supreme Court held that the juvenile court must respect the child's right to due process. Although the implications of this decision and others concerning juvenile proceedings are still being debated, it is apparent that the pendulum in juvenile justice is swinging from a "casework" or "therapeutic" model to a more "formalistic" or "legalistic" approach (Cox and Conrad, 1978). In his sociological study of the Los Angeles Juvenile Court, Emerson (1969) observed: "On a statutory and procedural level the court revealed elements of both models. Similarly, the working ideologies of judges and probation officers contained strongly legal and restrictive commitments along with the ideals of treatment and help" (p. 26). The resulting combination is often ambiguous and paradoxical.

Further complicating matters, the court also must consider the larger community context of its actions. What might be best for the juvenile may not be best for society. Consequently, although court personnel are generally more tolerant of juvenile misconduct than community members, a youngster may be incarcerated to protect the public (Cox and Conrad, 1978). Some juvenile justice officials view the court's role in crime control and social protection as more defensible than its treatment objective. Along with efficiently detecting and processing young offenders, advocates of this approach recommend greater emphasis on punishment, isolation from the community, and deterrence as legitimate functions of juvenile justice (Katkin, Hyman, and Kramer, 1976).

To encourage more uniformity and clarity in juvenile court practice across the country, the National Conference of Commissioners on Uniform State Law drafted the Uniform Juvenile Court Act in 1968. A growing number of states have revised their juvenile codes to conform to the standards of this act. Among other modifications, the Uniform Juvenile Court Act differentiates status offenders (labeled "unruly") from children adjudicated "delinquent" and generally requires greater legal accountability (see Cox and Conrad, 1978).

Procedures. Yet in spite of trends to administer juvenile justice more consistently, exactly how business gets done and what goals (rehabilitation, due process, social protection, and crime control) are pursued vary from setting to setting and even from case to case (Emerson, 1969). Hence, practitioners must acquaint themselves with the particular character of juvenile justice within their state and county. Much of this information can be gleaned from the state's juvenile code and from annual re-

ports of the juvenile court(s) in one's area. It may also be helpful to peruse an introductory textbook on juvenile justice (such
as Cox and Conrad, 1978, or Katkin, Hyman, and Kramer,
1976) as well as various legal and sociological studies of the juvenile court (for example, Emerson, 1969, or Stapleton and
Teitelbaum, 1972). There are also several journals, such as the
Juvenile and Family Court Journal, that provide information
about current trends in theory and practice in the delinquency
area.

In addition, it is strongly recommended that clinicians
seek information directly from police officers, judges, attor-
neys, probation officers (POs), and other juvenile justice personnel. Through these contacts, therapists not only can learn a great
deal about the personal qualities, beliefs, idiosyncrasies, and responsibilities of these individuals (such as whether they are
legalistic- or treatment-oriented, their pet peeves with mental
health professionals, or their theories of delinquency causation)
but also can begin to form the kind of collaborative relationship
with them that will facilitate therapeutic work.

Juvenile Justice from a Family Systems Perspective. It
should quickly become apparent while gathering information
about the juvenile court that the administration of justice to
children and adolescents is a complex and multifaceted process.
Perhaps most striking about this process from a family systems
perspective is that, in trying to meet the needs of both the child
and the state, court officials have until recently paid little attention to the needs of the most important system mediating relations between the two: the family. To their credit, the authors
of the Uniform Juvenile Court Act did recommend that the
child, if possible, not be separated from his or her parents. However, physically removing youngsters from their homes is not
the only way the child's relation to parental figures can be
strained. By benevolently assuming responsibility for the socialization and care of children who come within its jurisdiction,
the juvenile justice system risks forming a potentially problematic "cross-generational coalition," or what one judge has labeled a "mutual compact" with the child (Ketcham, 1962).
Parents are bypassed. Indeed, as Bell (1975) has aptly observed,

"Our laws and traditional procedures require individual work with the offender, as exemplified in probation, institutional placement, or parole. We do not place the family on probation, we do not institutionalize the family, and consequently, it is never on parole. Correctional relations with individuals are written into statute" (p. 252). Admittedly, the court's individual-oriented treatment of juveniles is sometimes needed and openly invited by many parents. However, the court does this routinely and often without regard for its effects on other family members. What little control parental figures have, for example, may be lost once the child enters the juvenile justice system.

I am not questioning that the court's tactics can alter the behavior of many youngsters. Placing a chronic school truant in detention where she is escorted by a guard to the court school can have a dramatic impact on her. However, it has little direct or predictable effect on the dysfunctional parental subsystem in the youngster's family and leaves her brothers and sisters at risk for court involvement as well. Moreover, even though the child may subsequently attend school, she may be conforming merely to avoid punishment, which, as social scientists have taught us, serves as a weak barrier against future misconduct.

Our goal as family therapists is to help family members learn as quickly as possible to relate to one another and their environment in a newer and more flexible fashion, thus creating a context in which the delinquent behavior is neither adaptive nor necessary (Haley, 1976). To the extent that behavior must be controlled or restrained in the course of therapy, we make every effort to find ways that the social network and family system of the court-involved youngster can appropriately serve in a "social control" capacity. This strategy, discussed in more detail later, is not pursued as an end in itself but, rather, as an intermediate step in the therapeutic process.

Changing Court/Family/Therapy Transactions

In view of their ideological and procedural differences, it is not surprising that family therapists and court officials often find themselves at odds. Though critical of the court, I am equal-

ly concerned about the contributions of the therapeutic community to the juvenile justice experiment. For example, in addition to supporting the court's traditional focus on the individual,
therapists of different persuasions, including family therapists,
have tried to implement their treatment strategies without sufficient regard for the context of the court. The contextually rela-
tivistic nature of any intervention requires that therapists learn
about their interconnectedness with the settings in which they
are working (see Chapter Four). Thus, rather than attribute
problems in the court/family/therapy relationship to any one
component, it may be more helpful to focus on the relationship
itself and on ways of reorganizing it to deal effectively with
delinquency.

In the remainder of the chapter, I will describe some ave-
nues that we have traveled with court officials, primarily POs, in
treating court-involved youths from a strategic and structural
perspective (Haley, 1976; Madanes, 1981; Minuchin, 1974;
Watzlawick, Weakland, and Fisch, 1974) and suggest other
paths that court/family/therapy transactions might take. Special
consideration will be given to how the context of the court
uniquely affects the following therapeutic processes: establishing a therapeutic system, assessing and reformulating the problem, goal setting, and restructuring the family. For ease of
presentation, these processes will be discussed individually, although in practice they are inseparable.

Establishing a Therapeutic System. In establishing a therapeutic system with court-involved youths, the therapist's first
task is to define his or her position in relation not only to the
family but also to the court. Unless this is done, the chances of
entering blindly into countertherapeutic, triangular interactions
with the court and family are extremely high. Many of these triangles, for example, are rooted in the therapist's tendency to
overemphasize the needs and dynamics of court-involved youngsters and their families in reaction to the court's concern about
immediate behavioral control. The therapist is then perceived
as "soft" or "permissive" by court personnel, who in turn are
seen as "restrictive" by the therapist—a process that may mirror
parental interactions in the court-involved youngster's family.

The converse of this pattern may also emerge. It is in the family's best interests that therapists and court officials develop a more cooperative relationship.

At the point at which the juvenile justice system or family pursues therapy for a youngster, he is often under the supervision of a PO. The functions of this person must be understood, as the therapist needs to form a working alliance with him. The PO works within the major component of the juvenile court that is responsible for meeting the special needs of youngsters and providing for their treatment (Lewis and others, 1973). Rather than continue to deliver services themselves, POs have increasingly become "social brokers," or links to community resources for their charges (Katkin, Hyman, and Kramer, 1976). However, even with this change, the demands of their job are excessive. Lewis and others (1973, p. 100) have pointed out that the PO functions as a "detective, psychiatrist, social worker, and parent." The resulting "role strain" (Lewis and others, 1973) is often exacerbated by large caseloads, poor pay, low status in the helping professions, and inadequate training.

Nevertheless, juveniles and therapists who think they have more influence or control than POs in the court setting are in for a rude awakening. Typically, the judge prescribes—or, more accurately, "orders"—particular actions by the juvenile offender, such as regular school attendance or counseling as well as compliance with the PO's directives, thereby empowering the PO with the authority of the court. Moreover, in further decision making about the youngster's status, the judge relies heavily on the PO's recommendations. For example, if conditions of probation are not met, then the PO can suggest that the child's probationary status be revoked.

Although the therapist is well advised to work closely with individual POs, it is useful to keep in mind that the PO is part of a hierarchical structure that in large court systems, such as the one in which we are working, typically includes the following individuals (listed in order of increasing power): the POs, the supervisor of clinical services, the chief PO, the referees, and the judges. The PO's behavior is constrained by these individuals and their policies. Countertherapeutic decisions by POs may have less to do with frictions in the PO/therapist relationship than with pressures they are experiencing in relation to their superiors. Remembering this fact may deter therapists from personalizing the PO's actions.

Recognition of the PO's position should also alert the therapist that he or she functions below the PO in the court hierarchy. Bypassing the PO to work out problems in the court/ therapy relationship can create the same sort of difficulties that arise when the court bypasses parents in dealing with children. Thus it generally is not wise for the therapist to problem-solve with the PO's superiors unless the PO is present. It is suggested, however, that the therapist join with clinical supervisors, chief POs, and judges by informing them of his or her services and interest in working cooperatively with the court. Knowing that their superiors approve of the therapist can greatly facilitate POs' willingness to collaborate. Another benefit of the therapist's relationship with higher-echelon staff is that it allows him or her to maintain a stable, ongoing connection with the court, since there is less turnover among these staff members than among POs. The therapist's relationship with court administrators also makes a difference when he or she testifies in court. Judges are more likely to listen to recommendations from clinicians they know, especially if the therapist and PO have worked together in developing a suggested plan of action. The initial investment of time and expense required of therapists to build the kind of ties I am suggesting will greatly enhance their ability later to handle predictable problems in the court/family/therapy relationship. (See Chapter Four for further discussion of the importance of the backing of administration.)

It can be argued that through these ties the therapist becomes an arm of the court, a role that is discomforting and objectionable to some. Our experiences and others' (Johnson, 1974), however, have clearly indicated that to pretend to be autonomous of the court is neither productive nor honest. Yet therapists can cooperate with the PO without abandoning their primary commitment to the family or serving solely as social control agents. In effect, therapists are both a part of and "meta" to the court and the family, a paradoxical relationship that gives them the latitude they need to work effectively (Haley, 1976). It is important, however, for the therapist, the PO, and the parents to clarify their different roles in relation to the court-involved youngster and to one another. For example, we have reached an agreement with the POs to share information about the youngster's attendance at sessions. Other information, unless it involves illegal or life-threatening behavior such as possession of a firearm by a minor, is shared only with the family's permission. However, even when we decide for ethical reasons that confidentiality must be violated, family members are always informed first and given the option of reporting the problem themselves to the PO. This agreement and other issues concerning case management and goals are discussed with the family during the initial session, *which is attended by the PO.* The boundaries between the different aspects of the court/ family/therapy relationship are thus clearly defined, and the parents' competence and power are respected.

In these sessions, POs often have a different experience of juveniles and their families. For example, family members who were earlier perceived as weak, irresponsible, or uncaring may be seen in a new and more positive light. The POs develop a greater appreciation for the context of their probationers' delinquency and for the value of a family-oriented treatment approach. By the same token, the therapist can benefit from the PO's observations of the family as well as from his or her knowledge of the local community and its resources. Unlike many therapists, POs also are not easily "conned." I remember one session in which the PO immediately recognized that the identified patient was high on drugs—an observation that led to confirmation of a serious but previously unidentified addiction. I am deeply indebted to this officer for teaching me the kind of "streetwise" knowledge about adolescents that I had not learned in years of close clinical supervision.

For various reasons, then, including the PO in the initial session is helpful. If problems in the PO/family/therapist relationship arise later, we typically call another joint meeting with the PO and the family. An example of such a meeting will be presented later. In some cases, however, we have been able to resolve the problem directly with the PO. For instance, consistent with his legalistic orientation, one of the POs closely monitored probationers for possible infractions of probation. Accordingly, he frequently called parents of children he had referred for counseling to check on therapeutic progress and on attendance at sessions. These contacts proved stressful for parents who felt their privacy was being invaded. The calls also tended to invite information from parents (such as dissatisfactions with therapy or excuses for missing appointments) that concerned the PO. He was especially troubled by new referrals who missed sessions initially. The PO and parents, in turn, complained to us about their conflicts with each other, sidetracking therapeutic work. We met with the PO. After sympathizing with him about the demands of his job, we offered to assume full responsibility for ensuring clients' regular attendance at therapy sessions. He acknowledged that this would help him but reminded us that he was responsible for his probationers' behavior and treatment, especially when treatment was compulsory. Nonetheless, he finally agreed to give us a month to iron out attendance problems with each new family, during which time he would not ask family members about their therapy. We eventually persuaded him and other POs to refrain from questioning their probationers about treatment and to ask us instead. In this way, we effectively interdicted recursive dysfunctional interactions that had begun to develop in the PO/family/therapy system. (For examples of interdiction techniques in other settings, see Chapters Five and Six.)

It is now clear to us and to the POs that the system operates best when we are seen as primarily responsible for the treatment and they for all court-involved actions (see Chapter Seven). Therapists can make recommendations to POs but cannot expect them or their superiors to always agree, although they are more likely to agree if a good relationship is established with them. The court/therapy system that I have described works especially well when the family are seen on a voluntary basis. It is not as easily implemented in cases of mandatory treatment, because the PO is expected to enforce the judge's orders. Yet we have been able to work out a satisfactory division of labor with

POs even in such cases. *Critical to sustaining the boundary, however, is the therapist's regular contact with the PO.* My staff and I have learned on more than one occasion how quickly the system can break down as a result of our failure to keep in touch with or to be available to the PO because of a busy schedule or a tendency to underestimate the importance of a brief telephone contact.

It is also important to avoid criticizing or blaming POs and other court officials when suggesting procedural changes. As illustrated in the preceding example, we usually frame recommendations as ways that we can help one another in carrying out our respective jobs. Moreover, just as we ask POs to avoid gossiping with families about therapy, we do not gossip about them in family sessions. Nor do we complain about their referrals. Administrators at the court were initially skittish about our project. Apparently, other mental health professionals to whom they had referred soon requested that they send them "less resistant" families. Of course, as one administrator explained to me, the court is populated by "resistant" families. Cooperative families would not be referred for treatment or, probably, involved with the court in the first place. Our attitude that recruitment of these families is an important part of the therapeutic process has been favorably received by court staff. But we had to modulate our initial optimism about being able to help difficult families, since some POs interpreted our positive outlook and early successes as evidence of our naiveté and beginner's luck—or, worse, of their failure. However, as a result of their participation with us as colleagues in the establishment of a therapeutic system, the POs are less cynical about treatment; and we no longer see them as merely potential obstacles to be manuevered around but, rather, as valuable coworkers. If POs and other court officials are expected to be difficult, then they probably will seem to be difficult.

As our relationship with the POs improved, so did our ability to effectively involve family members in the treatment process. The POs began backing us in our recruitment efforts. We have been careful, however, to avoid suggesting to family members that "the family needs therapy"—perhaps one of the surest ways of creating resistance. Rather, we have found, following Haley (1976), that it works better to use the parents' (and the court's) concern about the child as a lever for changing their interactions with him or her. Parents, siblings, and others are invited to sessions to help us understand and change the court-involved youth (see Chapter Six). It is critical that court officials grasp this way of working; if not, they may tell parents to attend sessions because of their part in the child's problems. POs and judges may also need help in understanding that family systems therapy does influence individual processes and that the youngster may be seen alone in the course of treatment. When first receiving referrals from the court, we discovered that the POs often had arranged for individual counseling to deal with the court-involved youngster's "internal" or "deep-seated" problems and family counseling to deal with his or her "family" problems. Many other youngsters were not referred to us because it was thought that their major difficulty was intrapersonal. Although this referral pattern partly reflects the nonsystemic orientation of the court's treatment ideology, we perhaps must also assume blame because of our tendency as family therapists to leave out considerations of the individual in presentations of our approach (see Rosman, 1979).

Assessing and Reformulating the Problem. In families of symptomatic youngsters, interaction sequences are such that an incongruous or inverted hierarchy often develops (Madanes, 1981). The child, rather than the parents, is in control of many, if not all, areas of his or her life in the family. Out of desperation, parents of these children may threaten court referral and even willingly relinquish total control to juvenile justice officials, who then understandably resent their status as a "dumping ground" (Janeksela, 1979). That the court may, however, become an essential part of the sequence of interactions supporting the child's delinquency or incorrigibility must always be considered.

In addition to possibly taking power away from parents and thus unwittingly feeding into their tendency to resign as parents (Madanes, 1981), the court's actions are often perceived by parents—correctly or incorrectly—in ways that further compound problems in the family. Adjudication of a child as "delinquent" or "unruly," for example, may label the parents, as well as the child, as "bad" or "sick." Often, mothers and fathers emerge from their child's hearing confirmed in their sense of parental failure and hopeless about being able to handle their youngster's problems. In the ensuing weeks, the child may be framed by the parents as "mental," "criminal," "dangerous," or "stupid"—attributions that help to absolve some of their guilt and sense of further responsibility. For family therapy to proceed effectively, these attributions must be changed. One way is to reframe the child in such a fashion that the parents again regard the problem as in their domain of expertise rather than in that of the juvenile justice system or mental health profession (Haley, 1976; Minuchin, 1974). It is one thing to view the court-involved youngster as emotionally disturbed or psychopathic and quite another to see him or her as "scared" or "immature"—behaving like a young child in need of parental limits and guidance.

It may be necessary to use a different tactic with families who grudgingly come to sessions, who show up because the judge or PO said they had to. Questions about the ethicality of mandatory treatment notwithstanding, therapy under these conditions can be difficult. This is further complicated for the family therapist by the fact that, except in the state of Florida, only the child can be ordered to receive counseling. Requesting the entire family to participate may be resented by family members. We have discovered that having the PO make a referral for a form of treatment that involves other family members can help circumvent family members' objections and confusion. Yet they may still deny having problems. Of course, these families do have a big problem that we and they acknowledge—the court is "on their back." Simply reframing their "problem" in this way and offering to help them cope with the court's involvement in their lives can often engage them in treatment (Watzlawick, Weakland, and Fisch, 1974).

The family's interactions with the court system may have other consequences as well that the therapist should incorporate into his or her definition of the problem. For instance, despite the juvenile court's attempt to reduce the stigma of its proceedings and procedures (for example, by using special terms such as *delinquency petition* instead of *indictment* and by holding closed hearings), the youngster may be stigmatized by teachers, classmates, employers, and others who learn of his or her court involvement. POs sometimes unwittingly contribute to this process by visiting youngsters at their schools or calling parents at their places of work. It also is not unusual for family members to cut off contacts with friends and relatives because of their shame and fear that others will find out about their court experience. The resulting isolation adds considerable pressure to family relations. We have found that simply supporting family members in their requests that the PO be more discreet and helping them to remain connected to their social network not only can provide them immediate relief but also can facilitate their willingness to work with us in tackling even bigger problems. (Berger reports similar issues with families of handicapped children in Chapter Six.)

POs and families may also become entrenched in repetitive sequences in which the PO attempts to help the youngster, the parents pull back, the PO fails, blames the parents, and threatens revocation of probation, the parents either give up or unsuccessfully intervene, the PO takes over again, and so on (Foster, Berger, and McLean, 1981; Haley, 1980). Unless relationships among adults—parents, POs, and therapists—are clarified early in treatment, as suggested in the previous section, the therapist can be easily drawn into this sequence by indirect, if not direct, requests to take sides.

In addition, we have observed that the stress of the child's court contact tends to exaggerate the family's characteristic style of interacting (Minuchin, 1974). Enmeshed families become more enmeshed and disengaged families more disengaged. Some families, however, undergo a qualitative change in their interactional pattern. Parents suddenly pull together and take charge of their children, long-standing marital problems are resolved, and so on. Whether the youngster's delinquency and court involvement triggers such changes or reflects adaptive shifts in the family is not clear. Nevertheless, unless therapists recognize that these changes do take place, they may develop a static, outmoded picture of the family.

A related point is that juvenile court involvement does not necessarily indicate personal or family dysfunction. *Delinquency* is a legal term, not a psychological one. Many argue that because behavior leading to referral to the court is endemic to adolescence, most court-involved youngsters do not need special services. Though sympathetic to this "radical nonintervention" position (Schur, 1973), we evaluate the need for treatment on a case-by-case basis. It is our impression that unruly and delinquent behavior that is serious (for example, assault, robbery) or repeated, even if it seems primarily peer-related, is usually part of a dysfunctional interactional pattern in the family. Yet we have discovered that not all families referred to us by the court need our services. To convert their normal difficulties into special problems requiring intervention would be an unwelcomed and possibly harmful intrusion into the life of the family (Lemert, 1970). Some of these families, however, have asked that we remain involved to help them cope with the stress of their court contact.

In other cases, especially chronic ones with more than one child in the family involved with the court, the juvenile court appears to be incorporated into the family structure as a part of the executive or parental subsystem. We have seen this pattern most frequently in single-parent families. The children are delegated to maintain court contact, thereby ensuring the family's stability. In light of their function, court-involved children in these familial contexts are usually not labeled negatively by their parents. The therapist, however, may seek to reframe the juvenile's behavior in ways that meet with the parents' disapproval.

Finally, in addition to assessing the role of juvenile justice in the problems of court-involved families, it is imperative that the impact of other external systems (for example, public housing, welfare, food stamps, schools, protective services) and sociopolitical conditions (race, poverty) be evaluated and considered in treatment planning. Inasmuch as poor and minority families are disproportionately represented in the court, these

factors often come into play, although they must also be considered in all families. See Aponte (1976b, 1980), Hines and
Boyd-Franklin (1982), Pinderhughes (1982), Colón (1980), and
Foley (1975) for helpful discussions of central issues in this
area.

The importance of identifying and working in a coordinated fashion with other agencies and service providers quickly
became apparent to us on the project. One of our initial referrals, Sally, a drug-involved school dropout, had successfully
avoided assuming any responsibility for most of her seventeen
years of life. Her mother, Ms. Barnes, had worked steadily until
she developed a neurological problem. Although it was finally
controlled through medication, she feared returning to work
and soon ended up on the welfare rolls. At the same time, her
relationship with her daughter became overly close. Along with
Sally's PO and mother, we decided that if Sally was not planning to return to school, then she should get a job. Drawing on
Ms. Barnes' previous work experience, we put her in charge of
the task. In the course of helping her daughter find employment, Ms. Barnes found a job for herself that she was excited
about taking until her welfare worker intervened. Rather than
resume working, which would have helped to establish a clearer
boundary between mother and daughter, Ms. Barnes was strongly advised to stay home to take care of her "needy" youngster—
which she did.

Goal Setting. Related to assessment and reformulation of
the problem is the task of setting goals for the treatment and
defining criteria of change. To accomplish this, the therapist
must do a juggling act. In addition to the therapist's own objectives, there are those of the family and the court. The therapy
may seem to be proceeding well from the perspective of the
therapist but miserably in the eyes of the court, especially if
their goals differ. The process of goal setting, therefore, requires
input from court officials.

As already mentioned, we invite the PO to our initial session with families, which gives us and the family an opportunity
to hear directly from the PO what the court expects of the juvenile. However, before requesting such information from the PO,

we *first* ask family members, including the court-involved young-ster, to convey their objectives as yet another way to support their competence (compare with Berger, Chapter Six). They usually have definite goals. So does the court, the exact nature of whose goals the therapist and the family need to clarify. For example, how many cuts from class in a quarter, if any, are allowable for a child who has previously missed school 80 per-cent of the time? What is expected of the parents? What other directives does the PO want the child to follow? What about marks in school? We have observed that many POs place greater emphasis on conduct grades than on academic grades.

During recent months, we have been writing the goals of the family and the court into a specially prepared "goals state-ment" that is cosigned by family members, the PO, and the therapist. We also ask the family and PO to work together in as-signing priorities within this list. This procedure serves a variety of functions, including concretizing and refining treatment ob-jectives as well as ritualizing and thus attaching importance not only to the objectives but also to the collaborative efforts of everyone involved.

The language of the court and its procedures may confuse the process of setting goals. Consider the concept of probation, for instance. One child I spoke to in training school was baffled by his incarceration for a series of petty thefts (stealing pencils and the like from stores); he pointed out to me, "I only got pro-bation for stealing that car" (his first offense). That probation can be revoked for a lesser crime than the one leading to a pro-bated sentence is a fact that youngsters may need help under-standing. In general, if family members as well as therapists understand court procedures and terminology, they will feel less intimidated and thus more competent in working toward their objectives.

It is also useful for therapists to remember that the court is most concerned that the individual court-involved youngster change, not the family. Telling the judge or PO that communi-cation patterns within the family have improved without a cor-responding change in the child's behavior simply will not do—nor should it. Yet short-term change in court-involved youths is unlikely to be stable unless their social environment changes. That they often resume their troublemaking activities on returning home from a stay in detention or in training school speaks to this point. Nevertheless, we have found that the court's objectives are reasonable with respect to the individual child and easily operationalized. The challenge for the therapist is to meet these objectives and those of family members while also pursuing other goals involving change in family interaction. Strategic family therapy (Haley, 1976; Madanes, 1981), with its clear problem focus, is especially well suited for this task.

Restructuring. For family members to relate more functionally to one another and to their community, they must be helped to find or to develop resources within themselves and others. Yet at the same time, relatives, children, helping and control agents, and other individuals who contravene parental decision making or to whom such authority is voluntarily relinquished must be encouraged to assume a more hierarchically appropriate posture. Of course, processes already discussed (establishing a therapeutic system, goal setting, assessing and reformulating the problem) constitute important ways of working toward this end and lay the groundwork for various other restructuring operations. Because of space limitations, I will present only a sampling of these interventions, particularly those aimed at directly altering the court/family relationship.

Handling Triangles. Despite the therapist's best efforts to prevent unproductive triangles from forming in the court/family/therapy relationship, they often do. If handled sensitively, these triangles can be broken up in a way that powerfully changes the family system without alienating court officials and family members. A few examples will illustrate this point.

Many families of delinquents have difficulty forming a functional parental alliance. In one such case seen through the project, asking the parents to collaborate with each other in disciplining their son proved quite threatening. Not coincidentally, they complained to their child's PO that therapy was not helpful. The PO, in turn, raised serious questions with us about our interventions, saying matter-of-factly, "If it isn't working, then I may need to recommend training school." He was feeling pressured not only by the family but also by his anticipation of the judge's disapproval for not revoking the child's probation sooner. Thus in this instance there were two interlocking triangles, which we managed in large measure by inviting the PO to the next family session. Although it was an emotion-laden session, all the adults finally pulled together in a meaningful way. Complaints about the therapy stopped.

In another case, we discovered that the PO had been inducted into the family system. The youngster involved, Jane, was a fourteen-year-old with a history of serious drug abuse, prostitution, truancy, thieving, and assorted physical problems associated with her life-style. Veins in her arms and legs had collapsed from repeated drug injection. She was described by a physician as having the body of an elderly woman with a short life expectancy. Jane lived with her mother and younger sister and consorted with a thirty-five-year-old "sugar daddy" friend of the family. After getting nowhere with Jane and her family in a month or so of therapy, we met again with Jane's PO. She was not surprised by our lack of progress with Jane. Previous therapy too had failed. The PO said realistically that Jane was "going down the tubes." She then told us stories of meeting "johns" who brought Jane to her regular appointments at the court. She also had information that Jane's family and friends were reinforcing her self-destructive behavior, making it unlikely that anything could be done.

Rather than confront the PO with her unwitting participation in Jane's difficulties, we asserted that Jane's future was much bleaker than the PO had surmised. We thought that she had at most six months to live before dying or getting killed and that we needed to prepare Jane's family and friends for her death. On hearing this, the PO radically changed her stance; she was suddenly prepared to muster all the resources available to her to alter the situation. For example, within forty-eight hours, the PO—following our directions—arranged a meeting of all the relevant figures in Jane's life at that point, some eleven persons, including a nurse-practitioner, the family's minister, the sugar daddy, and a counselor from a Big Brother/Big Sister program. In the meeting, the PO assumed a surprisingly authoritative and concerned posture—a posture we had not seen her take before in relation to this particular case.

Predicting Crises. In the course of family therapy, especially in the early phases, the family often experience considerable stress as they face the possibility of changing problematic but familiar patterns of interacting. Everyone has something to lose. The court-involved member, for example, must give up his or her exploitive or protective power, parents must learn to take care of themselves, and so on. As a result, the youngster's behavior may get worse before it improves. This is especially problematic in working with court-referred youngsters who cannot afford to make further trouble lest they be severely sanctioned by the court. Moreover, the kind of trouble they make is often dangerous. We sometimes handle this possibility by predicting it to the family, usually in terms of a novel construction of the family process, and then by prescribing less self-defeating and serious paths that such behavior could take. The alternative behaviors prescribed are legal and within tolerable limits for the parents; we determine this by directly asking them. For example, rather than detouring marital conflict by stealing another car, we might suggest that the youngster merely talk about further stealing when his parents fight. Or we might ask him to take a "vacation" from being the acting-out member of the family and to allow one of his siblings to be the focus of attention for a change.

In one family in which the court-involved youth's behavior expressed in part problems that both he and his older brother, James, were experiencing with their stepfather's rules, we recommended that, for the next week, James question rules in the household that he perceived as unfair. How he might do this without being disrespectful was discussed. In the process we learned that he had the ability to be quite tactful, in contrast to his brother's typically impertinent approach. To support the task, we used James' expressed concern about his brother's behavior to justify saying to James: "Your brother's ability to stay out of trouble depends on your taking a more active role in family affairs." The boys' parents acknowledged that this task would represent a big change, especially since James was so reticent around the house; however, they were willing to support it in the interest of their court-involved son.

Home-Based Detention. In some cases it is apparent that a "change in scenery" for someone in the family would help to deescalate a rapidly worsening family interaction pattern. Often the child is behaving in a blatantly delinquent fashion, incurring the wrath of parents, who may resort to throwing her out of the house. The court typically intervenes into this sequence by detaining the child, not the parents, for a short period (usually between three and ninety days) or by remanding custody of the child to the state, which may place her in a reformatory for an even longer stay away from home. In addition to having little, if any, effect in the long run on family interaction, these interventions may become part of a repetitive sequence (family conflict, delinquency, detention, family conflict, and so forth).

The court, however, is often quite open to alternative placements of the youngster, so long as she is appropriately supervised and stays out of trouble. This presents the family therapist with the possibility of helping parents to find someone in their social network to provide a "time out" away from home for their youngster. Consequently, parents do not abdicate control to the court, and family treatment can continue uninterrupted under the therapist's direction (see York and York, 1980).

We, for example, are currently seeing a family in which the youngster, John, aged fifteen, is staying temporarily in his aunt and uncle's home rather than in detention or training school. At the time we began working with him and his single-parent mother, he was (among other things) stealing her car regularly. Her efforts to stop him were ineffectual. She even removed the car battery; he simply replaced it with one that he stole from a neighbor's car. She finally demanded that John "get out of the house," something he planned to do as soon as he could find a place to stay. The PO was prepared to revoke John's probation in favor of institutionalization; however, he agreed to go along with an alternative strategy that we devised with the mother's help. When asked who might be able to keep

John on a short-term basis, she mentioned her brother and sister-in-law but did not think they would want to get involved. They not only were willing but were surprised that she had not asked for their assistance earlier. Our current focus is on how things will be different when John returns home in two months. The most sensitive part has been dealing with the aunt and uncle's tendency to side with John against his mother. Such a problem, which, of course, is an artifact of the arrangement, should be anticipated and perhaps predicted to adults who provide time-out for youngsters. That the aunt and uncle recently asked mother's permission to discipline John, however, suggests that our framing their help as assisting mother rather than rescuing John has taken hold.

Last Chancers. Many children, especially chronic offenders who frequently violate their probation, are referred to therapy as a "last chance" before institutionalization. In these cases there is often a definite time period, sometimes less than thirty days, in which prescribed changes are to take place. Although the therapist may understandably not "choose to accept this mission," the therapist who does must accurately represent the court's expectations in treating the family.

Even the most impossible conditions can often be exploited therapeutically, however. For example, with one "last chancer," where it was clear (as it usually is) that a direct approach would not work, we had success by first underscoring for the family the court's goals, along with the PO's skepticism about the child's ability to make necessary changes in such a short time span. We then suggested a more realistic objective: that the parents prepare their child to leave home to live in the training school. It was recommended that they make a visit to the school, buy him a new toothbrush, label his clothes, and so forth. In addition, the parents were encouraged to enjoy their youngster as much as possible before he left and essentially forget setting limits and imposing controls that well-intentioned POs, counselors, and others had advised them to do in the past. These directives were questioned by family members, who pushed the therapists to help them take steps to keep the youngster out of training school.

Strategic Use of Court Policies and Procedures. Implicit in many of the interventions we have described is the strategic use of court policies and procedures in helping families change. Numerous other features of the juvenile court can also be used therapeutically, including the court's atomistic focus on the child and individual responsibility.

For various reasons, many parents of court-involved youths have a long history of rescuing their youngsters from the natural consequences of their misbehavior. They often continue this pattern while the youngster is on probation, paying his or her restitution fees, negotiating with the PO for early release from probation, and so on. Therapists sometimes also participate in this rescuing game. Fortunately, the court usually frowns on such behavior, and this stance gives the family therapist leverage in helping these parents relate to their children in less overprotective ways. To facilitate this process, after establishing a workable therapeutic system we direct the parents to let their youngster handle all aspects of the probation. If the child needs help, for example, in finding a job to meet a condition of probation, then the parents are available to teach appropriate skills and provide coaching without actually taking direct responsibility for the task. I recall one youngster who said proudly to his mother that he finally had a chance to handle something on his own.

Another facet of the court that offers therapeutic opportunities is the child's appearance before the judge or referee at adjudicatory, disposition, or revocation hearings or preliminary conferences. In anticipation of these events, where the therapist's input is often requested in the form of testimony or written report, family members are usually much more motivated to follow through on therapeutic directives and tasks. In addition to discussing with the family what should go into our report, we make every effort to appear at these hearings to dramatize the event as a critical marker and possible turning point in the therapy. As Lemert (1970) has noted, the increasing administrative and perfunctory handling of cases in the juvenile court, due in part to the excessive caseload, has left the child's court appearance devoid of "affective meaning." Our input, therefore, is intended to challenge the family's, and in some cases the court's, complacency with the status quo. The amount of energy that we invest in this process is not lost on families. While sitting with us in the court, often for hours, waiting for their hearing or conference to begin, they frequently reveal themselves to us as they have not done before. They discover that we are committed to "going the distance" with them. Also significant is that family members and important friends whom we either have not been able to recruit or did not know about often accompany the youngster to court. On numerous occasions our presence has given us an opportunity to engage these individuals subsequently in the treatment process.

The child's discharge from probation presents the therapist with yet another opportunity for therapeutic ceremony. Special arrangements may need to be made with the court and family to formalize the procedure, as termination of probation is often handled informally. The discharge form, for example, may simply be mailed to the youngster. In one case, I encouraged the father of an adolescent being discharged from probation to compose a second discharge form of his own creation. Mr. Johnson worried greatly about his son, Johnny, during the probationary period, fearing that he would "get into more trouble." Johnny, however, handled the probation extremely well— so well, in fact, that his father's fear subsided considerably during the last few months of Johnny's court involvement. His son's discharge, however, reevoked Mr. Johnson's concerns. Would Johnny continue to do well, he asked, in the absence of the structure provided by the court? I was concerned that Mr. Johnson's fears would undermine his son's competence (as they had in the past), setting the stage for a self-fulfilling prophecy. Unless he could also discharge Johnny from probation, the court's discharge would be meaningless. By formally writing his own discharge paper, which addressed some important issues that he had not previously discussed with his son, Mr. Johnson was finally able to put his fears behind him.

We have also capitalized on situations in which the child's behavior is essentially seen as "bad" by the court rather than "disturbed." This label, which is suggestive of a discipline problem, can be used to motivate many parents to take charge of their youngster. However, we have discovered that with many youngsters and their families in which criminal activity is tolerated, if not encouraged, intimating that their behavior is "mental" or "sick" is more helpful in stimulating therapeutic movement.

It is important to keep in mind that every family is unique; each brings a particular set of beliefs, experiences, and interactions to the court/therapy relationship. It is necessary to assess carefully what both the court and the family give the therapist to create conditions under which change can take place. A court procedure or process that can be used in the interest of one family may be totally inappropriate for another.

I recall, for example, the case of Peter Bradley, a brash fifteen-year-old who had been referred to the court for theft and assault. His single-parent mother tended to infantilize him, which motivated the therapists, in spite of her protests, to put Peter in charge of handling all aspects of his probation. Peter, however, continued to live up to his mother's expectations—for example, by missing appointments with his PO. The extent of his overinvolvement with his mother became even clearer to the therapists several weeks into treatment when they received an early morning telephone call from the PO informing them that both Peter and his mother were in jail. Apparently, the day before while walking home from church, Peter had knocked a younger child, Bobby Lee McCoy, off his bicycle. The child told his older brothers, who threatened to beat up Peter. Peter ran home to his mother, who, on hearing what had happened, marched with Peter and his younger sister, Veronica, to the McCoys' house. A confrontation ensued. Two of the boys grabbed Peter; at Ms. Bradley's request, Veronica got her mother's gun. Ms. Bradley was holding the McCoys at gunpoint when the police arrived. Charges against Peter and his mother were later dropped.

After this incident, the therapists changed their tactics. They apologized to mother for not listening to her concerns about Peter's ability to assume responsibility for his probation. They noted that he was obviously a "frightened, immature youngster" who required even closer supervision than she was currently providing, as evidenced, for example, by his recent conflict with the McCoys. Thus she needed to help Peter as much as possible to meet the conditions of his probation. Ms. Johnson exclaimed, with a sigh of relief: "You finally understand!" Peter, however, was nonplused and set about to prove the therapists and his mother wrong. In this case, then, the tactic of explicitly encouraging the youngster to take responsibility for his probation, which we had successfully used in several previous cases, did not work. The feedback we received from the family led us to adopt a different approach to accomplish the same end.

Responsible Boundary Making. It can be argued that an implicit assumption underlying the various strategies discussed thus far is that parental autonomy in childrearing should be encouraged and protected. This is a relatively new assumption historically, closely tied to a Western, middle- and upper-class value system (Aries, 1960). Indeed, part of the impetus for the juvenile court movement in this country was the perception that poor, immigrant parents lacked the resources to function within such a value system, as evidenced by their children's delinquency, requiring the state to take control. *But the goal of family systems therapy is not to create totally autonomous family units.* As Colón (1980) reminds us, "In fact, no person or family system functions in the absence of supportive ecosystems" (p. 356). For example, establishing physical, let alone psychological, boundaries may be difficult for the "welfare family" living in a housing project where flimsy walls and delinquency-prone neighbors represent poor insulation against disruptive intrusions. Home visits perhaps should be mandatory for uninitiated clinicians, to acquaint them with pressures that countervail against changes they naively ask these families to make in therapy. If the therapist hopes to succeed in inducing them to break their ties to the court, then he or she must assume responsibility for helping them to develop or to use already-existing resources to function more independently. That may mean helping parents to find a job; directing family members to sources of help (for example, relatives, vocational training centers, community support groups, legal services, public education) and generally reconnecting them to their social network; helping them to ask for and to use assistance from others in a way that does not involve giving up control; and coaching them on how to deal with deleterious influences in their neighborhood, such as the parent who harbors runaways, the numbers man, the drug dealer, the pimp, the delinquent gang, the extortionist (Carl and Jurkovic, 1983; Milan and others, 1982; Colón, 1980).

In cases of gross injustice and maltreatment, especially when the family appears unable to alter the situation at the time, the therapist may need to directly advocate for the child or family (Clark, Zalis, and Saccho, 1982). Many parents, for example, simply have failed to develop basic parenting skills, particularly those parents whose family histories contain generations of biosocial disorder and stress: abuse, neglect, incest, poverty, chemical dependency, physical disability, criminality, deprivation, and so forth. On the basis of their work as members of an outreach family therapy team, Clark and his colleagues (1982) have raised serious questions about the applicability of conventional structural and strategic approaches with such families. Although more systematic research is needed in this area before drawing firm conclusions, we share their concerns, having experienced the most failure and frustration with youngsters living in such familial contexts. The ability to create and sustain a stable organizational structure assumes a level of differentiation that many of these families have yet to achieve. Expecting them to organize along more adaptive lines without having developed the requisite psychosocial resources is unrealistic. As Clark has pointed out, to help these families, the therapist must be prepared not only to broaden his or her therapeutic role to include functions such as direct education, socialization, and skills training but also to accept that change may occur slowly, provided family members can be engaged in treatment. We have found the work of Clark, along with that of Stanton, Todd, and Associates (1982), especially helpful in our efforts to reach out to these families. For example, in contrast to our stance early in the life of the project, we now initially accommodate much more, as by making home visits to families who cannot organize themselves to meet with us at the clinic, before asking them to accommodate to us (see Chapter Six).

Yet experience has also taught us that not all so-called multiproblem, disadvantaged families who frequent the court system have limited resources (see Minuchin and others, 1967). Such an assumption has contributed to the unnecessary institutionalization, foster home placement, and detention of their court-involved members. Although they do have undeniably grave problems, we have repeatedly discovered in our "search for competence" (Minuchin, 1974) that either they or their sociofamilial network (aunts, uncles, neighbors, ministers, friends, and so on) contain resources that can often be mobilized to facilitate and to support changes in their situation. Initially, we, too, assumed that this was not the case and thus had scores of volunteers available to provide ancillary services through our project. Fortunately, we asked family members who they thought could help before unleashing this volunteer force.

To work this way, as Lewis points out in Chapter Seven, the therapist may need to develop greater tolerance for the support that extended family members as well as children can and do provide to many parents. Rather than discourage their involvement, the therapist is advised to help them contribute to the welfare of the family in ways that do not undermine parental authority and competence (Minuchin, 1974). The following case example will demonstrate how this and other therapeutic strategies presented in this chapter can be implemented.

Case Example. * At the time of her referral to the project, Valerie Smith, age twelve, had been under court supervision for several months because of "unruly" behavior. She had missed some 100 days of school the previous year. The PO was concerned that this pattern would continue when school started again in a few weeks.

Valerie lived with her mother, who was in poor health and unemployed. The mother had lost three husbands through divorce or death. The family subsisted on Social Security payments. Other persons living in the home included Valerie's

*One aspect of this case example is discussed by Carl and Jurkovic (1983).

brother, John, age fourteen, her stepsister, Jane, age eighteen, Jane's boyfriend, and their eight-month-old baby. John also was on probation for truancy, runaway, and theft. Unlike Valerie's, his behavior had improved considerably following his court hearing. Although Mrs. Smith's two oldest daughters had married and left home, they lived nearby. Their children often spent time in the Smith household. Ten months before treatment began, Mrs. Smith's oldest son, age thirty, had returned home and within a few months had died of a neurological disorder.

The Smith family was organized in such a way as to lead Valerie's PO to say, understandably, that the "mother was weak and the children ruled the family." Information in Valerie's intake evaluation further supported this perception of Mrs. Smith. Although the background data indeed suggested that roles and responsibilities were not well differentiated in this family, the therapists (Michael O'Shea and Marsha Weiss) and I discussed in supervision before the start of therapy the importance of not drawing any conclusions concerning mother's personality. It was learned in the first family session, in fact, that Mrs. Smith had called the police to pick up John when he initially ran away and within a few days had requested that the school board deal with her daughter's truancy. The therapists quickly commented on these behaviors as signs that she was a "strong and concerned parent who knew when she needed help and how to get it."

When Mrs. Smith said later in the session that she had to devote herself to "keeping the children out of trouble," leaving her little time to develop a social life, the therapists again reframed the family's reality. They questioned whether she had no social life because the children got into trouble or whether their misbehavior gave her something to do. The children were told that an alternative way for them to help their mother would be to take her to a physician. Her last medical examination had been twelve years before. By the end of the initial interview, mother's parenting difficulties and the youngsters' troublemaking had been positively recast in terms of interpersonal processes rather than pathological personality traits. Family members seemed confused but willing to come back.

However, the family failed to show for their next appointment because of car troubles and canceled several more appointments. The children said their mother was sick; we were concerned that a functional therapeutic system had not yet developed. The therapists and I met with Valerie's PO to discuss the situation. Concerned because Valerie had already missed numerous days of school, days she would have to make up in detention according to the conditions of her court order, the PO suggested that we motivate family members to return to treatment by taking them food and clothing. This was something she had done. Our concern with this plan was that although it might indeed work, it would further reinforce the family's dependency on the court and undermine mother's executive power. It was decided instead that the PO and therapists would continue to telephone the family. During these calls the therapists joined further with family members and reminded the children that they could assist their mother by taking her to a doctor. The combined efforts of the PO and therapists paid off. The family requested another appointment.

Mrs. Smith informed the therapists in the second session that she had finally seen a physician: "The children made me go." That the PO and therapists had resisted the temptation to take care of the Smiths had apparently given them a chance to take care of themselves. Yet, during this session, it became even clearer that their caretaking exacted a heavy toll on their development as individuals and as a family. The onset of Valerie's truancy during the school year, for example, had coincided with her stepbrother's fatal illness. Valerie had stayed home to help her mother, who had become deeply depressed. Mrs. Smith also readily acknowledged that her children's growing up and leaving home was quite threatening. In support of her mother, Valerie said, "She knows that I can't leave 'cause I sleep with her." Valerie had not slept in her own bed since her father had died nine years before.

An important intervention early in treatment involved moving Valerie to her own bedroom, thus creating an appropriate boundary between Valerie and her mother and helping them to help each other more appropriately. This was accomplished in part by using the possibility of detention strategically. If detained, the therapists explained to the family, Valerie would have to sleep by herself—an event for which she could prepare by sleeping alone at home.

Consistent with our efforts to separate Valerie and her mother, another objective in treatment was that Valerie attend school regularly. This, of course, was of primary concern to the court. Our failure to address Valerie's truancy immediately would contribute to her punishment. After ruling out reality-based reasons for her truant behavior, we initially recommended that mother take her to school. Mrs. Smith, however, said she could not manage that by herself because of car problems; and even if she could, Valerie would simply go in the front door of the school and leave by the back. Mrs. Smith did say that Valerie's sister-in-law might be able to assist her. We then arranged a meeting at the school with Valerie and her mother, teacher, and sister-in-law. Before the meeting, the teacher expressed grave doubts about the therapists' ability to help. Her feeling was that "the mother doesn't care." In the meeting, the sister-in-law agreed to drive Valerie to school, accompanying her into the classroom if necessary. To everyone's delight except Valerie's, the teacher spontaneously offered at that point: "If you can get her to the front door, I'll make sure she doesn't leave." Mother's job was to make sure Valerie was up and ready to go in the morning. The therapists also helped everyone plan strategies for dealing with all the different problems that might arise in carrying out the task.

At the next session, the family proudly told the therapists that Valerie had attended school every day except one, when she was sick. It was also learned that Valerie had been sleeping in her own room since shortly after the second session, two weeks before. Everything was looking up until Valerie's reappearance in court a few days later. Because of the progress that had been made, the therapists and I asked the judge (through the PO) to consider waiving the consequences for Valerie's truancy at the beginning of the school year. However, we were reminded of our subordinate status in the court system. The judge ordered Valerie to be detained for a few weeks, saying that she had to maintain her credibility with other probationers who were under the same contract as Valerie. We understood. She did allow Valerie to continue her family treatment, however.

Feelings of hopelessness and victimization again began to develop in the family because of Valerie's detention. To combat this development, the therapists deliberately confronted family members in the fifth session with their part in Valerie's truancy and consequent detention. Because of the good relationship that the therapists enjoyed with the Smiths, family members could hear what was being said without feeling attacked. They wholeheartedly agreed to continue the program that they had successfully implemented before Valerie's detention when she returned home. The therapists also pointed out that Valerie would "really know" that she no longer needed to miss school if her mother began developing a part of her self that she had neglected for so many years—her social life. In support of the fact that mother could now turn her attention to this task was evidence that John was doing well academically and that Jane and her family were planning to move out of the house soon. Valerie, moreover, was being taken care of in detention. Mrs. Smith had "no excuse," the therapists playfully reasoned with her. She concurred. What had been initially framed by the family as a depressing setback, Valerie's detention, was used strategically by the therapists to foster further growth.

During the sixth session, three weeks later, the family reported a spate of changes. Valerie had been released from detention. In addition to going to school regularly without prompting from mother or assistance from her sister-in-law, she had made several new friends. John had a new girlfriend and his first job after school. Jane and her family were settled in their new apartment. Mrs. Smith had gone out with a friend to dinner and was planning to go dancing the next weekend—her first date in many years. The therapists met with the Smiths a few more times over the next four months. In these meetings, there was some reminiscing about the "old days" and sharing of feelings about the deaths of family members. Both Valerie and John were finally discharged from probation. A follow-up one year later indicated that the family were continuing to do well.

Generalizability and Implications

The services that we provide through the project are not a formal part of the juvenile justice system. Hence the issues taken up in this chapter have been considered largely from an "outsider's" position. "Insiders" from different courts and "outsiders" in public and private settings with whom I have collaborated, supervised, or debated theory and practice suggest that the ideas presented here have validity for them as well. Questions can be raised, however, about the generalizability of our observations to different treatment settings. For example, because the project deals exclusively with juvenile offenders from one court, we have had the advantage of an ongoing relationship with our referral source, resulting in a steady flow of information in the court/family/therapy system. This information has helped us to quickly modify our procedures and thinking when necessary. As our relationship with court personnel has grown closer over the years, so also has their responsiveness to our ideas. The therapist who deals with the court only sporadically often lacks both the credibility and the data to form such a connection. He or she may therefore have to work harder to establish a workable therapeutic system and to maintain it with each new case. Certainly, as my private work with court-involved youngsters has taught me, this can be done. Private practitioners may find it helpful to point out to families who object to reimbursement for the extra time involved that coordination with court personnel can shorten treatment and thus save them considerable expense in the long run.

Service providers working inside the system may also be at a disadvantage in that it can be difficult for them to assume a "meta" position vis-à-vis the court and the family (see Chapters Five and Six). I have found through the project and my private practice that neither the court nor the family know exactly where I fit in the court/family/therapy complex. This fact has expedited my maneuvering in the system—for example, using myself as a boundary between the court and the family.

Insiders, however, can benefit from their knowledge of and relationship to the juvenile justice system, especially if they have the support of their superiors. POs in particular are in a strategic position to use systemic principles to enhance their work. For example, my impression is that in their efforts to arrange services they often overlook obvious resources available in the juvenile's natural environment. The "professionalization" (Rosenheim, 1976) of the treatment of delinquency during the past several decades has diverted attention from informal socio-familial networks that can greatly help court-involved youths and their families. Along these lines, parent self-help groups represent a surprisingly untapped resource—a resource long used by parents of mentally retarded and learning-disabled children. Such "informal" intervention may not only effectively reduce the juvenile crime problem but also relieve POs of the kind of direct responsibility for their charges that has contributed to their high burnout rate. As one of the POs with whom we work said recently, "I'd like the parents to be the PO for a change instead of me." It would be interesting to observe the effects if an entire probation department staff were to adopt this attitude.

To the extent that professionals are involved, especially needed are legal and therapeutic services available on a voluntary basis when juveniles are initially brought to the court, rather than at their formal hearing days or weeks later or, worse, when they are on probation (Wald, 1976). It is during the initial contact that the family are typically in crisis and are most likely to seek help voluntarily. Predictably, we have found that the longer juveniles are involved with the court, the greater the chances that their families and friends have reorganized around their "delinquent" or "unruly" label.

Changes along these lines, however, will require additional training for court personnel, judges included, in family systems theory and practice and, ideally, broader-based reforms in the juvenile justice system. In light of that system's poor track record in rehabilitating troubled youngsters and its questionable legal base, lawyers, civil libertarians, parents, therapists, court officials, and others are calling for such reform (see, for example, Lemert, 1970; Rosenheim, 1976; *Task Force Report on Juvenile Justice and Delinquency Prevention,* 1976). Perhaps one of the most dramatic changes that already occurred in many parts of the country is the transformation of the juvenile court into a family court with jurisdiction over a variety of family-related legal problems (*Task Force Report,* 1976). Space does not permit further discussion of the complex set of legal and psychosocial issues being considered by reformists. It is important to note, however, that we as family therapists have an excellent opportunity to help reshape juvenile justice, although the question has been raised in some quarters whether the solution to delinquency lies in changing the juvenile justice system or the environment (see, for example, Tonry, 1976). Of course, as illustrated in this chapter, social agencies such as the juvenile court cannot be viewed separately from families and their environment. Change in one has implications for the other. Increased recognition of the juvenile court, along with the therapeutic community, as part of the ecological complex of delinquency promises to lead to changes that are not only more therapeutic but also more just.

9 Doris S. Greiner

Hospitals and Outpatient Clinics

This chapter describes features of the work of family therapists working in a physician's office practice and within a hospital. The first setting is a four-pediatrician group practice in a large metropolitan area. The second is a nonprofit 300-bed community hospital in a city of approximately 150,000. For both practices, Bowen family system theory (Bowen, 1978) provided the conceptual basis for working with clients, using the unique features of the setting therapeutically and for guiding the therapists' continuing work with self. The therapist was a nurse employed by the physician group in the first setting and by the hospital in the second. The therapist's educational background and employment status clearly center the therapy within, rather than outside, the medical setting.

The Medical Setting

People seek medical care for a variety of reasons, most of them related in some way to either actual or feared physical illness. Garfield (1970) has categorized the mix of people who de-

I would like to acknowledge with gratitude the help given to me by Janice Carr both in the preparation of this chapter and in sharing with me and allowing me to use her experiences in the outpatient setting described here.

247

cide they need medical care as consisting of the well, the worried well, the early sick, and the sick. It is in the physician's office or clinic that the initial assessment is often made of whether a problem situation that involves physical sickness exists—or whether problems in living have come to be conceptualized as sickness. It is in such an office practice, in this case that of a group of pediatricians, that family therapy was practiced. It is possible in this setting for a therapist to work with both (1) problems in living that have not yet escalated to sickness in a family member and (2) sickness in a family member that poses problems in living for the family requiring therapeutic intervention.

Garfield's categories coincide to some extent with the idea that some people have primarily a physical, some people a psychological, view of life. That distinction has proved useful in considering family work with people in medical settings, especially when they have found their way into hospitals. Though not universal, it is a commonly met point of view among clients and health care personnel that distress is physical. There is a problem and it is fixable. Thinking is directed toward solving the physical problem.

The medical model is at base a problem-solving effort applied to physical illness. Diagnosis, treatment, and care of physical ills (and, to a lesser extent, psychological ills) are what people have come to expect and, in fact, believe they have a right to have (Illich, 1976). The hospital as an institution seeks to deliver or provide services that do just that. The overt mission of the hospital is to assist patients through acute phases of illness. It is health-restorative. Similarly, although a pediatric practice is clearly focused toward health maintenance in infants and children, intervention directed toward curing illness or health restoration consumes a considerable amount of physician time, energy, and interest.

In general, hospitals are organized (1) to care for people when they are not able to care for themselves, (2) to centralize the often expensive technology needed to solve medical problems, and (3) for the convenience of the staff. Caretaking, a primary function of nursing services in hospitals, was organized in a traditional hierarchical fashion in the hospital where I worked. Staff nurses and their assistants were responsible to head nurses, who were responsible to patient care coordinators, who were responsible to the director of nursing. The director was responsible to the hospital administration and to the hospital board of directors. The technological aspects of hospital services currently affect all departments within the hospital, from microwave cooking in food service to laser techniques in surgery to computerized billing from the business office.

The convenience of the people providing services to patients is of special interest. Access to the use of the hospital and discharge from the hospital are controlled by the physician. The physician's relationship to the hospital is one of having admitting privileges. In the setting described here, physicians were not employed by the hospital but functioned interdependently with its facilities and its employed staff. This aspect of being separate from, yet in charge of, major aspects of the ongoing functioning of the organization in the patient's behalf poses interesting systemic variables. The physician's position in the system somewhat resembles that of the father in a traditional nuclear family of the recent past. The father is away from the central functioning of the family for most working hours and yet exerts control over what happens within the family during all hours. This control is rarely problematic when the system is calm and when roles of other family members stay clear. Distress, or simply change in the system, calls for action. In the traditional family structure alluded to, no member questions that the distant parent will react. The question is, when and how long. Similarly, in the hospital, the physician will react or will even be called in to react in the face of distress or simply change.

Unlike the traditional nuclear family, which has decreased in size over time, the hospital has increased in size and complexity, posing constant questions about roles and responsibilities for employees. Within the hospital discussed here, each nursing unit of ten to thirty patient beds had a head nurse, selected registered nurses who took charge for defined periods of time, and other nurses and nursing assistants. Together this staff planned and organized care for the patients assigned to it, each of whom may have been admitted to the hospital by a different physician. Although the roles of nurses within the hospital structure were relatively clear, as were doctor's orders for patients, specific goals of any unit of the nursing service that would help to define overall direction of care with each patient were often less clearly defined. Where a lack of definition and direction persists, anxiety is likely to be high. When problems occurred with a patient, staff members involved in dealing with those problems did not necessarily communicate directly with each other. Nursing staff members seldom contacted a physician directly; they would report problems to the head nurse. Similarly, when a physician perceived problems related to any aspect of a patient's stay on a unit, these problems were most probably discussed with the head nurse or the patient coordinator. The bigger or more annoying the problem, the higher in the organization a physician-initiated discussion was likely to begin.

The task for any therapist working thoughtfully within a hospital setting is to keep cognizant of the central focus of his or her work. A second task is to determine with whom one needs to communicate in regard to that work. When anxiety increases, the likelihood of direct communication between two persons involved in a particular issue decreases. The potential number of emotional triangles in which any one person could participate is awesome.

Theoretical Concepts. The major concepts of Bowen's theory, those involving anxiety and the differentiation of self, were central to conceptualizing the work described here. Although a thorough discussion of all the concepts of the theory is not possible here, these two will be described briefly before going further.

"The concept of triangles provides a theoretical framework for understanding the microscopic functioning of all emotional systems" (Bowen, 1978, p. 478). When anxiety increases between two persons, a third person or object is involved, decreasing the tension between the original two. If this move is effective, the anxiety decreases among the three, with one of the original pair in a more outside, or distant, position. If that position becomes too distant, anxiety will increase and the outside person will move toward one of the other two or will tri-angle in yet another person or object, forming a set of inter-locking triangles. Emotional triangles function in repeated pat-terns in family systems. During periods of high anxiety, the usual triangles available within a system are not adequate, and outside individuals and agencies are brought in. Consequently, one working hypothesis with patients in medical settings is that the move to seek help from the physician may be a way that family anxiety is being handled.

Since patterns of emotional triangles are active in any on-going system, relationships in the work system also function in understandable and predictable triangle patterns. During periods of high anxiety in work systems, patients and their families are vulnerable to being triangled into staff anxiety in an attempt to achieve greater emotional comfort among staff members. Hence, a working hypothesis of the therapist's when asked to see a hospitalized patient was that staff anxiety needed to be assessed in order to determine when to devote attention to staff concerns and when to involve herself directly with the patient and patient family.

A third working hypothesis was that a therapist is con-tinually vulnerable to becoming involved in triangles in anxious emotional systems. The work of the therapist thus continues to involve identifying anxious personal issues and working with these issues in his or her family of origin. There are probably other ways to approach this particular aspect of working with families. I know of none as effective. The freer one becomes of the patterned responses in one's own family, the freer one is to think about emotional issues and to make choices about behav-ior in regard to them. Moreover, the freer one is to consider hu-man behavior in terms of the concepts of this theory and to continue to question the theory.

The concept of differentiation of self describes the inter-action between emotional and intellectual functioning within a person. Each person exists at a level of differentiation that is fairly constant over time, although during periods of calm a per-son might seem to function at a level considerably higher or lower than the basic level. People at a low level of differentiation function in automatic ways that are emotionally dictated most of the time. Emotional and intellectual functioning are fused. Behavior is directed toward achieving some degree of emotional comfort within the ongoing emotional systems, family and societal, within which the person exists.

At the other end of the differentiation continuum, emotional and intellectual functioning are relatively separate, and people are freer to remain independent of the emotionality around them. The higher the level of differentiation, the more likely it is that the power of the intellect can be brought to bear on decisions and that choices can be made based on thought-out positions rather than simply a need for emotional comfort.

Bowen described people for whom emotional and intellectual processes are more fused as experiencing more life problems and recovering more slowly from them. People who have a higher degree of differentiation are better able to pursue life goals, can relate with others in more satisfying ways, choose more freely to be independent of emotional reactivity in systems, and recover more quickly from life problems that do occur (Bowen, 1978, pp. 362–373).

Careful assessment of the level of differentiation of the families with whom one works is a detailed process that requires knowing a system over time. In the work described here, a careful assessment of differentiation in the clinical families could rarely be done, since people were seldom seen over long periods. However, a working hypothesis about the level of differentiation was useful, especially in trying to formulate realistic goals for work with families. Hypotheses about level of differentiation were formed during the usual initial questioning. When a standard genogram format is used, information about chronic relationship difficulties becomes apparent through data such as the number of divorces and numbers of persons in the extended family about whom the patient has little or no information. Questions about illnesses will usually give some information on whether chronic diseases or numerous surgeries are part of the life history of one or more family members. A few questions about alcohol and drug use can be useful in estimating the extent to which these chemicals are a part of long-standing patterns of dysfunction. The initial work in assisting family members to think about their current problem is not changed appreciably by a hypothesis regarding level of differentiation. Goal setting for future work is. I find that staying focused on anxiety centered on an immediate problem is most useful with less differentiated patients. By contrast, an assessment of a higher level of differentiation would lead me to work toward setting goals beyond immediate symptom relief.

In the hospital setting, the therapist did have an opportunity for ongoing contact with some staff members. Head nurses are in a unique position to affect the emotional climate on nursing units. With head nurses who were freer to think about emotional issues, alternatives to usual triangles could be considered and some differences in staff functioning on those units observed. The concept of differentiation was thus central to defining the work in this setting.

The hierarchical issues were of less concern in the pediatrician's office practice. Each physician referred cases directly to the therapist. The work of the therapist and the work of the physician with the family seldom needed to involve the other physicians in the practice or other aspects of the health care system. Communication stayed relatively open and direct between each physician and the therapist. Patient families would seem to have been a likely target of anxiety had communication not stayed open, but this was not observed, probably for several reasons. One was the autonomous action orientation of the physician practice. Each professional was goal-directed in his or her own work with patients and patient families. Very little team effort or consideration of issues as a group was expected or required. The second reason was that the physicians with whom the therapist might have had more difficulty staying in open communication were less likely to refer patients.

A third factor that may have masked some of the triangling that did occur related to the therapist's observation that the families that were seen tended to be child-focused. These families always had children with serious physical problems that the physicians were concerned about. It was not clear how much potential emotional reactivity was channeled into concern about the physically sick children as a focus for system anxiety.

Framing the Work. In both the office and the hospital

practice, the usual way of framing the work with families was to offer to think with them about the problems they were having and what those problems had been like for family members. The decision to involve other people in sessions with the therapist and the referred patient was made on the basis of the assessment of each family system. This involved sketching out in genogram form who family members were and making a beginning assessment of whom, if anyone, it might be useful to include in future sessions, should further work be indicated and agreed to by the family.

Involving additional family members was, at times, the decision of the family member first seen. When the therapist thought another family member's presence was important and communicated that request directly, it almost always happened. This request was not made by the therapist as a general practice but, rather, with a particular rationale for involving whole family units or particular family members. The medical setting lends itself to this kind of cooperation. Patients, to some extent, do try to do as they are told, and many patients and family members hunger for information that will help them deal with the mysteries of illness or hospitalization.

Four particular premises about anxiety in systems guided all therapy described here: (1) Thinking about one's situation with an objective outsider who is alert to emotional pulls and able to keep from reacting in usual system ways can be useful, even if the time together is limited to a single encounter (Bowen, 1978, p. 342). (2) Anxiety or emotional reactivity is evoked by identifiable developmental issues or concerns within each person's life and within the life of a family. (3) Anxiety or emotional reactivity is evoked by major life events that may or may not be related to developmental issues. In either case, physical illness or concern about illness may be a way of trying to manage the anxiety and regain some degree of emotional comfort. (4) Each person within a given family is involved in key relationships that are primarily supportive or primarily distressing to that person. Examination of issues in these key relationships can shift the anxiety focus from physical symptoms, resulting in more openness in the system and possibly reduction in physical symptoms.

The first and third premises are illustrated by an in-hospital patient situation. A head nurse contacted the therapist about the needs of the family of a dying patient. The head nurse and, by her report, some other staff members thought that the wife of a patient they had been caring for was not facing the reality of her husband's impending death. The therapist arranged to see the patient and his wife. She found them open to each other and to talking about their situation, much more directly than she had expected. When she commented on this, the wife agreed that although the situation was extremely difficult, she thought she was managing. She did have some concern, however, about the nurses, especially the head nurse, who seemed to the wife to be having a hard time caring for her husband as his illness progressed. She also had some concern about one of their teenage daughters and wondered whether the therapist might want to meet with the daughter. The therapist saw this request as an attempt to involve her in a triangle. Instead, she asked for more information about the mother's concerns about the daughter and the nature of the communication between them. The mother had some ideas about talking with the daughter that she had not carried out. The therapist's assessment was that the concerns could most effectively be dealt with between the mother and the daughter, and the therapist encouraged the mother to do what she had described.

The therapist offered to see the couple again if either felt a need to discuss further concerns. The therapist's assessment was that the family was dealing with a highly emotional and difficult event in a relatively open way, one that for that family seemed effective. The wife's comment on concerns about the head nurse was also explored briefly with the wife. On the basis of the wife's observations, the therapist chose as a next step an assessment of staff anxiety regarding this patient. She suggested to the head nurse that the therapist meet with the staff at a regularly scheduled planning conference when this patient would be discussed.

At the conference, the therapist invited staff members to talk about their concerns in caring for this patient. The head nurse expressed some ideas about what should be done by and with the dying patient that were extremely difficult for her to implement, especially since so much of her energy had been focused on returning him to at least a limited life outside the hospital. She needed to shift her focus from keeping the patient alive to helping him die. The patient's wife had already made this shift, and that very fact further increased the nurse's anxiety. With the help of questions posed by the therapist, staff members examined their own position and saw the direction that their work now needed to take. The therapist empathized with the difficulty that the staff had in continuing to provide care for the man, knowing he was terminally ill. She also validated the staff's assessment of the work that they now needed to do. Interestingly, once this work was accomplished, staff members no longer raised concerns about the wife's lack of coping; rather, they now saw her as someone who might herself be in need of staff support. It was as though once the staff dealt with their own issues about the man's terminal illness, they both stopped focusing on the wife's anxiety and were clearer about the kinds of physical care the man needed.

The therapist saw no need for additional scheduled sessions with either the patient's family or the staff. Both were told she would be available if there were further issues they wished to talk about. Later, the head nurse commented on how much the therapist had helped that family. This comment suggests that shifts in anxious triangles involving both the patient family and the nursing staff had been made.

In the following example, developmental issues and key family relationships were important considerations. A pediatrician referred a six-year-old boy and his mother to the therapist after the mother had told the doctor that the boy had fears in the night. The fears had developed after the boy heard sirens in the night. He was certain that the sirens would return and wanted his mother to be with him to calm these fears. A brief family history revealed that the mother was in a second marriage of two years' duration and that she had given birth to a daughter within the last six months. For much of the time between marriages the mother had worked, and her son had spent his days with the mother's mother. In discussing the family relationships with the mother, it became clear that an anxious relationship existed between the mother and her mother, rather than between the mother and the father of the son or between the mother and her current husband. (The referring physician had mentioned the latter two relationships as possibly troubled.) It seemed to the therapist that the sound of the siren that had actually been heard represented a signal of distress for the family. Although these other relationships were being investigated, some time was spent in talking with the boy about different sounds, what they were like for him, and what he could do, with an emphasis on his action in response to them.

The mother's concerns in the relationship with her mother were detailed, and by the end of the third session, the therapist invited her to bring her mother into the next session. The mother decided that it was very likely that she could talk with her mother directly, and although she was not certain what had kept her from doing that before, she resolved to take her concerns directly to her mother. She did, however, want to schedule a next session with the therapist. To this session she brought her son and her husband. Having begun the work of clarifying issues in the relationship with her mother, especially those related to childcare, she was apparently ready to face some of the childcare concerns she had in the current marriage. The session was spent talking about childcare, the therapist monitoring the anxiety and intervening as necessary to increase listening, decrease blaming, and assist in clarification of responsibility. The boy's night waking had not yet entirely ceased, but by the end of this fourth session, the mother expressed confidence that she could manage her childcare responsibilities and appreciation for the supportive role that her husband was taking.

However, she wanted to return alone for one last session, which she did. The time was used to do some infant development teaching that she requested and to review her family situation. Her relationship with her mother was much calmer. She described herself as less likely to react to her mother's comments as criticism and as feeling more support from her mother. She also noted that recently she had become so preoccupied with her own obligations that she had seemingly forgotten that her mother had a life and concerns of her own. It also was obvious that she and her husband were cooperating more in parental tasks and were talking more directly with each other. She indicated a willingness to return, although she said she did not feel a particular need, and the therapy ended.

The therapist saw the recent birth of a child into this family as an event that had increased anxiety in the nuclear family group. Shifts in role responsibilities and relationships were happening as a result of practical necessity as well as anxiety. The influence of practical necessity was somewhat clear to each family member, including the six-year-old boy. The influence of anxiety was much less clear. When the mother was helped to examine current responsibilities and relationships, the anxiety decreased sufficiently to allow family members to think about alternatives to the less satisfying behaviors.

The Nurse's Role: Hospital. Both an accepting familiarity and a nonspecificity are always inherent in the place of a nurse within any particular medical setting, since nurses do a wide variety of tasks. The quiet endorsement of an effective and trusted nursing leader, such as the director of nursing in the hospital described here, can support hospital nurses in involving the therapist with patient problems they define as family-related and with problem patients. Quiet endorsement is that which does not unnecessarily evoke authoritatively mandated responses in staff members. Some staff members will respond to everything the leader says as a mandate. A hierarchy encourages obedient behavior.

In both the hospital-based practice and the physician's office practice, collegial trust of the nurse-therapist had developed over time. In the former setting, the nurse was employed by the hospital as a master's-prepared clinical nurse specialist with postgraduate training in family therapy. She had administrative responsibility to the psychiatric units. Within these units she worked directly with patients and their families and also consulted with patients and staff in other parts of the hospital. She had been hired by the director of nursing to fill an existing position. Although family therapy had not been a specific focus of work by former occupants of the position, nurses who had held the position had achieved the respect of physicians and hospital staff. The fact that the position had a positive reputation in the hospital system was part of the history of the organization that the therapist learned about and capitalized on in developing her own role.

Sobel states that "striving for optimal functioning in an organization is based on the same principles as optimal functioning in a family" (1982, p. 21). She goes on to mention a number of variables to learn about in any position. The history of the organization, particularly the history of your own position, heads the list. (Friedman, in the next chapter, also makes this point.)

The importance of this therapist's holding a line position (one in which she had subordinates for whom she had administrative responsibility as well as superiors to whom she reported), rather than a staff position (one in which she would have had superiors to whom she reported but not subordinates) is unclear. This particular position included administrative responsibility for the psychiatric service, each unit of which was managed by a head nurse who reported to the therapist holding this line position. In other hospitals, therapists have held staff positions with no administrative responsibilities, consulting with patients and staff and reporting only to the director of nursing. In this setting the advantages of the line position as a base of operation were that it was understood within the organization and that it formed a natural link to the world of family therapy. The disadvantage was that the therapist had administrative responsibilities that consumed her time and energy, especially during times of high anxiety in the psychiatric units.

Within the psychiatric unit of the hospital, the therapist was known to and in daily contact with the admitting physicians, most of whom were not family-oriented. In this setting they became familiar enough with the way she worked that they often referred patients directly to her for doing "whatever you do with families," or she would suggest to the physician that family issues were a concern and offer to see the family and make an assessment and work with them through the hospital stay. It was unusual for this offer to be turned down.

For example, one forty-year-old woman was admitted to the psychiatric unit with a diagnosis of depression and prior hospitalizations. Her physician customarily treated the depression with medication and used the hospital primarily as a safe environment during the most intense periods of the depression. This time the physician asked the therapist to see her. In talking with the woman, the therapist learned that she was very concerned about her twenty-year-old daughter's behavior and was trying to exercise control of the behavior by rigid but ineffective rule making. Exploration of this woman's relationship with her own mother at a similar point in her own life revealed a remarkably similar pattern. Her mother and father continued to take responsibility for her. Anxiety was high in the triangle involving the three, in part because of concerns about her mother's increasing age and illness. Her parents and one of her mother's sisters were identified as key family members to be invited to family sessions. After two sessions, the patient's husband, who had always remained distant and unavailable, according to previous hospital records and the patient, confronted the therapist angrily over not being involved. Subsequent sessions were held with the husband and wife in which issues between them and in his family of origin were discussed. A final session with the patient and her mother occurred before the patient's discharge. Anxiety in this family had decreased considerably since the patient's admission. The patient had identified ways in which she had been participating in the family emotion and had begun to question exactly what responsibility she wanted to take for the behavior and happiness of her nuclear family and her family of origin.

In evaluating the work with this family, two differences from previous hospitalizations were noted, both related to developmental themes. The fact that the patient's only child was trying to make changes in her relationship with her parents and develop a life separate from them increased the mother's established vulnerability to dysfunction but also increased the pressure for change in the parental relationship. This daughter's behavior could hardly be described as rebellion, but it fits with Hoffman's observation that "perhaps adolescent rebellion serves not only to establish beginning independence for a child, but offers an issue that the parents, who by a natural process will one day be child-free again, can use to test out the nature and strength of the bond between them" (1980, p. 66).

The second difference was postulated as a developmental change on the part of the patient's physician. Although his own work remained individual-oriented and involved medication maintenance of most patients, he was interested in other ways of viewing patient problems. He had recently become more open about his growing respect for other treatment approaches and about his expectation that others respect his approach and not require him to change or try to change him. This attitude facilitated an openness between the therapist and physician that seemed advantageous for all concerned. Each pursued different, but not mutually exclusive, goals.

With other services of the hospital, nursing staff, usually the head nurse, requested the consultation. The therapist's operating principle was that the physician was treating the patient's symptoms in a medically responsible way. However, direct communication between physician and staff or physician and patient was not assumed. The therapist also assumed that because staff members have an ongoing work relationship into which patients come for relatively short periods, increased anxiety in staff members about a patient may have more to do with work-system issues than with the patient. Therefore, clarifying the nature of the work each staff member is doing in relation to the patient may be what is needed to free the patient from staff triangles and start staff members thinking about work-system concerns that seem to have clouded that awareness. In most instances, the physician's input is not necessary to this process, at least initially. However, when anxiety among staff members is high, they are likely to involve the physician. This often takes the form of asking the physician for written orders for a nursing consultation rather than informing the physician of the staff need and the plan to deal with it. I read staff behavior of the sort just described as a cue that the target for intervention was staff members rather than the patient or the patient's family.

The Nurse's Role: Outpatient. In the office setting, the

therapist was employed part-time by the physician group. She initiated the idea of the position because she believed that many problems that family members view as medical problems can be more effectively treated in a medical context than in a psychiatric one, thus precluding the need for these problems to escalate to less manageable proportions that would warrant formal psychiatric diagnoses and treatment. Her further belief was that these physicians' interests, training, and time constraints placed them in a position to be open to providing for this further assistance to families without getting caught in issues about competition. The nurse had first become known to the physicians as the mother of two of their patients. As her career developed by way of a graduate degree in nursing, she became known as "the nurse who knows about working with families." In addition, she had worked for a number of years as a head nurse on a child psychiatric inpatient unit. Unlike the family therapist role, the head nurse role was familiar to all the physicians and seemed to have an influence in their decision to work with her in the ways she suggested.

Limits on Family Therapy in Medical Settings

Power and competition and conflicting beliefs are the major limits to approaching patients in medical settings as families. They have little to do with the direct work with families but a great deal to do with realities of medical settings.

At this time the physician exercises explicit power in medical settings. Historically, this has not always been true, and one can envision a time when redistribution of explicit power and responsibility in the health care system will take different standard forms, as seems to be happening in the functioning of some family units. For example, although change occurs slowly, in dual-career families in which both parents work outside the home and each takes significant economic responsibility for the family's functioning, redistribution of power and responsibility over many aspects of family life is occurring. For now, recognizing the position of the physician in the lives of patients is a first step in working with people for whom a medical diagnosis is or might become a reality.

In both therapy practices described, the therapist respected the position of the physician in patients' lives and structured her work in recognition of it or aligned herself with it. In both settings, as the therapist's reactivity to system pressures decreased, and as the usefulness of family intervention was demonstrated, many more opportunities for direct therapy were available than the therapist's or the physician's practice could absorb. This translates into a basically noncompetitive stance that had implications both for the therapy and for the fiscal economy of the patients, therapists, and physicians. In the hospital setting, the therapist's most apparent institutional link was to the psychiatric inpatient unit. It was in this setting that more direct referrals from non-family-oriented psychiatrists occurred. This fact is important, because the position itself involved considerable freedom and required daily choices about where energies were to be devoted (unlike a scheduled private practice). The decision to work with the family of a hospitalized psychiatric patient was obvious and straightforward, in comparison with the decision to work with the family of a patient in another part of the hospital. With the former, the initial assessment and entry into a working phase of therapy were the rule rather than the exception. The difficulty in working with these families in this setting was that the family work terminated after discharge. The hospital's administrative structure permitted the family to continue in family therapy on an outpatient basis, but coordinating this effort with the individual outpatient practices of the psychiatrists was not possible, mainly for what seemed to be economic reasons in this community: There were more therapists than the market could bear. Without a direct commitment to family therapy or a full caseload of patients, physicians were unlikely to refer. In other communities where economic competition for patients has not been an issue, continuing family work at the hospital after inpatient discharge has been established (see Chapter Three).

Economic issues for patients and therapists and the degree to which they influence the treatment offered or received are seldom dealt with in the literature on direct family therapy practice (but see Chapter Two). The hospital-based practice described was within the budget of nursing services, not a service charged specifically to the patient. In the pediatric practice, the sessions were charged as follow-up office visits under the auspices of the referring doctor and at the doctor's usual per-visit rate. Since this rate was not connected to time spent, the revenue to the practice from the longer amounts of time the therapist spent covered costs, but the sessions were not easily demonstrated to be cost-effective when only the physicians' usual ways of accounting were considered. The fact that the therapist's position was part-time contributed to the difficulty. A cost/benefit approach to evaluation would have been useful.

Fagin (1983) argues that, in facing current and future reimbursement realities, nonphysician therapists either must compete to provide services already offered or must clearly demonstrate that their services are substitutable for services presently provided by others. In either case, nonphysician services must be cost-effective. A number of studies report that decreases in use of medical services have resulted from psychotherapy (Office of Technology Assessment, 1980). Studies have also shown the effectiveness of psychological intervention in medical crises (Mumford, Schlesinger, and Glass, 1982). A case for substitutive services could be taken with regard to the work described in this chapter and would seem to be the most useful approach for nonphysician therapists working in medical settings.

In working in a medical setting, a family systems perspective conflicts with prevailing beliefs and functions of the healers in major ways. The most obvious is the belief that problems are experiences within individuals. This belief is reinforced, for example, by surgical scars, lab tests, and the fact that tubes injecting and removing fluids are usually inserted into only one family member. Another such belief is that healing occurs through the efforts of a staff team, headed by a physician who is in charge. If asked, most team members would say that the patient is part of the team and is involved in his or her own care. When behaviors of team members are examined closely, however, the concerns or requests of the patient are often not elicited, and the patient's attempts to communicate them are often missed totally. Staff members are more likely to characterize a family member as "interfering" than as "a key system member with whom the patient has emotional business." Family members, even those who are not particularly anxious but merely eager for information, are quickly labeled as "interfering" by an anxious staff simply for asking too many questions. It is easy for a medical professional to get reinforcement for a belief that one's work with patients could be done more easily and effectively if it were not for the family.

Working in settings so consistently individual-oriented required careful thinking and planning by the therapist. Meeting regularly with other professionals who shared her theoretical orientation was extremely useful to her in that such meetings raised questions that were not being raised in their work settings. These discussions were invariably enlightening and particularly useful for clarifying situations in which an individual view of problems had taken over. Bowen (1980) describes a ten-year process in which he purposely sought out case presentations from an individual perspective to sharpen his own thinking. These work settings required reversing that process.

The Work Compared

Working within a system that is not exclusively a therapy system forces a continual search for key family and institutional-system interaction points. The challenge of designing interventions that influence both is endless.

Of the two practices described, the outpatient physicians' office practice was in many ways similar to a private practice in which strong professional ties have been established, thus ensuring referrals. A major difference between such a referral system and the office-based practice was in the continuing direct tie to the medical-model system. No conceptual shift was required for the patient and family to label themselves and their problems in a different (psychiatric, or "crazy") way before seeing the therapist. Although maintaining a medical diagnosis and condition over time may be destructive and may support a dysfunctional system, to work with the issues as the client sees them is most important as a starting point, as has been amply demonstrated since Bradt and Moynihan's (1971) early work.

The hospital practice offered endless possibilities for thinking creatively with people about their situations. It also raised interesting questions about the boundaries of therapy. For example, if the terminally ill patient discussed earlier had had to pay for the therapy, then the therapist would have had to see him even though, in this particular case, it was more useful to work with his wife and with staff members. Such questions become very practical if therapists wish to be reimbursed for their work and the criteria for documenting one's work do not fit with the work one is doing.

In the hospital, a highly useful and theoretically enlightening process developed for working with the referral of patient problems from the nursing staff. The therapist would respond as quickly as possible to the staff member's request to talk. When the assessment of the concern suggested that internal staff relationships seemed to be triangling the patient rather than vice versa, further discussion with key staff members was requested.

Usually a request like "Tell me about what you are doing with this patient" or "Tell me about how you usually handle patients like this" would bring forth as detailed a discussion as time allowed, leading toward clarifying the direction that staff members were taking. The therapist would then suggest that she return later that day, or preferably the next day, to see the patient but that she would call first. Most often when the call was made to the identified key staff member, the therapist learned that the patient had settled down considerably, if he or she had been upset, or that the patient was much more alert and responsive, if he or she had been withdrawn. In such cases, the therapist would then offer to come if additional problems developed. Interestingly, although in many such cases the therapist never saw the patient, informal feedback from staff members frequently focused on how much she had helped the patient.

On a very practical level, when one thinks about the complexity of scheduling time with a patient in a hospital, compared with a private practice, humor helps. Hospital procedures are carried out by personnel in a multitude of departments on schedules that are certain to change, particularly if an attempt has been made to work around them. Somewhat surprisingly, given the complexity of scheduling, family members do seem to manage to be available, especially if the need for them to come has been accurately assessed and clearly stated to key members of the family system. Since the hospitalized patient might have disappeared to the far reaches of the radiology department fifteen minutes before the appointed meeting time, it is especially useful to be working from a theory base that clarifies the purpose and direction of the work and is not dependent on having every family member present in order for work to proceed.

A last point in comparing work in the hospital setting and in private practice is to note the usefulness of high but semi-focused anxiety in combination with a tendency to view life's problems as physical in effecting family-system shifts. For most of the families seen in the hospital practice, a deliberate decision to consult a therapist for psychological problems had not been required. This meant that families could be seen earlier than in situations in which fixed, unproductive patterns become established while unsuccessful attempts to solve problems are tried in an effort to forestall actual contact with a therapist.

Future Directions

Some consequences for the settings have already been described. The presence of a family therapy in each setting served as a consciousness-raising experience for physicians and other hospital staff members. Even though it was known by administration and staff members in the hospital that the nurse was a family therapist, it was never stressed as a way that employees must think about her. Problem patients were often described individually with no consciousness of family issues apparent until the therapist raised questions about the family. In both settings interest was generated among some staff members in knowing something more about theory, although the more usual indicator of raised consciousness was in informal discussion, when a problem would be described individually, followed by the question "Do you think something else could be going on here?"

Consciousness raising has many implications. It was striking that in both settings the structure itself conveyed an action orientation. Comfortable spaces conducive to talking at length were not readily available. Changes in space allocation and decor in both settings, to provide for just that, not only enhanced the work of therapy but reinforced awareness of thinking and talking with families as an option.

For the pediatric practice, the most striking difference was the ease with which referrals were made to the therapist. The doctors described themselves as previously having tried to do something, even though feeling ineffective in their efforts, rather than referring to a private psychiatric practice or a mental health center. By their descriptions, such referrals were often not effective in saving them time, since at the next visit the parent would take even more time to describe why an appointment had not been made or kept or how unsatisfactory the experience had been. The obvious need for communication within the health care system required a greater effort than the doctors were making. Even infrequent experiences like those they described were highly effective in keeping their system closed.

A next step in expanding the family therapist's practice in the pediatric setting would be to develop in-hospital consultation with these pediatricians' patients and their families. This would be done to intervene directly at high-stress times, capitalizing on the availability of the family for work that may not be present once the family system has reorganized around a diagnosis of disease in the child—for example, in the case of a newly diagnosed diabetic. (The importance of working with a family before family organization crystallizes around the diagnosis of a family member is also discussed in Chapters Six and Eight.) Some of the intervention would necessarily be focused on keeping open system communication between the hospital staff and the family. The economic base for this form of practice would need careful and imaginative development, since some of the obvious and usual indicators of success—for example, decreased length of hospital stay and decreased use of medication—could decrease income somewhere in the system. A number of studies already report decreased utilization of medical services resulting from psychotherapy (Office of Technology Assessment, 1980). Given current third-party reimbursement upheavals, just where this income decrease would surface is difficult to predict.

The last comment has particular implication for the inpatient practice described—in this case, potentially positive. If the prospective payment plan using a formula diagnostic group approach recently proposed by the Secretary of Health and Human Services for hospital reimbursement becomes a reality, approaches that help patients and families to detriangle from the hospital system sooner and more effectively in any given episode of physical illness could become sought-after commodities.

Given the complexity of the medical setting, many professionals often entertain the idea of cutting off from it completely rather than remaining within it. Emotional cutoff is a concept of Bowenian theory that describes one way people have of handling their unresolved emotional attachments to parents as they make the effort to establish their own lives in the present generation. Rather than remain in emotional contact with the family and work with resolving difficult issues, they separate themselves from the family, believing that the issues are a part of their past. The theory proposes that the same issues will recur in new settings (Bowen, 1978). As in family systems, cutoff is not an effective solution for professionals having difficulty functioning effectively within the complexities of the system. It may appear to change the most obvious symptoms of distress for a time. Meyer (1982, p. 23) suggests three principal factors that contribute to personal achievement and professional freedom in the workplace, based on eight years of working in one agency where the administration remained unchanged: "(1) the degree of clarity an individual has regarding the principles and objectives which underscore his work, (2) the degree to which an individual meets job expectations, and (3) the degree to which an individual maintains relationships throughout the work system." These factors are helpful in thinking about working within a system. They are also useful, especially the first, for therapists who work outside the medical setting to consider in thinking about how they might involve themselves in traditional medical settings if that is indicated as a way of working effectively with families.

Family therapy as an approach to working with disease or dysfunction in a family system is much more recent than the medical practice with which it has been connected in this chapter. Both are developing systems, as are the practitioners within each, as are the family systems that seek assistance. It is an exciting time to be part of the developments in all three systems, especially as medical care shifts its focus from illness to health.

10 Edwin H. Friedman

Churches and Synagogues

All members of the clergy are family thera-
pists. Whether they are considering the emotional lives of their
congregants, their congregations (which also function as families), or their own marriage and parenting, the family is the context of the clergy's being. This is an ecumenical concept; it
holds true no matter what the faith or denomination. Even for
unmarried, Catholic clergy, the rectory or the order functions as
a nuclear or extended family system.

The family model therefore offers clergy a valuable ma-
trix for understanding the interlocking emotional forces in
which they are constantly engulfed. What makes this possible
is that the three families of the clergy—their own, their congregations, and those of their parishioners—connect in such a way
that problems in any one can produce symptoms in one of the
others, while deeper understanding of any one provides a better
grasp of how to function in the others (Friedman, 1984).

For example, by applying the family model to a church
or synagogue when terminating employment, members of the
clergy can gain more insight into the emotional process of separation than can be gained from reading books on the emotional
processes of death and divorce. Conversely, the family model
can take the understanding of separation that clergy gain in the
course of their ministerial duties during death and divorce and
draw from it a complete strategy for how to leave a congrega-

tion in a manner that leaves the least amount of unresolved residue in either "partner."

A full exposition of all the ways the family model can be useful to the clergy would have to discuss a wide range of family issues from marriage counseling to geriatrics, from visitation of the sick to rites of passage. It would have to touch on the nuclear and extended families of the clergy themselves and the manner in which congregations function like families, particularly during periods of change or in response to leadership (see Friedman, 1984, for a comprehensive depiction of how family process affects the clergy's personal and professional existence). Instead of trying to cover the waterfront, this chapter will concentrate on one aspect of the clergy's responsibility: premarital counseling. No other mental health profession has as much opportunity to encounter the emotional forces characteristic of this passage. In addition, the position that clergy occupy in families during courtship will serve as a metaphor for the source of their real healing power: their unique entry into families, a constant, almost natural availability not given to others—although, as will be seen, application of the family model to couples in courtship can be of use to other members of the helping professions as well. The entree is more difficult, but the rules are the same.

Most writing about premarital counseling has not been in the context of the family model. The literature has thus missed the opportunity to show members of the clergy how that model offers them predictive power, as well as a built-in file system for future contacts with the couple, if not with the entire family. It will be my purpose here to correct that omission.

This chapter has four parts. The first section explores the notion of courtship as a family phenomenon. It describes important aspects of the courting process overlooked by counseling that emphasizes the couple's relationship alone. The second section establishes a theoretical basis for the clinical sections that follow by outlining a family systems understanding of marriage. The third part describes three representative examples of the application of the family model to courting couples. The fourth is also clinical but does not focus on problems. Another advantage of the family approach to premarital counseling is that it offers an overall strategy toward all couples whether or not they are experiencing difficulties. This section shows how the construction of family genograms can teach much about the couple's emotional heritage, can provide some guidelines for predictions about their future life together, and because it is generally less threatening than questionnaires or pointed advice, tends to bypass much of the resistance couples present when all they want to talk about is "the ceremony."

This "research" approach also reduces the degree to which clergy counselors project their own anxieties through too much advice giving. Expertise always creates too much reliance on the healing power of the expert, and future marriage counseling by clergy is hindered by magical association when the couple goes back to the minister who "tied the knot."

Finally, a family approach to premarital counseling is a good example of the aforementioned insight-crossover between different aspects of the clergy's many-dimensioned existence. A family approach to courtship can tutor clergy on how to select new congregational partners and how to develop their own relationships in those professional marriages.

The Failure of Premarital Counseling

It was not long ago that the number of books on premarital counseling being published for the clergy almost appeared to exceed the number of couples being married. This emphasis in the pastoral field reflected both the growing anxiety in our society over the divorce rate, then accelerating, and the awareness that this phase of the marriage cycle was a natural special interest. But the pastoral movement, with its roots deep in the psychoanalytic model, produced this literature from the point of view of individuals coming together rather than from the perspective of the interlocking of family systems. It was like trying to explain molecules in terms of nuclear forces alone. Just as chemistry is not reducible to physics, so the forces at play during courtship (or, indeed, marriage) are not reducible to indi-

274   Practicing Family Therapy in Diverse Settings

vidual psychodynamics as much as they contain them. The intrinsic relationship of two "atoms" in any context can never be understood apart from a larger force field. Or, to go from the microcosm to the macrocosm, the nature of the marital bond can no more be isolated from the emotional systems of the partners' families of origin than the marriage of the earth and moon can be understood without taking into account the gravitational effects of other members of the solar system. The thrust of such an analogy is not to the materialistic atoms or planets themselves but to a way of conceptualizing relationships. Field theory is a way of thinking, and whether one is considering objects or people, there is no such thing as a two-person system (Friedman, 1977).

Premarital counseling that ignores this vital fact will tend to focus on the content of symptoms rather than the underlying emotional process that generates them.

There are also several other reasons for the inadequacy of the individual model as a basis for premarital counseling. All are related to the courtship process itself.

1. Relationships change qualitatively after commitment.
2. Unless they are experiencing extreme difficulties, during the courting period individuals are *least* able to hear advice about their relationship.
3. The capacity of individuals to create strong but flexible bonds is determined primarily by the nature of their previous separations, and this is as true whether the previous separations involved divorce, death, or leaving home.

Commitment. When I first began to perform weddings twenty-five years ago, one of the most surprising phenomena to me was the number of couples who had been living together in blissful harmony, sometimes for years, who began to experience conflict from the moment they decided to get married. The frequency of this occurrence over the years has not diminished. Aside from raising questions about the usefulness of trial marriage, this connection between commitment and compatibility sheds light on the very nature of the human bonding process. Almost all couples lose some flexibility when they get married;

some lose it from the moment of engagement. This seems to be related to a shift in responsibility from "self" to the "other" or to the relationship. Even though it was the "self" of each partner that attracted the "other," once individuals think in terms of marriage, they begin to shift their focus away from preserving the "self," which attracted the other, to the "other."

An extremely voluptuous woman once came in complaining about her inability to "hang onto a man." Attracting men was no problem, but they all distanced within months. "Funny thing is," she said, "if I don't care about them, I can't keep them away. But once I start to like them, they run away. It's almost as though I lose something in myself when I begin to care."

Existentially this shift in focus is experienced as seriousness. Witness the phrases used in our culture for getting married: "How long have you been dating *seriously*?" "They are *serious* about each other." "I hope your intentions, young man, are *serious*." When individuals begin to think in terms of "getting hitched" or "tying the knot," they shift their primary focus of concern. The resulting fusion process changes the relationship qualitatively.

Courtship and Advice. A second reason for the failure of most premarital counseling is the effect of the courting process on the capacity of individuals to hear.

Years ago a psychiatrist (Protestant) and I were given an opportunity by the local archdiocese to run an adjunct program on marriage for those who participated in its compulsory "pre-Cana" program. A letter inviting couples to participate in a short series of about five sessions, at a very reasonable cost, written in a style that attempted to bypass known resistance to such guidance, and showing that the program could be fun rather than threatening, was sent out on archdiocesan stationery to more than a thousand couples from every class and caste. We received one response. People do not hear you when they are moving away from you. Since individuals engaged in courting are moving toward each other and, relatively speaking, away from everyone else, with a speed approaching that of light, messages from others, no matter how they are transmitted, just do not catch up.

If this is true generally, it is all the more true to the extent that the forces leading to any impending union are energized by efforts to escape unresolved issues in other systems (particularly families of origin). Every mating must include at least 30 percent of that type of emotional energy, but some have close to 100 percent. The obvious paradox, therefore, is that the more individuals need advice about marriage, the less capable they are of hearing it during courtship.

Actually, many first marriages seem to serve as halfway houses. They permit individuals to escape or at least get some distance from their families, to act out their problems in a less important system, to dump their transferences on their first mate, and then to go out into the world and find a more suitable partner. Not only can those couples not take advice before marriage, maybe it should not be offered to them. Why interfere with a natural abortion?

Ironically, clergy have an experience in their own professional lives that parallels this inability to hear before experiencing commitment. This is the advice given to them in the "prenuptial state" of seminary training about how they should function in the relationship systems of church and synagogue. Over and over clergy in the field lament that what they learned in postgraduate workshops should have been taught while they were still in school. It was.

Couples during courtship are no more capable of hearing advice on how to fight, budget, communicate, and have sex than clergy are capable of learning how to deal with unjust criticism, triangles between congregants, or separation anxiety when their charges cannot find them in the office until they have spent some time in the committed responsibility of their own post.

Engagement and Disengagement. How people engage with each other may have less to do with their own compatibility potential than with how they disengage from their previous associations. The capacity of any relationship to "take," whether it is a personal marriage or the match between a member of the clergy and his or her congregation, is primarily a function of how these partners left their previous relationships. Elsewhere (Friedman, 1980) I have illustrated how the time periods between such leaving and entering can themselves be indicative of how much baggage individuals are carrying with them.

This principle holds true no matter what the cultural background and irrespective of whether the important previous relationship was with a former spouse or a parent and whether the disengagement was precipitated by leaving home, divorce, death, or a psychotic break. Actually, the reciprocal processes of engagement and disengagement do not end with a marriage ceremony but continue throughout the course of the new union. Almost all nuclear family problems get stirring within six months of a major change in the family of origin of one of the partners. Moreover, as will be seen, they often have multigenerational roots.

And all this can also be true in churches and synagogues where the sudden resignation or suicide of a minister, or a bitter struggle that precedes the ousting of a particular minister in one generation, affects the selection and the congregation's relationship with another minister, several ministers later. Hospitals and mental health clinics are, of course, immune from such problems.

The horns of the dilemma are these: Individuals who break too abruptly with their past will transfer all the intensity of their unresolved issues to the new relationship system (marriage or congregation, spouse or minister); but individuals who do not differentiate themselves distinctly enough from their families of origin will also have little flexibility in their new family.

On the one hand, this relation between engagement and disengagement seems to suggest that the only form of premarital counseling guaranteed to be successful is working with the parents of the couple when the bride and groom were about age five. On the other hand, this reciprocity between entering and leaving suggests that the rite of passage of marriage is not to be equated with the ceremony itself. Like all such nodal events, it probably begins in earnest six months to a year before, and ends six months to a year after, the ceremony. *Anything, therefore, that can be done during the courtship phase to help facilitate* leaving *in a manner that avoids the extremes of cutoff or intense unresolved feelings will do more for the future of a couple than counseling that focuses on their own relationship.* In this sense divorce counseling can also serve as premarital counseling and may be most productive when the focus during the separation period before remarriage is on still-remaining issues with family of origin rather than with estranged spouse. To the extent that such unseen encumbrances are dissolved, any new bond in the process of formation is given maximum opportunity to establish itself in the same natural way that mating has occurred for millennia. Premarital counseling that emphasizes the personality traits of the partners and their transactions totally misses this crucial aspect of bonding.

In sum, traditional approaches to premarital counseling have been largely ineffective because they have failed to take into account important aspects of the courtship process that are not reducible to the psychodynamics of the bride and groom. Such counseling has wound up stressing symptoms rather than emotional process and, worse, perpetuating into the union the myth that a marriage relationship can be isolated from the broader influences of the partners' extended family fields.

Family Theory and Premarital Counseling

A theory of premarital counseling must begin with a theory of marriage. Our approach to couples before marriage depends on what we consider a good marriage to begin with. Family theory always sets the marital relationship within the context of the nuclear family and the extended families of both partners. Regarding the nuclear system, it is just too easy to misread marital harmony by failing to note a focus on a child—too simple to say, "The marriage was a success; it's too bad one of the partners died early." Marital harmony achieved by projection to a child or the sacrifice of integrity—that is, the "dis-integration" —of one of the partners can disguise itself as concern for togetherness or humility, but its eventual cost can range from dysfunction in an offspring to cancer in a parent.

To avoid such subterfuge, successful marriage is not defined in terms of good feelings or the absence of conflict or even the longevity of the relationship. Instead, a continuum is established that states that all marriages are successful to the extent that the entire nuclear family is symptom-free, with the idea that no human marriage achieves a rating of better than 70 percent. Such a perspective covers all three of the previously mentioned locations in which family symptoms can surface in a nuclear system, and it helps us keep in mind that marital disharmony is only one of the three. This nuclear-system model for evaluating marriage has two advantages.

First, it suggests that criteria for change in a given marriage relationship must take into account whether the entire nuclear family became less symptomatic. Did the symptom disappear from the marriage relationship only to recycle elsewhere in the family several months later, perhaps as a pregnant daughter or as a husband's heart attack? From this perspective, marital conflict and even infidelity, two of the primary foci of most marriage evaluation, may be among the *least* pernicious symptoms in families.

Second, this systemic perspective makes it easier to keep in mind that when using a family history to evaluate the success of a future marriage, its potential cannot be judged by looking only at the marriages of earlier relatives. Unresolved issues in previous generations could have surfaced as dysfunctional children or spouses instead. The key questions when making predictions, therefore, are not how much marital conflict but how much unresolved pathology in any form is on its way down, and how family members in previous marriages tended to deal with or displace their problems.

The family system model thus also sets marriage in an even broader context than the nuclear system alone. Logic suggests that a given nuclear family can be fully understood only within the entire network of nuclear families, the extended systems, of both partners.

Many, if not most, nuclear family problems can be influenced, perhaps eliminated, by focusing the spouses on unresolved issues in their own families of origin *instead*. This is to some extent a different use of the past than in psychodynamic therapies. It is not just how "the past" affected us while we were growing up but also how we are still a part of it in the present. This way of viewing our "past" also plays havoc with the widespread sociological convention that the family is breaking down. It may really only have gone underground and is always most likely to surface again during rites of passage (Friedman, 1980).

The major ramification of the concept of the extended family field for premarital counseling is that focusing a prospective bride and groom on their positions in the path of the multigeneration transmission processes is one of the most healing, and one of the most prophylactic, measures that can be brought to bear on the experience of bonding. It is here that we can see most clearly how disengagement is the other side of engagement. (In this context it should be mentioned that "eloping" is usually connected to unresolved issues that the parents of the bride and groom still have with their own families of origin. Couples often "elope" for their families.)

All this is not to say that the couple's own relationship is unimportant. But that too must be understood in systemic terms, not only because their functioning is symptomatic of their respective positions in their families of origin but also because "it takes two to tango."

In traditional, psychodynamic theory, the way a person functions or dysfunctions is primarily the sum of his or her own past experiences, with particular emphasis on the earliest ones. Family theory, however, suggests that a symptom in either partner may have more to do with the nonsymptomatic partner's past. The reasoning for this is, first, that symptoms do not materialize out of thin air like Pallas Athene. They are more likely to be the crystallization of patterns of interaction that have been going on for some time. Second, for something to remain chronic, there must be feedback. Third, everyone brings into marriage more pathology from his or her past than could possibly become manifest in a lifetime. It is therefore the *other partner's response* to presymptomatic behavior that is most likely to determine the extent to which any given behavior will become an occasional or a perpetual phenomenon. This is why working with nonsymptomatic partners in regard to their anxiety over the other's behavior, by having them understand where that anxiety emanates from in their own family of origin or how it is perpetuated by their position in extended family triangles, can often do more to prevent or reduce symptoms than focusing on the nature, meaning, or origin of the symptom itself or on the symptomatic partner.

In this regard two implications of family theory for counseling technique should be mentioned by way of introduction to the clinical material that follows. The first is that family therapy is not to be distinguished from individual-model counseling by how many come to the session. It is possible to do family therapy while seeing only one member. The differentiating characteristic of the family approach is the focus on the system rather than the person, not the quantity of counselees seen simultaneously.

Second, the criterion for which family members should be seen is who is most motivated rather than who has the symptom. That may or may not be the same person. This choice of persons to see is an emphasis on strength rather than weakness that has important evolutionary consequences, and it robs the symptomatic person of his or her power to retard change.

One cannot judge the future success of a marriage by quantifying the amount of personal problems each partner brings into the union. Everyone has a right to bring as many idiosyncrasies as he or she wants into a relationship (doors securely locked at night, gas jets triple-checked when leaving the house, thermostat always exactly at 67, all dishes always stacked neatly in the cupboard, the safety on the cruise control always turned off with the motor). What partners do not have a right to do is to try to make the other responsible for their own anxiety.

Three Case Histories

This section will present three examples of how family theory can be applied to problems during courtship. In the first two, the issues surface in the couples—one previously married, the other never married—and in the third, the issue begins with the parents. In all three, however, the approach is directed to emotional process in and around the couple, rather than to the content of their focused symptoms, and to other members of the family network beyond their own connectedness.

Lois and Keith. Lois and Keith came to see their minister struggling with a relationship that had become stormy from the time they fell in love. After several efforts to make Keith commit himself, Lois finally broke off completely. Then after six months, just as she had finally managed to get him off her mind, he called. Within two weeks they were living together. Three months later they were talking about marriage and began to discuss arrangements with their minister; then Keith again began to drag his feet. He also became symptomatic (chronic sore back). Once more, Lois began to think of leaving, but a friend suggested she avoid the either/or extremes and discuss the problem with their minister.

Lois' complaint was that she had to initiate everything. Keith's response was that they just thought differently. Lois said it had to do with their different backgrounds; her German stock, she explained, gave her a proclivity for order and neatness. Keith, having had Irish ancestors, was "naturally" less concerned with such values. Keith objected, however, that his Dublin-bred mother was more concerned about his perpetual tardiness than Lois. (Friedman, 1983, points out how blaming cultural factors for the emotional process is one of the most common ways in which family members avoid responsibility for their own contributions and dupe therapists into thinking they are hearing important causal information.)

The transactions in this couple's relationship involving an overfunctioner and an underfunctioner, each of whom adapts progressively to the other's extreme by becoming more extreme in the opposite direction, is one of the most common relational patterns found in partnerships. It is as likely to show up in the relationship between the clergy and their congregational partners as between husband and wife. When it goes beyond certain bounds, a threshold is reached in which the increasing stress on the overfunctioner or the total loss of integrity of the underfunctioner will do one of them in. It is therefore a relational style to be concerned about, and when it surfaces as a problem in courtship, a couple are lucky if they are thus forced to deal

with it then. The need to marry at a particular time (in order to
defuse issues with one's family of origin) often makes such partners hope things will get better afterward. They generally get
worse. Usually a couple like this cannot change by simply discussing their issues, and rarely can underfunctioners begin the
process of change by trying harder to take initiative. They
might try for a while, but usually they will slip back within a
week, and the overfunctioner's anxiety will preempt the initiative before the underfunctioner gets a second breath. It is with
the overfunctioner, therefore (who is usually the one who calls
and almost always the one who suggested the counseling), that
the counseling process must primarily be focused.

The process has two phases. First, disrupt the two-step
between the partners and help the overfunctioner learn to default. Second, try to focus each partner, but particularly the
overfunctioner, on emotional processes in his or her family of
origin and on how that partner's position in the transmission
keeps him or her in predictable patterns.

One method of helping such couples get free of their
straitjacket is the use of paradoxical techniques apparently
aimed at pushing them in the direction of their extremes. Such
an approach, when implemented playfully, has the added advantage of reducing the terribly serious tone with which all over-
functioners color all their efforts, activities, and goals.

Minister: Lois, how come you haven't been able to shape Keith
up?

Lois: He's just stubborn.

Minister: Well, maybe you should try to out-stubborn him.

Lois: I try, but I get tired after a while.

Minister: Perhaps you just don't try hard enough.

Lois: Are you kidding?

Minister: I'm just trying to help. But maybe the point at which
you quit is just when it would have worked, if only you had
given it more effort.

Lois: I've given it all I have.

Minister: Besides, if Keith really loved you, he'd know what you want him to do without your having to express it.

Keith: I think she really thinks that.

Minister: Keith, what do you think would happen if Lois over-functioned less?

Keith: Well, for one thing, I would be less tense. I never know when I'm going to be criticized for not doing something the way she wants it.

Lois: That's not true.

Minister: Well, Keith, maybe if you just did everything the way she wanted it, there wouldn't be any problem.

Keith: No, that won't work either; I've tried that.

Such an approach can give both partners some distance from their patterned response. It will not, however, change the basic nature of this type of relationship. The overfunctioner/underfunctioner equation will surface again and again with each other and with the children, mainly during periods of crisis and anxiety. Well-intentioned advice by the counselor, pointing out such dangers, will be totally ineffective.

It is here that a family approach to premarital counseling based on partners' positions in families of origin can affect the future of this emerging marriage on a fundamental level.

Many would see Lois as controlling; she really has very little control over the way she controls. She is as caught as Keith, but she is also more motivated to see change, in part because the overfunctioner usually winds up with the stress for the relationship.

Lois was therefore seen separately and encouraged to understand how she had got programmed to be such a rescuer. She thought it had to do with being a chip off the old block. Her mother had overfunctioned with regard to her father, whom Lois described as extremely passive. In fact, she had always vowed that she would never be like her mother, whom she saw as Dad's castrator, and she was shocked to see how much she had fallen into similar patterns. She also added that her mother's overfunctioning with respect to her docile father had kept her from ever getting to know him. She could not remember one time when he had written to her on his own or had ever stayed on the phone with her alone. It was suggested that she invite him down for a weekend alone. "Mother would never let him go." "Then enlist her aid."

Lois called mother and asked her for help in getting to know her father better, adding that she would like to have him come for a visit by himself. She waited for all the excuses mother would proffer. Instead, mother immediately called to her husband, "Your daughter is on the phone; she wants you to come for a visit."

By the end of that weekend Lois no longer saw her mother as controlling but, rather, as hoodwinked. Father took no initiative the entire time for either conversation or activity and asked Lois' advice on every move. The climax came at dinner when he asked her whether he should pay by cash, check, or credit card. During this visit Lois asked father to talk about his younger days and learned that over and over he had purposely avoided promotions because he did not want to get into trouble.

With a new awareness of her parents' relationship, Lois was able to get closer to her mother and engage her in conversation about the overfunctioning pattern of almost all the females in her family. As nearly as they could tell it, it had begun with great-grandmother, whose husband was an alcoholic and a chronic roué who left her precipitously and forever with four girls, whom she raised by herself.

Soon Lois found it easier to outwait Keith on just about everything from standing still at green lights to catching a bottle on its way off the table. At first Keith appeared to get even slower, but eventually he expanded his functioning into the vacuum left by his fiancée's purposeful recalcitrance. Lois was helped to continue in this direction of default by having her put most of her thinking into her own personal development rather than the relationship. In direct proportion to this change, conflict disappeared, Keith's back got better, and the groom made a formal proposal, which, with greatly restrained alacrity, Lois accepted.

The idea, of course, is not just to get them married but, rather, to launch them in an attitude that will also be good for the whole trip.

Charles and Donna. Charles and Donna both had unresolved issues remaining from their previous marriages. Each had custody of his or her children, and each was still in conflict with the former spouse over property rights and some custody issues. They were both, in short, already divorced but not yet separated. Their early dating discussions with each other had been filled with mutual commiseration over their exes. Such victim-portraits of oneself can be splendid substitutes for aphrodisiac dialogue and help many second marriages get a head start. When couples come together in this manner, however, the pseudo mutuality that results will prove fragile in crisis.

They had met one Christmas season shortly after separating. Donna's husband was already living with his paramour from the previous year. Charles' wife had found an apartment, said she was considering a lesbian life-style, and left him with the kids so she could go back to law school, an ambition she had dropped when she married.

By June, Charles and Donna were considering setting up house together and, if things worked out, getting married in about a year. But matters had become so difficult over the previous month that Donna was balking. A long-time member of her congregation, she asked her minister what to do. She did not want "premarital counseling" because it was not clear that they were really going to marry, but she needed someone who had some expertise in this kind of thing to help her sort out what was happening.

The minister, who had known her since she was confirmed but who had not officiated at her previous marriage because it had taken place in another town, suggested they come in together.

My own tendency in such situations is to tell the couple that I see them as stuck, that I have no personal preference concerning whether they should get married or not, that I have not the foggiest idea of how to judge the success potential of their relationship, but if they are interested in trying to get unstuck, then whatever decision they come to will probably be right for them. It is rare that I see a couple work on this type of problem in this way and decide to break up.

On the surface, Donna and Charles simply had become impossibly fused. Neither could make a comment without the other's jumping in to correct the record. The issues between them were legion. She wanted more cooperation; he wanted more affection. She wanted him to work less at the office; he wanted her to stop correcting his faults. She wanted him to stand up to his former wife; he wanted her to understand that he was working on the problem in his way. He wanted her to discipline her children more; she wanted him to understand her children more. They simply needed to separate so they could get married.

They might hear their counselor's advice in the office, but back home they would not be able to maintain the changes. The major reason for this leaky phenomenon is that all their issues were symptomatic of the various triangles in which they were caught rather than anything endemic to their relationship. Focusing on their own relationship alone, the couple looks simply like Figure 1. A more accurate diagram of the emotional system in which their relationship is embedded, however, would look like Figure 2. And this does not even begin to take into account other influences and triangles with members of their extended families (Figure 3).

For example, Donna's mother had died several years earlier, and her father was remarried to a woman who, in Donna's eyes, stayed so hoveringly close to him that she was unable to get close herself. In addition, this woman and Donna's younger sister were at serious odds over the way dad's wife treated sister's kids, and each would periodically call Donna and complain about the other.

Charles was in a more subtle, multigenerational triangle, one that produces what I have come to call the "family standard bearer." The person who occupies this position (usually

Figure 1.   The Couple in Isolation.

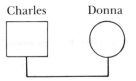

Figure 2.   The Couple in the Context of Their Previous Marriages.

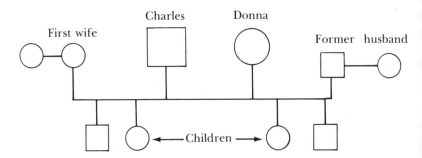

Figure 3.   The Couple in the Context of Their Extended Families.

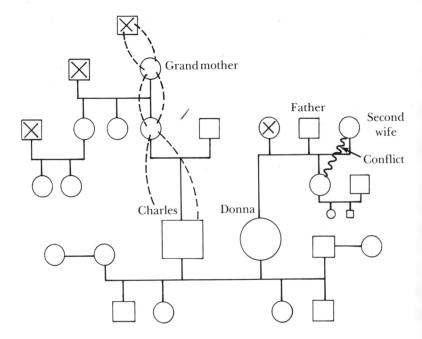

male) has been catapulted out of his family to achieve. Whoever becomes emotionally involved with such a man should not expect too much help around the house or with the children. He will have great difficulty committing himself to marriage or anything else except his career. In fact, every male I have ever seen pull out on a wedding after the date was set occupied this position. Unless such men are willing to understand the multigenerational emotional forces that have been transmitted to them, they cannot change. Such transmission usually comes down through mother's mother. In Charles' case, his grandmother had been taken away forcibly from her adored father, had failed to produce a male offspring herself, and had selected this firstborn, male grandchild as the replacement.

To appreciate the broader view afforded by this genogram, one must understand the concept of an emotional triangle. The relationship between Charles and Donna is a good example of how emotional process can spawn content issues and how change on the process level will make those content issues atrophy. Generally speaking, previously married individuals creating a so-called blended family are not experiencing something qualitatively different than other couples do, with one exception. The emotional triangles are far more complex and active. When the bride and groom who are also mother and father can come to understand how emotional triangles function, as well as what makes them setups for getting caught in triangular binds, things usually go pretty well no matter whose children or how many are being brought into the new union.

To put it another way, I could, with better than 90 percent effectiveness, teach such couples how to destroy their relationship within weeks: Become involved in your future mate's previously established relationships and try to rearrange them. Constantly push advice on how to do things differently, or inject yourself into the middle between your future mate and his or her former mate (or child or parent) and try to be the referee, arbitrator, fixer, or therapist. This approach will get the others closer together through the process of ganging up on you. In one case it succeeded in getting a man back together with his former wife. (Why the fire when I can have the security of the frying pan?) All this can be true in first marriages, of course, where the party in the background is not a former spouse but a parent, a job situation, or even a hobby.

Most couples grasp the basic laws of triangles pretty quickly. They can be spelled out using a blackboard to diagram the network, or one can simply say, "In the history of the human species, no member of a family has ever said to a second member of a family, regarding a third, 'I think you should do it this way instead,' and have the third respond, 'You're right, honey, I don't know why I didn't see it that way myself.' "

An emotional triangle is any three persons in a family or any two and an issue or symptom. The basic rules of an emotional triangle are as follows (Friedman, 1981).

1. It is not possible to change a relationship you are not a part of. If you are at A, you cannot change B-C directly.

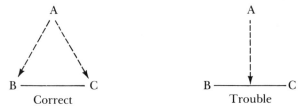

2. You can bring about change in B-C only by working on your own relationship with B or C one-to-one.
3. All efforts to change B-C from the position of A will generally be converted to their opposite intent; pulling B and C apart will force them together, and trying to force them together will drive a wedge between them.
4. The person trying to bring change to the relationship of two others will often wind up with the stress for the entire system.
5. Any one triangle in a network interlocks with others. Thus, sometimes the best way to bring change to a triangle in one network (a nuclear family, a congregation) is to work on triangles in the extended system.

Both Donna and Charles were able to see the patterns fairly quickly. Each was able to avoid commenting on the other's relationship with his or her children, former mate, or anyone else in the other's previous life. Almost overnight the conflict between them subsided, and the symptomatic issues atrophied.

To cement these gains, both were also encouraged to disengage from the tugs-of-war in which they were respectively engaged with their former spouses over the children. It was clear that their former partners used issues around their offspring to keep Donna and Charles from disengaging from the earlier marriages. Instead of trying to hug their kids away from their former mates, therefore, the counselor encouraged Charles and Donna to push them closer. Within no time Donna's former husband moved out of town, and Charles' former wife dropped all legal threats.

Both were also encouraged to work on the triangles in their respective families of origin by, among other things, dropping responsibility for the relationships of others and becoming more playful about the most intense issues.

After several months of detriangling and disengaging elsewhere, Donna and Charles found their own relationship to be so rewarding they decided they would not have to wait the trial year before they were married.

Jack and Claudine. Jack and Claudine came to see their minister, furious about their son's choice of a mate. The son was a hardworking steel foreman at the factory and always did an honest day's work. He was about to be snared by some uppity college girl from another town, another religion, and another world. Jack and Claudine wanted their minister to talk some sense into their kid. Although they had disagreed with her talks on the generation gap, they figured that since she was closer to their son's generation, maybe she could get through.

The situation in which parents come to a minister to straighten out their child is a complex triangular trap. When ministers counsel families, it always involves their position in the congregational "family" as well. On the one hand, the parents are paying the minister's salary, and he or she cannot go

round all the time being an ombudsman for the next generation. On the other hand, too obvious support for the older generation on personal matters, and the minister will lose his or her
credibility with the younger generation, who will dismiss the
minister as an Establishment fink no matter how progressive his
or her ideas on politics or society.

The best way out of this dilemma (which happens to fit a
family approach) is not to get caught in the triangle. This can be
accomplished with either of two systems approaches: seeing the
couple with their child (future in-laws may also be present) or
seeing the parents alone and trying to redirect their focus.

If the couple are seen with the parents, the minister never
has to, and probably never should, take a position one way or
the other on the advisability of the forthcoming marriage. The
minister need "only" try to maintain a nonanxious presence in
which he or she asks dozens of questions designed to facilitate
more self-definition between the various family members. This
approach not only protects the minister in the congregational
family, it fosters definition in the parishioner's family. Three
interconnected emotional coordinates will always determine the
family's emotional context at such crises, no matter what content issue is being raised—race, religion, social class, economic
status, age, or previous marital status. These three interdependent factors are—

1. Lack of differentiation of self between the reacting parent
    and the child about to be married.
2. Important unresolved issues in the parents' marriage which
    are causing Factor 1 to be so intense). Parents do not be-
    come severe in their objections when their own marriage is
    satisfying.
3. An important unresolved emotional issue in the reacting
    parent's family of origin, usually involving responsibility of
    some sort, in which that parent is caught. (This family-of-
    origin factor is usually behind Factor 2.)

It can be categorically stated that when relatives object
vehemently to their child's marriage, no matter what the grounds

of their objections, any counseling that is guided by these coordinates rather than the content of the issues, whether it is with the parents or the children, will be premarital counseling at its best (Friedman, 1980, 1983).

An episode early in my own experience convinced me of these connections. A young woman in my congregation came in to get married, saying her parents were violently opposed. I suggested a meeting with all four. The couple were reluctant; the family had all been to see a therapist for several sessions a couple of years before, but "mother would have apoplexy and father fell asleep."

I always suggest to the future in-law that this is not his or her problem, even if he or she is the focus—that is, the displacement—and that during the session I want to redirect the focus. The presence of the future in-law will help the fiance stay loose, but not if the future in-law becomes too engaged in the issues.

When the parents came in, I immediately told mother (a major force on my synagogue's board of trustees) that there were three hospitals within five minutes of the building. She naturally inquired why I was telling her that, and I answered, "Because your daughter told me that you were given to apoplexy at such family meetings, and I wanted you to feel free to express your feelings."

Throughout the session, she answered all questions with reserve and reason, expressed her doubts logically, and had some solid, mutually respectful interchanges with both her daughter and her future son-in-law.

Father, however, the one who usually fell asleep during such sessions, without his wife overfunctioning as his defense, was out of his seat every five minutes saying things like "Well, isn't that enough now?" or "I don't think we need to go any further" or "Excuse me, I need a smoke."

Mother called back the following week and came in about her own marriage.

With Jack and Claudine the displacement had another twist, one that highlights a different dimension of family process at nodal events and is particularly prone to surface near weddings. They had had an older son who died at eighteen. He was the college student in the family, the child the parents had sacrificed for. But the night after graduating from high school with many honors, he had been killed on his bike by a hit-and-run driver. The same minister had officiated at the funeral and said it was one of the most bizarre funerals she had ever attended. It had been clear that the loss was a major shock to the entire family, yet all seemed to be outdoing one another to maintain a stiff upper lip. From the day of his death, the son was never mentioned again, and the only noticeable remembrance of the lad was a small picture, isolated on the TV, of the two boys playing as youngsters at the beach. On several occasions when the minister had visited this family, mostly during extended illnesses (which had become frequent in recent years), she said the picture would remind her of the funeral and the absence of natural remembrance.

Now, it is a fundamental rule of all rites of passage that unresolved issues from one passage are likely to surface in the midst of another disguised as anything from conflict with relatives to perseveration over etiquette. This can happen with any two rites, but it is most likely when the unresolved issue is from death and the current passage is marriage, which, far more than baptism or bar mitzva, for example, again involves "loss" (although a funeral may be seen as a marriage, with death often "courted" for some time).

During the session, the minister got the discussion around to the dead son and confessed her own surprise about the lack of emotional expression at the funeral and the total burial of his memory ever since.

Mother and father immediately denied it was true, but son took advantage of the opening. He mentioned that his parents never talked about his brother and that they seemed to have become more isolated since his death. He added, "Though they never say it out loud, I think I'm expected to take his place."

The future groom, on encouragement to say more, told how he had become a perpetual disappointment to his parents, not because of anything wrong with him but because he had expectations grafted onto him that were not natural to his own being. "My brother was a brain. I'm just good with my hands."

Mother started to weep, but still the parents remained silent, simply looking at each other.

Then the flashpoint was touched.

When asked why he thought his parents had responded to his brother's death in this denying manner, the groom responded, "Because of Grandma." Dad's mother was a mind-over-matter person, and dad, in deference to her, had squashed his wife's emotions. He immediately said he hadn't, but mother agreed that was true, adding, "I guess I just fell into the habit." Mother also expressed guilt over their having cut their older son's memory out of their lives, and dad over the fact that he had fought with this son the night before the accident over a girl he had been dating who was not going on to college.

With the displacement returned to its rightful place, the issue of their son's choice never surfaced again. The parents were encouraged to visit their elder son's grave to confess their guilt. And shortly after, they held a party to introduce their "lovely daughter-in-law" to their friends.

The only time an in-law problem surfaced again was several years later when, after finishing medical school, the young woman decided to go into research, and Jack and Claudine started pressuring her, through their son, to "hang out a shingle" instead.

Premarital Counseling with Couples
Not Experiencing Difficulties

In the previous section we saw how a family model of courtship can be useful in helping troubled couples. A family approach to premarital counseling can be equally useful with couples not experiencing difficulties.

Some ministers regularly use procedures that vary from written questionnaires to a litany of personal questions designed to ferret out hidden problems or to find out whether the couple are well matched. This approach tends to be pontifical and irrelevant. There is little connection between the original reason a couple get married and whether or not the union takes. The worst reasons can be superseded by the bonding process, and the best reasons can be sabotaged by emotional forces in the extended families. Although hidden problems can sometimes be brought to the surface in this way, the assumption that anyone knows what is good for another couple is presumptuous. And often the effort to help, well-meaning as it may be, will have the effect of distancing that couple from the minister.

As a general approach to premarital counseling, the taking of family histories brings many benefits not available in the prescriptive approach while simultaneously avoiding some of the dangers just mentioned. It also bypasses the resistance mentioned earlier under "The Failure of Premarital Counseling."

Another major advantage is that it establishes a tone that is inquisitive rather than inquisitional. It conveys "I want to understand" rather than "I know what is good for you." In addition, its multigenerational emphasis conveys historical processes and suggests that the viability of a relationship is not totally the couple's own responsibility. Rather than making couples feel helpless or pessimistic, the usual result is that they feel less burdened with unrealizable standards. And the historical approach does uncover patterns from the past that couples can be taught to be wary of. The minister can therefore give genuine advice based on the couple's potential need (as foreshadowed in their emotional heritage) rather than advice dependent on his or her pet concerns or projected anxieties and needs. If, in addition, the genogram research does spawn discussion of issues directly related to the couple's own transactions when they take place in a multigenerational context, such discussion is less likely to be mere elaboration of symptomatic issues.

Last, but hardly least, the research process requires that bride and groom talk with their own families. A prime by-product of such contact is not only information—and often it is information they would never have thought to inquire about—but also a deeper intimacy with those relatives. In fact, nothing seems to aid parents more in letting go of their children than talking about, thinking about, or reexperiencing their own separation experiences from their families of origin. Such reencounter with their own past almost always comes naturally in the history taking.

Other advantages of the extended family focus for the

minister are that it does not run up against the usual resistance to premarital counseling; couples actually enjoy it (some resist anything, of course, and that usually is a red light for the future). Usually, humorous stories come out, and the overall effect on the relationship of couple and minister is increased camaraderie. Naturally, the minister often has known the parents and other relatives of the bride and groom; thus family history taking cannot help making the minister more understanding of those parishioners also. And he or she will find a file system of such genograms particularly helpful as the family goes through other passages in the future, since multigenerational forces are most likely to materialize again during such transition periods.

The way I have put this practice into operation myself is to begin by telling all couples that despite my broad experience with marriage and family problems I really do not know what to advise couples before marriage. I tell them that, high as the divorce rate is, if we add all the marriages that failed but stayed together by displacing their problems onto a child, the success rate is even worse than we think. I then describe my notion that it is the nuclear family that should be considered as a context for evaluation, not the relationship taken in isolation, and I describe how extended family still influences individuals after they marry. I say that I have been experimenting with a new approach, which I do not make compulsory. I explain what a family genogram is and say that "recent evidence has shown" that issues have an uncanny way of surfacing throughout the generations of a family. Then I add, if they would be willing to create such genograms, "I believe I could make some educated guesses about when in your future life together things might get rocky."

I spend one session with each partner on his or her own family and ask the other at the end of the session to comment on where her or his thoughts had been going while learning more about the future partner's family; I leave some time for any mutual discussion that might follow.

Since the couple usually do not have all the information at their fingertips, and often what they do not know but should know (parent's age, birthplace, basic information about parent's family) is itself telltale, they are scheduled to return anywhere from two weeks to a month later. At that point they report the additional information and analysis is made. Sometimes the couple do not do their homework; other times they find out exciting information they never knew. Sometimes they want to continue with the process; sometimes they are challenged by their parents' resistance to talk about their origins. Sometimes facts from the genogram or the fearful fantasies they promote become fertile ground for counseling of the couple around hitherto unseen issues. But always the entire experience teaches the couple a way of thinking about their marriage that focuses on emotional process rather than the content of symptomatic issues. The process is gentle, interesting, and often extremely productive. It also takes the burden off the clergy, who generally tend to assume that they have to do all in their power to make this marriage work.

For a full explanation of how to construct a genogram, see Bradt's (1980) handbook. Briefly, it is a way of putting all the important constituents of an emotional system together in a form that easily shows their interrelationships and creates a model that can be simply remembered. It is both a map and a system of coding emotional process. Important information recorded is the following: the members of the family, including those who have died, for as many generations back as one can go, ideally through the great-grandparents; the dates of change (marriage, divorce, birth, death, retirement, and geographical relocation); extreme illness and dysfunction; causes of death; extremes of cutoff and fusion. Correlating the dates can be helpful in observing who is connected to whom.

Some examples of the kind of prediction possibilities that genograms afford are as follows: If for several generations in a row marriages broke up, one way or another, around the birth of a child, it is worthwhile to note this fact and tell the couple they might find particularly difficult sledding at such a juncture in their own relationship. Sometimes the standard-bearer transmission processes show themselves, in which case the ramifications of that issue for a family can be mentioned. (It would be best to initiate such a discussion with some playfulness, perhaps something like "You're really lucky to find a wife who is not going to make any demands on you, considering that you have so much to accomplish in your lifetime.") For women, a big issue is always the preservation of their integrity after marriage; and patterns of adaptiveness, of loss of self after marriage in females in their family, will always show through. Other multigenerational patterns worth watching are those connected to fertility, illness, child focus, methods of leaving home and marital dissolution, cutoffs, gender of offspring, and sibling position.

A side benefit accrues to both the clergy member and the couple from the genogram approach to premarital counseling. With a practiced eye, the minister will sometimes pick up dangerous binds now existing for other members of the family, who are often also his or her parishioners, and he or she can thus encourage the bride or groom to initiate some process to change that malignant condition in the family. During courtship, through the construction of family genograms, members of the clergy have an unusual opportunity to get to know and help the entire family system, although the concepts and methodology for premarital counseling explored here can be useful to some extent to any therapist who encounters the same opportunity.

Finally, everything said here about courtship can be applied to members of the clergy entering or leaving congregations. To the extent that the "divorce" from the previous position is difficult, the next relationships of both partners will have more to work through. Conversely, considering or having to enter a new congregation, ministers can learn an extraordinary amount about what to expect from their future partner by doing a "family history" of the congregation, which, like any genogram, notes the nature of its origins, its previous relationships, the dates of change, and the manner of previous separations. Similarly, noting what is happening in the extended system of that congregation (the local community or the hierarchy) can also be extremely helpful in understanding just what one is marrying into.

Last, but hardly least, whenever clergymen and women enter new posts, the coming union is analogous to a blended family. One is always marrying into an established system complete with its own internal sibling rivalries and interpersonal as well as intergenerational transference issues. As in any blended family, the fastest way to get yourself kicked out of a new congregation is to try to rearrange the established relationships or the memories of your partner's "former mate." Flak that comes in the wake of administrative changes you initiate, however, is probably really symptomatic of what that change augurs for the congregation's relationship system rather than the false issue of the specific change.

Once again, all the same can be useful to any therapist entering or leaving a clinic, hospital, or teaching institution. For the clergy, however, the intimacy of the connection between the personal and the administrative families is always more profound, always more entangled, always more enlightening. And this is why, for the clergy especially, a family approach to premarital counseling can be as personally helpful to the minister, priest, nun, or rabbi as it is for the couples being counseled (Friedman, 1984).

11 Thomas C. Todd

Family Therapist as Administrator: Roles and Responsibilities

This chapter is based mainly on the author's personal experiences and observations drawn from several treatment systems (including public and private inpatient and outpatient facilities) in which family therapists have been the major architects in designing the programs. I will focus on three major areas: (1) aspects of program design that are critical for the success of family therapy as a primary modality, (2) pitfalls that seem particularly attractive to family therapists as administrators or program designers, and (3) some of the inevitable compromises and conflicts with the larger system. The chapter concludes with a set of summary recommendations that can be used for individual programs or larger treatment systems.

Existing Literature

There is relatively little in the existing literature to guide the administrator who wishes to implement a clinical program consistent with family therapy principles. The literature includes references to difficulties encountered when trying to implement family therapy programs, particularly training programs, in hostile environments, but these references say little about how to design a more favorable environment.

Haley (1975) was one of the first to write about the potentially far-reaching implications of adopting a family therapy orientation in a clinical program. Although his article was written tongue-in-cheek as a warning about why clinics should avoid family therapy, most of his cautions are quite real. He describes the profound changes that can occur in several areas:

- Changes in the theory of causation—abandoning psychodynamic theory; shifting from the unit of one person; abandoning the theory of suppressed emotion; deemphasis on history.
- Changes in the diagnostic system—traditional diagnosis based on the individual is irrelevant; dropping traditional diagnosis means radical changes in intake procedures.
- Changes in the theory of change—change is no longer seen as a consequence of insight or other internal process; rather, increased emphasis is placed on the actions of the therapist, who is responsible for making change occur.
- Change in training procedures—even experienced staff members need training; supervisors and other staff members are much more exposed.
- Changes in professional hierarchy—blurring of professional lines, particularly a loss of status for psychiatrists.

Haley correctly notes that it is foolish to expect an institution to undergo such profound changes simply to improve the outcome of treatment.

Framo (1976) has described his efforts to establish a family unit in a community mental health center (CMHC) in the late 1960s. He saw clearly that family therapy provided a valuable conceptual model for treatment systems, and he correctly perceived that the community mental health movement lacked a clear theoretical rationale for treatment. He noted the practical implications of family treatment—better coordination of treatment, potential impact on other family members, and ability to reach hitherto inaccessible segments of the population. He recommended two immediate changes in treatment, conducting family diagnostic interviews and emphasizing short-term family crisis therapy, intervening with the whole family while the crisis was still acute.

Although Framo's original proposal called for establishing a separate family unit, he quickly saw that the implications were much more radical: "Out of my enthusiasm for what the family approach had to offer . . . I recommended a daring concept. I proposed that CMHCs become family centers, and that diagnostic family evaluations, where possible, become a routine part of the admission procedure to a CMHC, no matter how the problem was presented or who presented it" (p. 31). It is important to note that Framo made a fundamental distinction between family therapy as a treatment technique and as a conceptual framework. Confusion about this distinction continues to cause difficulties even now. He was not recommending family therapy as the treatment of choice in all situations. Instead, he was advocating that it is always important to view the symptom in its broader context, which includes, but is not limited to, the family (compare Chapter Ten in this volume).

Framo encountered difficulties on numerous levels, many of which are still encountered at present. For example, the National Institute of Mental Health indicated that his proposal would be viewed more favorably if it were oriented to the treatment of children or drug abusers, presumably on the grounds that children or adolescents are more readily seen as the appropriate targets of family therapy. State funding sources expressed concern that the family unit might violate the CMHC act, which requires treatment for psychiatric illness. They suggested that it might even be illegal to treat family members without psychiatric problems or at least that such individuals definitely were not eligible for treatment. At the level of the CMHC, there was a lack of support when difficulties were encountered such as complaints from family members about mandated attendance of the whole family (Carl, in Chapter Four, reports similar experiences).

Overall, Framo was "not sanguine" about the receptivity of mental health agencies to family therapy, and he questioned whether the systems model of therapy can be mixed or integrated with an individual-illness model. Although most CMHCs "do family therapy," considerable resistance to the broader implications can be expected: "When some of the full implications of the systems viewpoint become apparent—in terms of effects on diagnosis and treatment procedures, admission policies, status, and so forth—establishment mental health finds it too threatening" (p. 36). Despite this pessimistic conclusion, Framo did not blame CMHCs for their resistance: "As in a family, CMHCs are not 'bad' systems, and no one, really, is to blame. People get caught up in organizational structures with their rules and guidelines, and these systems develop a life of their own, with their own regulatory powers" (p. 36).

Liddle (1977) has described problems encountered in introducing family therapy in a relatively traditional academic psychology department. Several issues he encountered are also applicable to clinical settings: (1) Family therapy was seen as threatening because it represented a degree of specialization that conflicted with the prevailing emphasis on generalism. (2) Family therapy introduced a threatening new ethos of sharing supervision and therapy openly, using one-way mirrors and videotapes, with pressure on senior staff members to show their work. (3) The excitement of students, who became "enthusiastic disciples," was particularly threatening to established staff members who emphasized more traditional modalities. (4) When Liddle began running the counseling clinic operated by the department, there was widespread alarm lest it become a "family therapy clinic."

Once again, a major issue was whether family therapy was just another treatment modality or represented a fundamental paradigm shift. For Liddle, the shift was a pervasive one in which psychopathology was defined as a relationship event. Other faculty members found it much more comfortable to raise questions about who should receive family therapy and whether students were seeing enough individual patients. "Family therapy was viewed as another method of treatment, rather than an orientation to human problems. It was seen as another procedure or technique in the therapist's armamentarium, as opposed to a new way of conceptualizing symptomatic behavior" (p. 5).

Liddle offers several recommendations for implementing family therapy training, which include these: (1) Trainees should be sensitized to the sociopolitical nature of family therapy training. (2) Family therapy trainees should anticipate predictable resistance from staff, rather than seeing themselves as scapegoats. (3) It is important not to try to convert colleagues and to avoid "outward displays of evangelical fervor." Liddle quotes Kopp (1976): "The Truth does not make people free" (p. 13). (4) Any change in attitudes that occurs will probably be slow and will ultimately be based on the demonstrated effectiveness of family therapy. (5) Family therapists working in hostile environments need a support network of others who are encountering similar adversity. (This point is elaborated in Chapters Two, Three, and Nine.)

Viaro (1980) described a novel approach of "smuggling in" family therapy without the knowledge of the sponsoring agency or its clientele. Rather than allow himself to be discouraged by extreme obstacles to implementing family therapy, including lack of space, insufficient time allocation, and lack of staff to perform psychotherapy, he decided to try something different, "to deal with the absence of these 'ideal' conditions by trying, contrariwise, to exploit them for our own benefit" (p. 36).

His work began with a careful analysis of the context of treatment. The parents came to the agency with the familiar "fix my child" agenda. Their clear expectation was that the professional would find the causes for symptoms within the child, although there was also the fear that the parents would be implicated. In actual functioning, the agency performed diagnosis almost exclusively, with the diagnostic process culminating in the "verdict" of the consultant. This contextual analysis led to one crucial and unavoidable conclusion: "In a context like ours . . . the consultant runs the risk of increasing the resistance and therefore of missing the therapeutic possibilities exactly when he has reached the stage of recommending family therapy as useful, advisable, or necessary" (p. 37).

This analysis led Viaro to adopt a treatment strategy with several unusual features. Family sessions were defined as "preliminary," with the sole purpose of gathering information. Individual interviews were used together with family sessions to fit the parents' expectations and to gather additional information to generate hypotheses about the symptom. At a later stage, the family were reconvened to give the "answers."

During this process, the consultant stated explicitly, "This is not family therapy." In addition, several contextual characteristics seemed to support this assertion: There was no treatment contract. It was clearly stated that therapy was not indicated, and efforts were made to restrain the family from changing. The time interval between sessions was varied in an irregular and apparently purposeless manner. There were none of the usual "trappings" of therapy, such as therapy offices or one-way mirrors. The therapists referred to themselves as experts in child pathology.

The results of this strategy were interesting and apparently different from some of the usual results of attempting to implement family therapy: No one (out of twenty cases) rejected the initial family meeting. The dropout rate was not high. The families did tend to discontinue treatment after symptom resolution. There were often changes in symptoms early in therapy (after one or two sessions), especially if the symptom was not entrenched. (Berger, Chapter Six, has adopted a similar strategy in working in special education settings.)

Stanton, Todd, and their associates have written extensively about implementing family therapy for drug abusers (Stanton and Todd, 1981a, 1981b; Stanton, Todd, and Associates, 1982; Van Deusen and others, 1980). Their work illustrates the difficulties in engaging such a "resistant" population in treatment, as well as the results that can be achieved if an agency is willing to have skilled clinicians devote considerable energy to the recruitment process. Despite the difficulties in working with this population, therapists were able to recruit over 70 percent of the families into treatment. The estimated cost of their recruitment efforts was only $89 per engaged family (Stanton and Todd, 1981b). To achieve this, however, required considerable program flexibility and the creation of incentives (rather than disincentives) for therapists to do this difficult work. Measures recommended by Stanton and Todd

(1981a) include flexible staff scheduling, easy access to the telephone, provisions such as beepers and travel money to facilitate recruitment, and providing concrete incentives for recruitment.

Woody and others (1982) and Stanton, Todd, and Associates (1982) have outlined the program changes necessary to conduct effective family therapy in a multimodal drug treatment program. Considerable effort is needed to place the family therapist in a central and meaningful role in such a program, since typically family therapy is only one of many modalities offered and participation in family therapy cannot be mandated. There are also particular problems created by the central importance of medication (methadone) in such a drug program. Unless the family therapist is seen as having meaningful input into medication decisions, he or she will be viewed as impotent and disregarded by the addict. Many of these problems can be circumvented if the family therapist is given the dual role of drug counselor and family therapist and if the family therapist is assigned to the case immediately on the patient's entry into the program.

Anderson and Stewart (1983) have offered pragmatic suggestions for dealing with "resistance" in the helping system. They describe ways in which the resistance of family members, therapists, and the larger system can interact cumulatively. Those recommendations that deal explicitly with the larger system are presented here in outline form. (For further details, see Anderson and Stewart, 1983, pp. 230-245.)

Problem: Systems Resistance Based on Unfamiliarity with Family Therapy

1. Enter the system carefully—through the power structure.
2. Avoid evangelism and hopeless power struggles.
3. Prove to be helpful and of goodwill.
4. Bring up family issues at every opportunity.
5. Don't use family therapy jargon.
6. Make analogies.
7. Present cases.
8. Avoid discussions of the therapist's own family.

Problem: Resistance Caused by Administrative
Nuisance Factors

1. Evaluate the source and level of nuisance-related resistance in the system.
2. Get a commitment from the administration.
3. Visit the gatekeepers often.
4. Volunteer to revise forms.
5. Send memos.

Problem: Resistance Generated by the Turf Issue

1. Keep the hierarchy sorted out.
2. Define treatment goals and methods.
3. If all else fails, confront triangles.

Problem: Special Resistance Produced by Inpatient Units

1. Establish contact with the family immediately.
2. Be the family's representative to the staff.
3. Work to move the system to a family perspective.

Conceptual Underpinnings

Before proceeding with the rest of this chapter, it is wise to warn the reader of the author's conceptual bias. Since many of the generalizations drawn in the chapter depend heavily on my personal experience, it is important to keep in mind my strong commitment to a structural/strategic model of treatment. Although many of the conclusions and recommendations may be representative of the field in general, there are definitely some situations in which other models of family therapy lead to radically different conclusions and recommendations. Where possible, these differences will at least be mentioned.

My structural family therapy training at the Philadelphia Child Guidance Clinic has definitely colored my style of administration. As in structural therapy, the family therapist as administrator is willing to have clear goals and to try to move the system toward these goals. Although these goals may be explicit and openly acknowledged, and although that is seen as ideal, they need not be. Familiar structural techniques can also be very useful in administration—joining and accommodation, paying careful attention to hierarchies, and shaping boundaries and communication patterns. Further, it should come as no surprise that a structural therapist turned administrator tends to be comfortable within a hierarchical structure and to exercise a fair amount of power.

It is equally important to acknowledge the more strategic component of the orientation to therapy and administration. This has included a willingness to work in indirect and even somewhat devious ways, especially in situations that offer only modest ability to affect the outcome through a direct exercise of power. Over the last several years my orientation toward treatment and administration has become progressively more strategic, partly in response to the obvious limits of power. Within the strategic orientation there has also been a shift. Initially my approach was primarily manipulative and goal-oriented. It has progressively evolved to a greater respect for the lawfulness of the system, a sense that "the system knows best" (Jurkovic, in Chapter Eight, notes a similar shift in his thinking). Coupled with this is a skepticism about any unequivocal notion of "progress." Instead, it seems that there are inevitable trade-offs, in which achievement of even the most laudable goals has a definite price in other areas.

Brief Description of Program Contexts

Material for this chapter has been drawn from direct observation and participation in several treatment contexts. These contexts are described briefly here to give the reader a better understanding of ways they may have shaped the observations and the conclusions drawn. All these settings have one unusual feature in common: In each a family therapist was granted his or her wish to be in charge of a major agency or program and to have the power to shape policies and practices to fit a family systems orientation. The programs are specifically identified, since it would be impossible to disguise their identities. For this reason, I hasten to add that all conclusions drawn are mine alone and in no way represent the viewpoint of the agencies. As far as mistakes and pitfalls are concerned, I was a direct participant in all those listed.

The first example is a newly created inpatient service and psychoeducational day program for children, developed at the Philadelphia Child Guidance Clinic (PCGC), a prominent family therapy training institution. At the time the inpatient service was established, the PCGC had been operating only community-based outpatient services and training programs. The move to a much larger new building with connections to a prominent children's hospital provided an unusual opportunity to design an inpatient and day treatment program that was consistent with the overall family therapy focus of the institution. This was an undertaking of some magnitude, since it was to consist of a twenty-five-bed acute inpatient service and educationally focused day programming for 100 children and adolescents.

In the second setting, two well-meaning family therapists (Stanton and Todd) were given considerable freedom in designing the family therapy component of an existing outpatient methadone maintenance program and later in developing similar adjuncts to two other drug treatment programs. Major research grants provided the means for doing this. Although the exploits of this duo have been described extensively elsewhere (Stanton, Todd, and Associates, 1982), the painful lessons learned have been important sources of material for this chapter.

The third setting was established when a nonmedical family therapist seized the opportunity to create a family therapy training program and to emphasize family therapy in the outpatient mental health services of a general hospital (Bristol Hospital, Bristol, Conn.). There were similar but less radical opportunities to influence the direction and practices of a twenty-five-bed inpatient psychiatric program.

In the final example, the author was given considerable latitude in creating a comprehensive network of outpatient services as part of the community services of a state psychiatric hospital, the Harlem Valley Psychiatric Center (HVPC). The area to be served, Putnam County, New York, is an exurban area that had few existing mental health or social services.

It seems important to note that all the programs described

were developed during roughly the same period, from the late 1960s to the middle 1970s, the heyday of innovative mental health programs. Some of the "backlash" phenomena to be described are undoubtedly part of an overall pattern of conservative reaction to a wide variety of nontraditional mental health and other social programs. This backlash is a complex mixture of political, fiscal, and professional conservatism that seems to be having a pervasive impact throughout the mental health system.

Critical Aspects of Program Design

Examination of these and other treatment programs run by family therapists reveals a number of critical areas in which administrators have felt it necessary to shape program policy and practice. For the most part, the choices made have been very similar, despite the considerable variability in the types of programs studied. These broad trends will be described, as well as factors that may contribute to diversity.

Intake Policies. It is clearly necessary to begin to involve the family at the point of inquiry about treatment and intake. Guidelines of standard practice are usually established that determine who will handle the initial inquiry, how the necessity for family involvement will be determined, which family members will be scheduled for the intake interview, and how to deal with resistance to family involvement (compare Chapter Four). In some programs, family involvement is mandated by the program or is a necessary condition to be eligible for treatment. Obviously this makes the screening task much simpler.

Programs show wide variability in the type of staff assigned to intake scheduling and screening and the handling of family recruitment and resistance. To some extent this assignment seems to be determined by several factors, including how "doctrinaire" the program is about family involvement, whether there are other constraints that dictate family involvement, and how much resistance is expected with the particular treatment population.

At one extreme is the work of Stanton, Todd, and Associates (1982). Research constraints dictated that the family must be involved in order for the case to be included in the study; clinical experience indicated that the difficulties in recruitment would probably be enormous. For these reasons, experienced therapists were used for all phases of recruitment, and considerable time and energy were expended to engage families in treatment. Similarly, in the family-oriented inpatient service at PCGC, accepting a case meant committing significant treatment resources of a specialized nature. This made it desirable to use skilled family therapists to conduct preintake "contracting" with the family before the case was accepted for treatment. Such contracts routinely specified the goals of treatment (both inpatient and family therapy) and roles and expectations of the identified patient, family members, the outpatient therapist, and various inpatient staff members.

More typical practice in most outpatient programs is to use specially trained paraprofessional or clerical staff members to deal with preintake inquiries. They are taught how to elicit information about family involvement in the problem and indications of willingness to participate in treatment. Usually they are told to recommend routinely that the entire family come for the intake interview; they are told to instruct the family to discuss any issues about family involvement at the intake interview. Such intake workers are not expected to deal with extreme resistance themselves. Either they are told not to force the issue, or they are given clinical backup to allow a clinician to cope with the family's concerns. The clinician will then use a variety of strategies to ensure family involvement. (See Stanton, Todd, and Associates, 1982, pp. 76-102, for specific clinical principles in family recruitment.)

The outpatient procedure outlined above will be sufficient for most program needs and is usually the most cost-effective. It is important to recognize the key role of the paraprofessionals coordinating intake and to select these persons carefully. It is also definitely worthwhile to spend considerable time and effort with these individuals explaining the rationale for family involvement and giving specific suggestions for handling typical situations.

Scheduling of Treatment and Staff Time. In any program, it quickly becomes obvious that making a serious commitment to involving families in treatment has major implications for scheduling of therapy sessions and other staff scheduling. To begin with, considerable amounts of evening time for treatment are required, since the working schedules of all family members should be considered. Less obvious but almost as important is the fact that session scheduling becomes more unpredictable and cancellations more likely, because of the increased number of participants whose illnesses, schedules, and other commitments may conflict with therapy appointments.

A variety of measures have been used to deal with these issues. If an administrator has a real commitment to family therapy, it is probably inevitable that he or she will mandate evening hours for clinicians and some adjustment of clerical and support schedules. Flexible scheduling should be encouraged, using some mechanism such as granting of compensatory time. Hiring part-time employees who can work a high proportion of evening time is also helpful (compare Chapters Four and Six).

Diagnosis, Treatment Planning, and Philosophy. If an agency or program is to make a major commitment to family therapy, this typically means changes in the emphasis on diagnosis and in the process of treatment planning. At the same time, subtle changes occur in the underlying assumptions about treatment that can have far-reaching consequences.

As Haley (1975) has indicated, a family therapy focus usually means significantly less emphasis on diagnosis and a shift to the use of milder diagnoses such as "adjustment disorder." Accompanying this deemphasis on diagnosis is a corresponding shift to a greater concern with planning treatment strategies rather than spending time in diagnostic case conferences.

Adopting a primary emphasis on family therapy usually includes a reduced emphasis and devaluation of other, more traditional treatment modalities. These often include individual therapy, various group modalities, and chemotherapy. Although none of these treatment modalities is truly incompatible with family therapy (see Chapter Three for examples of collaboration between practitioners using different treatment models), they are usually discouraged in subtle or not-so-subtle ways during treatment planning. Conflict is apt to be particularly dramatic when hospitalization is discussed. Those who emphasize family crisis intervention typically see hospitalization as something to be avoided if at all possible, and they tend to advocate extremely brief hospitalization if hospitalization is unavoidable. This stance obviously contrasts sharply with a more traditional psychiatric orientation.

Other changes are less obvious but quite important. A systems view emphasizes the importance of coordinated planning and clear lines of authority and thus argues against using multiple therapists for different family members. Emphasizing these values and considerations inevitably means giving less weight to such factors as individual confidentiality and autonomy (but see Chapter Two for strategic ways of handling the issue of multiple therapists).

Case Management and Responsibility. Writers such as Haley (1980) have emphasized that the family therapist must have overall responsibility for the case and all important treatment decisions. In all the programs discussed in this chapter, the family therapist was given considerable responsibility for overall case management. Other treatment modalities were considered part of an overall family treatment plan.

Implementation of such ideas in an inpatient context often results in complex models of responsibility and division of duties. Since the hospitalization is usually regarded as a brief episode in an outpatient treatment program, an effort is made to keep the family maximally involved and to keep the outpatient family therapist in charge. Although this objective is laudable, it places extreme time pressure on the family therapist. Instead of weekly sessions in the therapist's office, the therapist may be expected to conduct the family sessions at the hospital and to meet separately with the inpatient team once or twice a week.

If these demands cannot be met, a compromise solution is to have an inpatient staff member brought in as a cotherapist in the family sessions. This staff member can be given responsibility for communication with other inpatient staff members and can also provide whatever individual therapy is required. This model works well as long as the cotherapists can work well together. It has the particular advantage of making obvious the almost inevitable split between inpatient staff, who tend to view reality through the eyes of "their" patient, and the parents or other family members. The outpatient family therapist is cast in the "outsider" role along with the family and can be very supportive to them in their efforts to understand and influence the inpatient treatment. This point also makes obvious the primary potential drawback of this model—it works only when there is the underlying assumption, mentioned above, that the hospitalization is a brief episode in a basically outpatient treatment plan and that the primary locus of change will be the home. If this assumption is not met, or if the hospitalization is lengthy, both family members and outpatient therapist will feel like "fifth wheels," unnecessary and with little power (but see Chapter Three for some ways of alleviating these difficulties).

Coordination with Other Agencies and Programs. Other agencies and treatment programs may be involved that do not share such enthusiasm for family treatment. It is therefore necessary to tread lightly in dealing with them, particularly around the issue of overall responsibility. Plans that imply that one agency out-ranks another will consistently be resisted. The most successful way around this dilemma is to put the family in charge, with the family therapist merely the helper. This is particularly likely to succeed when the identified patient is a child. For example, in conducting a home and school interview (Aponte, 1976a), the therapist can publicly adopt the benevolent assumption that of course the school wants the parents to be involved and to be supportive of the child's educational plan (although there may be considerable covert hostility) and that the parents feel similarly; the role of the family therapist is simply to prevent miscommunication, since everyone has the child's best interests in mind.

As long as the family therapist avoids appearing militant, other agencies are often surprisingly cooperative. For example, as the need to spend extensive amounts of time in case coordination becomes obvious, other mental health practitioners (at least those who work in agency settings) are often quite willing to give up the case to the family therapist (Berger, in Chapter Six, reports a similar experience in his dealings with special education and medical agencies). Similarly, experience has shown that other agencies rarely oppose having the family therapist organize a multiagency conference on the case, as long as the agencies see the family therapist as adopting this role merely for the sake of convenience and expedience. If this action by the family therapist is seen as a power play, however, resistance and trouble are virtually guaranteed.

Staff Selection and Training. It is probably not coincidental that all the programs under consideration in this chapter were characterized by a very strong commitment to training in marital and family therapy. Regardless of the mission of the agency, there was a heavy emphasis on the training of agency and program staff. This training emphasis has been extremely successful in reinforcing the programs' commitment to family therapy. It allows a peaceful, gradual transition in which many staff members are "coopted" through training, rather than forced to do something. It works best when staff members can be selected who are relatively inexperienced and eager to learn new techniques. Other tactics, discussed later, are usually necessary to deal with psychiatrists and senior staff members who are strongly committed to other orientations.

Typically the family therapy training programs were open to personnel from other agencies, often at little or no cost. Dissemination of training to other agencies has greatly facilitated interagency cooperation, collaboration, and referral patterns. Giving away family therapy training is often the most successful intervention in the overall service delivery network that an administrator can devise. The quality of family therapy referrals goes up, and referring agencies are more supportive in handling resistance from families. There is also considerably greater understanding of the goals of the family treatment and much greater cooperation in developing joint plans for services that will mesh well. Examples have included guidance personnel, social service workers, and alcoholism counselors. At a later point, it is still necessary to formalize interagency policies on issues such as sharing of cases, even though there may be some resistance to doing so when things are already working smoothly at the line staff level.

Typical Pitfalls

Family therapists who have the opportunity to exercise wide latitude in program design and policy making seem prone to a number of predictable errors. These pitfalls seem particularly seductive to family therapists, including the author. The illusion of administrative power can mask such problems for long periods. Though unseen, these problems can have powerful effects on treatment, the functioning of the agency, and even agency survival.

Administrative Structure. As mentioned earlier, programs run by family therapists seem to give rise to complex administrative structures. This may occur when different types of programs are involved, such as inpatient and outpatient, or when treatment is split for other reasons, such as a division between child and adult agencies. To keep the treatment integrated and well coordinated, there is usually an effort to give the family therapist overall responsibility for the treatment.

It is difficult to object to this line of reasoning or to suggest more satisfactory solutions, but the results can be quite problematic. When the programs involved are on relatively good terms, coordinating the treatment can be very time-consuming and can place a considerable burden on the family therapist. When the programs or agencies involved are in conflict, case coordination becomes a diplomatic nightmare.

Medical/Psychiatric Responsibility. Opportunities abound for difficulties in the area of medical/psychiatric responsibility when an attempt is made to implement family therapy systematically. For example, unless the family therapist happens to be a psychiatrist, trying to give him or her overall responsibility for the case will often result in conflicts over medication and inpatient admission or discharge.

These conflicts are not new. Faced with such recurring

problems, family therapists have often wished for greater power so that family treatment would not be undercut by psychiatric decisions. In all the programs I discuss, the family therapist administrator tried to give such power to the treating family therapist. (It is noteworthy that in most instances the administrator was not a psychiatrist; although this certainly did not help matters, it does not seem to have affected the overall outcome.) Every effort was made to give the family therapist maximum responsibility for the case, within the constraints of medical responsibility. Often, however, the results were far from ideal. In some cases, the psychiatrist rebelled openly and stated flatly that the responsibility inherent in his medical degree could not be removed. At times the psychiatrist simply refused to meet with the other team members and continued to act completely independent of team decisions. Compliance appeared greater when the family therapist administrator had considerable power, but usually this simply meant that the resistance was underground rather than overt.

Haley (1980) has offered a typical example of the frictions encountered when family therapy ideology conflicts with psychiatric authority. He describes a case conference in which a psychologist stated, "If we need to medicate someone, we can always bring in a psychiatrist." An irate psychiatrist responded, "A psychiatrist has more to offer than medication!" Haley comments that "the anger of the psychiatrist seemed inappropriate unless one takes into account the shift in the status of the professions which comes about with the introduction of family therapy" (p. 185).

As will be discussed at greater length below, the use of raw power in dealing with psychiatrists should be avoided wherever possible. When confrontations are unavoidable, it is crucial to assess carefully the degree of organizational support for the nonmedical administrator. In my experience the most successful approach has been to be clear about my own need for cooperation from the staff psychiatrists. It was then possible to support the status of the psychiatrists where their knowledge and importance were clear. This included having psychiatrists conduct training in areas such as DSM-III and the assessment of suicidal risk and insisting that the nonmedical staff on the crisis team work closely with the crisis psychiatrists. Although staff resentment definitely existed for what was seen as placating the psychiatrists, this approach nevertheless provided the staff with an effective model of how to deal with psychiatrists.

Other Treatment Modalities. Haley (1975) has correctly noted that it is naive to think of introducing family therapy as if it were simply another treatment modality. In many settings this is exactly what is attempted, with the kind of results Haley describes—either the family therapy efforts are extremely crippled or abortive, or they begin to have radical effects on agency practice. What happens, however, if a key administrator adopts family therapy as the predominant modality?

Before examining the lessons from such examples, it should be reiterated that all the programs studied had an important advantage—they implemented family therapy in programs undergoing rapid growth, making it possible to add staff members who would support the family therapy emphasis. Whatever problems were encountered undoubtedly would have been much worse in programs where there was a sizable existing staff that resisted this orientation. (Carl, in Chapter Four, also stresses the need for assessing the economic condition of the therapy setting when attempting to introduce a family therapy orientation.)

On one level, all the programs examined were quite successful in establishing a programmatic emphasis on family therapy, together with most of the necessary structural modifications mentioned earlier, such as intake policies and staff scheduling. All the programs became well known for the high quality of their family therapy. Problems were nevertheless encountered within the program, in the agency hierarchy, and in the larger community context.

Internally, one of the major problems concerns other treatment modalities. Even in an agency with a hand-picked and hand-trained staff, there will always be staff members with a strong commitment to other modalities, such as individual or group psychotherapy. Psychiatrists, though the most vocal advocates of other modalities, are by no means the only ones.

Rather than engage in endless theoretical arguments about appropriate treatment, the administrator may be tempted to mandate marital or family therapy. The obvious danger is that this will merely drive the disagreements underground. At the HVPC clinics, for example, the author attempted to solve this problem by taking charge of the case disposition meeting. Various treatment recommendations were discussed, but irresolvable differences were usually arbitrated in favor of family therapy. This tactic created problems primarily when the "minority view" (individual therapy, group therapy, chemotherapy, and so forth) was not aired sufficiently or when those offering this view did not feel respected. The author therefore went to considerable lengths to have such views expressed and taken seriously. (Of course, doing so often displeased the more committed proponents of family therapy.)

Taking charge of the case disposition meeting had other clear benefits. It had a major impact on typical practice of both telephone screening and intake interviewing. When crucial information about the family context was missing, usually because a key family member had not been part of the intake, case assignment was often postponed while the presenter did an extended intake and re-presented the case. Intake workers quickly learned to take care of such issues immediately, rather than waiting to be told in the meeting.

Over a few years, the case disposition meeting clearly filled its desired educational and organizational function. This does not mean that all staff members were "converted" to family therapy zealots or that family therapy was always used. The desired effect was more subtle but was quite pervasive. All staff members, even psychiatrists and other resistant personnel, became much more sensitive to examining each case within a much broader context, which included the family and other helping agencies. Treatment recommendations became more sophisticated in taking such factors into account. (See Chapter Nine for other ways of increasing staff knowledge of family issues.)

Involvement of the Whole Family. A current quip about family therapy observes that family therapy is enjoying widespread popularity with everyone but the families themselves. Although this is somewhat overstated on both sides, it is often true that one or more family members will oppose being seen conjointly. Considerable difficulty with referring agencies and with the superiors of the program director may result. For example, when a guidance counselor or school psychologist referred cases to the clinic, it was not unusual for the parents to drop out of treatment when the therapist insisted on seeing the whole family. The school personnel then became upset, feeling that months of preparation had gone down the drain.

Can such disasters be prevented? The author concurs with Framo's conclusion (1976, p. 35) that it is rarely possible in a public agency to insist that the whole family attend. (Unlike Framo, I rarely so insist in private practice either.) At the HVPC clinic, clinicians were discouraged from taking a hard-line position early in therapy about the attendance of resistant family members. Forcing the issue was supported only when it was obvious that nothing could be accomplished if a key family member continued to remain absent from sessions. Even then, therapists were encouraged to get back to referral sources and explain this stance carefully, so that the referring person would support the family therapy referral and help deal with the family's resistance.

Before deciding when and how much to push for family therapy, it is crucial to examine the program context, which strongly affects the degree of militance about family therapy that can be sustained. In the HVPC clinic, for example, children could be treated only if seen with their parents, since HVPC is an adult agency. It was therefore possible to insist on family involvement or to refer resistant cases elsewhere. However, HVPC has a major mandate to serve severely disturbed adults, particularly those at risk of hospitalization. Such cases could not be refused service if there was resistance to family therapy or to including the spouse in therapy.

Other programs offer similar examples, showing the importance of a careful analysis of factors influencing the treatment context. At PCGC, for example, it was difficult to refuse treatment to anyone within the catchment area but possible to be much stricter about conditions for accepting cases from outside the catchment area. In the drug program, close scrutiny of the real "rules" that were operative made it clear that cases could not actually be dropped from the drug program or referred to another program if the addict refused family treatment, even though that was sometimes threatened. One reason was the rights that these addicts had as veterans; other drug programs not hampered by this constraint have been able to mandate family involvement.

Particular Problems with Inpatient Settings. For a variety of reasons, implementation of a family therapy orientation often runs into particular problems in an inpatient setting. Many of these problems seem to stem from the incompatibility of the two orientations. It may not always be true, but a significant proportion of family therapists seem to believe that inpatient hospitalization is to be avoided at all cost or at least minimized. Instead, outpatient therapy is more highly valued, with inpatient hospitalization seen as an unwelcome interruption in the outpatient treatment.

It should come as no surprise that such thinking does not meet with a favorable reaction from inpatient staff members. At times they have accused the family therapist of regarding them as little more than babysitters and seeing the family therapy as the only "real" treatment. As outlined above, there are good reasons for seeking to put the family therapist in charge of the case, yet doing so feeds into this perception of the devaluing of inpatient treatment.

Other powerful factors exacerbate these conflicts. Even in inpatient units run by family therapists, it is obviously necessary to give other modalities a prominent place, since having family therapy sessions once or twice a week hardly constitutes an adequate inpatient treatment plan. Giving increased importance to individual therapy, group modalities, and chemotherapy, however, reduces the importance of family therapy. The responsibility for admission to and discharge from an inpatient service also increases the power of the psychiatrist, accentuating that potential source of conflict.

Given all these issues, it is not surprising that attempts

have been made to find a form of inpatient hospitalization that would be more compatible with a family therapy orientation. At several prominent family therapy centers, such as PCGC, there has been experimentation with hospitalizing the whole family (Paolino and McGrady, 1976; Steinglass, Davis, and Berenson, 1977; Brendler, 1983). This is done on a selective basis (roughly two out of twenty-five beds) at PCGC; in most other settings, it has been used mainly for research.

Implementing such a system creates perplexing problems of payment for the hospitalization, since the other family members are not recognized as patients by insurance companies and other third-party payment sources. Family hospitalization is unlikely to be used on a widespread clinical basis unless it can be implemented in a manner that results in reduced cost, as has been done with the "village" system in Nigeria, where the relative assumes considerable responsibility for the care of the patient (Asuni, 1976; Jegede, 1982; Williams, 1983).

As mentioned earlier in this chapter, I take an unmistakable structural/strategic emphasis. Other family therapy models can lead to somewhat different recommendations concerning the problems mentioned in this section. For example, some family therapists emphasize the analogy between behavior in the family and relationships that develop with inpatient staff. Whitaker and his coworkers (Stern and others, 1981) have reported such an approach to the inpatient treatment of anorexia. It describes the parallel process between staff and parents and between parents and child. In this model, the therapeutic staff act as "good-enough parents," not only for the patient but also for the whole family. Such a conceptualization offers another approach to integrating family treatment and inpatient hospitalization. It has other implications that differ from those of a structural/strategic orientation. It tends to require somewhat longer hospitalization, since it requires more working through of issues while the child is still an inpatient. Similarly, it is much more focused on process rather than goals. (For yet a different way to conceptualize and use the isomorphisms between patient/staff and patient/family transactions, see Chapter Three.)

To make the contrast clearer, my own paradigm for in-

inpatient treatment will be outlined briefly. It is not markedly different from the inpatient component of the anorexia program described in *Psychosomatic Families* (Minuchin, Rosman, and Baker, 1978). Hospitalization is avoided whenever possible and kept brief when unavoidable. (For anorexia, for example, it was necessary to hospitalize only half the cases, and then only for an average of two weeks.) Hospitalization has well-defined and somewhat limited goals; the "real action" is seen as occurring at home. A strong effort is made to involve the parents and family to the maximum extent possible, using a contractual agreement usually closely related to the family treatment. To the maximum extent feasible, the parents or the spouse are given considerable weight in the decision making around home visits and readiness for discharge. Many of the usual trappings of inpatient programs are deemphasized or absent; to encourage a quick return to the family and the community, it is important that the inpatient program not be too "fancy" or the cathexis of inpatient staff to patients too strong. Inpatient staff are given a thorough orientation to family systems thinking and are taught to give community survival the highest priority. Using this approach, it is possible to return patients home quickly and with minimal disruption to their community adjustment; similarly, the tendency of inpatient staff to hold onto cases is minimized.

"We Do It Better." One recurrent problem is a direct consequence of the zealous advocacy of family treatment. All the mental health programs examined—PCGC, Bristol, and HVPC—went through a period when a large number of cases were "taken over" from other agencies in order to provide family therapy. This happened in a variety of ways. At PCGC, family therapy was mandated for all inpatient cases, theoretically to be provided by the outpatient therapist making the referral. In many instances, however, the referring therapist and agency could not provide family therapy, or the quality of the family therapy provided was judged inferior by the PCGC staff. In the early days of the inpatient service, particularly before some of the problems mentioned later became obvious, many of these cases were assigned outpatient therapists at PCGC, even though

these cases were from outside the catchment area. At both Bristol and HVPC a similar phenomenon took place. Both clinics became identified as high-quality providers of family therapy. Many cases were referred to these clinics on the grounds that they needed family therapy, even though they should have been seen at another agency according to catchment areas, agency mandate, and so forth.

This is a very seductive situation for a well-meaning family therapist. After all, what could be better than to have cases needing family therapy get the services they deserve? Unfortunately, this reasoning ignores several long-range problems that quickly became obvious in each clinic. During the early period when staff and services are growing, taking on nonmandated family therapy cases does not appear to create a problem, but as soon as the staff stabilizes or even shrinks, therapist overload quickly develops. At PCGC this effect was exaggerated because the inpatient cases created much more work for the outpatient therapist than typical outpatient cases require. (Eventually therapists had to be given extra statistical credit for such cases.) At Bristol and HVPC requests for family therapy were often thinly veiled excuses to "dump" difficult multiproblem cases. Accepting such family therapy referrals eventually creates major distortions in the overall service delivery network. Agencies that should be providing family therapy are under no pressure to do so. At the same time, the family-therapy-oriented agency usually does not get sufficient credit for exceeding its mandate, since the cases are from the wrong catchment area, are of the wrong age group, and so forth.

There is a straightforward solution to this problem that will eventually pay off. In addition to offering family therapy training, as outlined earlier, the family-therapy-oriented agency can offer to provide family therapy jointly with the "host" agency, as long as the host agency provides a cotherapist and continues to take overall responsibility for the case. Although this solution requires considerable staff time and presents obvious problems of logistics and case coordination, it eventually will go a long way toward ensuring that those agencies that should provide family therapy will eventually learn to do so.

The System Fights Back

All the treatment systems described have reached their "high-water marks" of the degree of emphasis on family therapy and have receded somewhat. A variety of fiscal and bureaucratic factors have combined to make this slippage inevitable. Although these factors are described below as if they operated independently, in fact their effects are multiplicative, since each factor makes the others worse and each is often used as an excuse or justification for the others.

Recordkeeping, Billing, and Statistics. Outpatient clinics nationwide are experiencing increased pressure to meet the standards of accrediting bodies, such as the Joint Commission on Accreditation of Hospitals, and to show increased accountability with respect to issues such as fee collection and accounting for staff time. These changes have significant consequences for those wishing to do family therapy in public settings. This is a direct result of the fact that most of the accountability systems have been established to handle more traditional services, such as individual psychotherapy and inpatient hospitalization.

Family therapy often falls into a bureaucratic no-man's-land between individual and group psychotherapy. Although many individuals are seen together, as in group therapy, the fact that they are all in the same household makes it difficult to charge each member for services, as would be done in a group. Family therapy is comparatively expensive to provide (especially if cotherapy is used), since sessions typically run longer, are more demanding, and often require more systems work with other agencies between sessions. None of these factors is considered in a typical system of accountability for staff time. In addition, attendance is usually more irregular, and more flexible scheduling is required.

During an earlier, looser era it was sometimes possible to circumvent some of these problems, but this has become increasingly difficult. The major tactic has been to register all family members as patients but bill for only one session. Now, however, most systems require a close link between billing and number of sessions. In addition, recordkeeping systems have become more fanatical, sometimes even requiring a separate chart for each family member.

Drug treatment agencies present unique problems. Most methadone maintenance programs are funded on the basis of the number of maintenance "slots" occupied by patients on maintenance. Because their funding is not based on the amount or kind of services actually provided, they are discouraged from providing expensive, time-consuming services such as family therapy. There is little incentive to cure patients, and if too many improved patients are removed from the rolls, staff members can become worried about their jobs.

This analysis makes it clear that a variety of factors combine to make family therapists look unproductive by usual work load measures and to make family therapy appear more expensive than other treatment modalities. Ultimately this is inevitable unless the system is changed to focus on outcome and particularly to value positive outcomes achieved by fewer sessions. Only then will the true cost-effectiveness of family therapy become obvious (Carl, in Chapter Four, stresses this point with regard to chronic patients).

Emphasis on Diagnosis. There have been parallel shifts to an increased emphasis on more precise and typically more severe diagnosis of patients. As noted earlier, family therapists tend to deemphasize diagnosis and favor milder, interpersonally oriented diagnoses such as adjustment disorder. This practice has run head-on into an increased emphasis on more severe diagnoses in order to obtain third-party payment and in order to demonstrate that the agency is serving a high-priority treatment population. For family therapists, the problem is further complicated by the fact that other family members often do not have diagnosable symptoms, especially not ones that would support a severe diagnosis.

For the time being, there seems to be little alternative other than to have family therapists "bite the bullet" and agree to play by DSM-III rules. If we really believe that family therapy provides an effective treatment for severe disorders such as depression, psychosis, and drug abuse, then we deserve to get appropriate credit for treating such syndromes. Treating other family members will always be a "fringe benefit" of family therapy, somewhat akin to prevention. A case for the desirability of such preventive efforts needs to be made separately; trying to count all family members as if they had equal qualifications as patients will weaken the case for family therapy as a treatment modality.

"Remedicalization" of Psychotherapy. It appears to me that the mental health field is experiencing a pendulum swing back toward increased status and authority for psychiatrists. There has been a considerable exodus of psychiatrists from the public sector, which probably goes as far back as the beginning of the community mental health center movement in the sixties (Light, 1980). The loss of psychiatrists has occurred at a time of increased need for psychiatrists to perform functions required for accreditation, third-party payment, and so forth. Increased emphasis on accountability, malpractice, and so forth has made psychiatrists less willing to rubber-stamp the actions of non-medical colleagues. Clearly psychiatrists have thus gained a better bargaining position, and even when they have not pushed for greater status, they appear to have been given greater status by anxious administrators fearful of a critical shortage of psychiatrists. Unfortunately, this same shortage has made administrators more willing to settle for psychiatrists who may have a shaky command of English, extremely part-time availability, or other obvious limitations.

For those faced with such an impossible situation, the author's advice as a strategic therapist turned administrator is quite clear-cut: Administrators and nonmedical staff must be prepared to treat situations involving psychiatrists as if they were clinical cases. At the same time, they must never acknowledge that this is going on. There are abundant opportunities to practice such skills, such as finding graceful ways around language difficulties or personality quirks, having psychiatrists spontaneously choose the desired course of action, and relabeling situations to avoid power struggles. Teaching such skills to novice family therapists should receive as much priority as teaching other vital clinical skills.

Increased Emphasis on Needs of the Bureaucracy. Every

programmatic context examined for this chapter has contained a considerable degree of administrative "backlash" against family therapy. In particular, this has included replacing family therapist/administrators with other administrators who are much more bureaucratically minded and often have not been clinicians. I have no intention of attributing such incidents to a vendetta against family therapy. Nontraditional programs of all kinds have suffered a similar fate, and the trend toward nonclinical administrators is widespread.

At the same time, it appears that I have been somewhat naive, as have some of my colleagues, about the warning signals, believing that virtue, greater treatment effectiveness, and so forth will prevail. An ostrichlike attitude makes the ultimate disaster (viewed from the narrow perspective of a family therapist) more cataclysmic. There is, unfortunately, no alternative to applying our skills in systems analysis and change to the institutional context of the program.

In particular, it is a mistake (or at least not very useful) to think of one's immediate superiors as the villains. It is more useful to analyze the organizational context in which these superiors are embedded. It is then easier to find ways to convince these superiors that it is in their best interests to be more supportive of family therapy. (Examples of the utility of this approach can be found in Chapters Three, Eight, and Nine.) An administrator who remains ignorant of details such as billing systems, work load measures, and indicators of program effectiveness will almost always find that these systems work to the disadvantage of family-therapy-oriented programs.

Epilogue: Structures Erode, Learning Abides. It may seem that this chapter has had a generally pessimistic tone. It is true that many of the apparent accomplishments of the late 1960s and early 1970s have been considerably eroded in the recent climate of conservatism. Family therapy and other innovative programs have been particularly affected, and staff members from these programs have been widely dispersed. It is possible, however, to take considerable consolation from the knowledge that all these staff members and others who have received family therapy training have been irreversibly changed

by the experience. Although they may not practice family therapy with such fanatical zeal (and would not survive in most organizational contexts if they did), they will never stop thinking
in systems terms.

Conclusion: A List of Do's and Don't's

- *Do* take a careful look at the overall context of the program
  or agency.
- *Do* try to identify factors in the context that would support
  family therapy.
- *Don't* expect that family therapy will prevail simply because
  it is more effective.
- *Do* carefully examine agency structures that will hinder the
  implementation of family therapy.
- *Do* keep working to change policies and procedures, funding
  mechanisms, and other factors that emphasize individual
  therapy and the medical model to the detriment of family
  therapy.
- *Do* work to make accountability systems outcome-oriented,
  rather than rewarding short sessions, regular appointments,
  and so forth.
- *Do* make a clear distinction (at least in your own mind) between family therapy as an orientation and family therapy as
  a treatment modality.
- *Don't* expect to establish family therapy as the exclusive modality of treatment.
- *Do* make a particular effort to understand the potential contributions of other approaches and practitioners, especially
  the contribution of psychiatrists.
- *Don't* use brute force in dealing with psychiatrists, even if
  the administrator appears to have sufficient power.
- *Do* attempt to build on strengths of the psychiatrists and
  model for staff members how to deal with M.D.s.
- *Do* train intake workers to encourage family attendance.
- *Don't* insist rigidly on family attendance unless it is obvious
  that the agency will support this stance and referral sources
  have been well briefed.

- *Do* give away family therapy training to other agencies and work to change those agencies, rather than trying to take on all family cases.
- *Don't* mistake the enthusiasm of students and junior staff members for genuine acceptance from above.
- *Don't* expect to achieve permanent success (and keep watching for important changes in the context).

12

Gregory J. Jurkovic
Michael Berger

Conclusion: Implications for Practice, Training, and Social Policy

A variety of therapeutic approaches have been developed to help symptomatic individuals change by altering their family relationships (see Gurman and Kniskern, 1981). As we discussed in Chapter One, however, there is no reason that family therapists should limit themselves to working with families or subsystems within families. Indeed, it is becoming increasingly obvious that therapy may fail unless attention is given to the family's linkages to other systems in society (for example, schools, hospitals, and courts).

As our perspective on families grows to include their ties to the community, so must our perspective on therapists. The major premise of this book is that the therapeutic system involves not only the therapist and the client (family) but also the larger social context in which treatment takes place. This idea is implicit, if not explicit, in the writings of various theorists (for example, Aponte, 1980; Auerswald, 1968, 1983; Haley, 1976, 1980; Hoffman, 1981; Minuchin, 1974). However, its significance is easily lost when trying to implement systemic principles in various community contexts. The imaginary lines separating the therapist, the client, and the treatment setting may be seen as real rather than arbitrary divisions, creating the illusion of the therapist plus the client as a closed system and contributing to the view that social service agencies are "resistant" to family approaches.

As illustrated repeatedly in the foregoing chapters, once one views the therapist, the client (family), and the treatment setting as parts of a mutual process, then one both views problems within a unit that includes all these interacting parts and seeks to integrate them into a workable therapeutic system. That is not to say that service agencies will easily accommodate to a systemic approach. The experience of the contributors and others (Auerswald, 1983; Framo, 1976; Haley, 1975) suggests just the opposite. If this book is any indication of the growing maturity of the family field, however, rather than avoid institutional contexts as settings in which to practice systemically, it is time to consider seriously and creatively how systems therapy might become a more integral part of the community without unacceptably compromising its own position or endorsing the current social service establishment.

Implications for Practice

One of the most important practical implications of this view is that the therapist must actively create a functional therapeutic system in each case rather than taking for granted that such a system will exist without his or her efforts. This task involves, in part, developing predictable ways in which information is exchanged among the different components of the therapeutic system (for example, among the therapist, the family, and other agencies) and constructing a definition of the treatment unit and the problem being treated that allows the members of the system to collaborate. Usually there are sufficient degrees of freedom within the system to accomplish these tasks (Haley, 1976), although, as Todd aptly points out in the preceding chapter, compromises probably cannot be avoided—nor, we hasten to add, should they be. Clearly, there is no one correct way to implement systemic approaches in different settings, although it is important to be politically astute.

Working in this manner affects how therapists view themselves and other members of the therapy system. To solve the client's presenting problem and to contribute to his or her family's welfare, it is helpful if the therapist regards the other helping agents involved with the family as allies and collaborators. Several of the authors in this book (see Chapters Two, Three, Six, and Eight) have noted a shift in their thinking from viewing these other professionals as obstacles to be ignored or maneuvered around to viewing them as valued colleagues who truly have something helpful to add to the therapeutic process. We do not conceive of this shift as the addition of a "positive connotation" of these other helping persons that enables the therapist to maintain control. Rather, it is a recognition of the interdependence of the various components of the therapeutic system. Such a recognition leads the therapist to speak a language of cooperation and to focus on doing what is necessary to solve the client's problem rather than to concern himself or herself solely with matters of control (compare de Shazer, 1982). Indeed, from the therapist's perspective, one often does not feel in control of the situation in this way of practicing; rather, one feels like a part of a larger system.

The focus on working cooperatively with others to resolve problems often requires that the therapist abandon many of the conventional trappings of therapy. For example, one may function at times like a traditional therapist but at other times as a social broker or a liaison (Hobbs, 1982). In some settings, such as the educational system, it may be more useful not to speak of doing therapy or to talk about oneself as a therapist but, rather, to present oneself as someone who is somehow helping to solve the problem. And as Greiner (Chapter Nine) has noted, it may be more useful at times for the therapist to work with staff members than with clients and their families.

The therapist must also learn to cooperate with higher administration. The authors in this book are clear in their conviction that treatment programs will fail unless supported by upper administration. To obtain such support, it may be helpful to stress the efficacy (see Gurman and Kniskern, 1978) and the preventive value of working with families (see Chapters Two, Three, Five, Eight, and Eleven for some examples). It will certainly be necessary to demonstrate the cost-effectiveness of systemic therapy (this point is considered in more detail in Chapters Nine and Eleven), and it will be crucial to stress any utility that systems therapy has for meeting the administrator's goals.

Finally, to establish the kind of cooperative treatment system that we are describing, the therapist must not only collaborate with administrators and other professionals but also involve families much more centrally in solving their own problems and in making decisions for themselves that agencies or therapists have traditionally made for them (Coopersmith, 1982). A common thread throughout this book is the need for therapists to help empower families and for agencies to relinquish some of their authority and control over families. As this happens, it may be important for the therapist to assist families who have become dependent on social service agencies in developing or gaining access to alternative sources of support (see Chapters Seven and Eight).

How the therapist goes about establishing the treatment system is influenced by a number of factors, such as who will be directly worked with in the treatment system, how the treatment situation and the presenting problem will be framed, and what kinds of interventions the therapist will use. For example, the various authors differ in their view of who should characteristically be engaged directly in the treatment process. Many of the authors indicate that they sometimes work directly with just the family, with just the other professionals involved, or with both the family and the helping persons (see, for example, Chapters Five through Eight). Others generally work with one particular unit. Dammann and Friedman, for instance, usually work only with the client and his or her family, although Dammann, at times, will collaborate with another therapist who is seeing one of the family members, and Friedman pays close attention to the effect of the therapist's work setting on his or her therapeutic involvement with a particular family. By contrast, although Greiner is sensitive to interconnections between two systems, she generally works with either the staff or the family but not both, while Reamy-Stephenson's and Jurkovic's tactic is always to work with both systems. These differences may reflect the authors' idiosyncratic styles or may result from their differing theoretical orientations.

The structure and function of the agency in which the problem is being treated affect how the treatment situation and the presenting problem will be framed. On one level, this means that the therapist tends to talk about the problem in the language that is characteristic of the agency—in schools one treats educational problems; in hospitals, medical problems; in mental health facilities, psychiatric problems. There are, however, certain interesting nuances here. For example, in mental health settings, therapists must be careful to share a common psychiatric language with others in the setting while not stressing their theoretical differences from these colleagues (see Chapters Two, Three, Eleven). This is not a problem in other settings, since there the therapist seldom talks about his or her theoretical orientation to psychiatric problems.

It is also apparent that the kinds of interventions described by the different authors varied as a function not only of their treatment context and theoretical orientation but also of whether they were insiders in that context. For example, it is clear in reading Greiner's chapter that her status as a nurse employed by the hospital allowed her to intervene with nursing staff in ways that would have made them defensive had she been a nonnursing outsider. By contrast, Foster, in discussing the advocacy function of the therapist at educational staffings, notes that an outside therapist can serve as an advocate for the family against the treatment setting with an intensity that is not available to a therapist inside the treatment setting.

Thinking of the unit of treatment as therapist/family/treatment setting also affects the kinds of intervention the therapist will use. In this way of thinking, effective interventions, ideally, will not create untoward effects in any part of the system. For example, Lewis (Chapter Seven) appropriately cautions therapists against offending the other professionals involved with child welfare families through the use of interventions they find strange or offensive, such as symptom prescription. Other authors—Reamy-Stephenson and Todd—stress the importance of avoiding the common trap of defining the administration of a setting as the enemy and note that interventions designed on that basis not only will fail but are likely to get the therapist expelled from the setting.

There are times, however, when optimal interventions cannot be devised, times when clients are in danger of being harmed by the actions of agencies or of other clients (for example, when children are in danger of being abused by adults). The therapist may then have to side with the client who is in danger and run the risk of destroying his or her relationship with the agency or other clients involved. Chapters Five through Eight discuss such situations.

Implications for Training

Teaching others to do systemic therapy in context depends on several factors. Trainers must be skilled in working in this style and able to teach others to become at least equally skilled. Training also must occur in a setting in which students can work in different therapy contexts. This will happen if trainers work in these contexts or have connections to them that will enable trainees to be placed there. Family therapy in context cannot be learned solely from books and lectures, because it depends on the therapist's knowledge of particular treatment settings and professionals in those settings, knowledge that can be gained only through firsthand collaborative experience. Haley (1976) has noted that an effective family therapy training program will expose students to a wide variety of clients and presenting problems. We would add that training programs must be organized so as to allow students to work in a wide variety of therapy settings.

The various chapters in this book speak to the kinds of content issues that should be addressed in training students to work in this fashion. For example, trainees must learn to evaluate social service systems, their network of relationships with other service systems, their possible role in the family's problems, and their utility as resources to help solve the problems (see Chapter Four). It is important as well that trainees know when to advocate for families who are dealing with a particular service system and when to coach family members in dealing with that system themselves.

The importance of hierarchy suggests that trainees must also learn how to obtain the support of higher administration and to take administrative functions seriously before proceeding to do systemic therapy in a particular setting. In addition to developing skills in relating to and understanding administrators, trainees need to learn how to join with other professionals and agency staff in the same way they join with family members; that is, it is important that they learn to see the world from the perspective of these other people, to speak their language, to share their concerns, and so on. In the process trainees may notice that these other persons have a reasonable point of view and at times can be more helpful to families than therapists. Failure to learn how to work competently and flexibly from a one-down position and with a variety of people in different contexts will seriously limit the therapist's effectiveness, even in private practice settings, as illustrated by Dammann in Chapter Two.

There are also several important issues that transcend questions of working in any particular setting. The first is that the student must develop the ability to think *meta* to the setting in which he or she works. This is analogous to the need for the therapist to join the family system while also remaining one step removed from it. A number of authors have stressed the importance of collegial support to achieving a higher-level perspective on their setting. Helping students learn to identify when they need support and how to get it is an often-ignored training issue and requires that such support be available to them during their training experience.

A related point is that in this kind of therapy the question of who is the client is no longer simple (compare Monahan, 1980). Is it the problematic individual, the family, or society and its institutions? This question is especially complicated for the student/therapist working in an agency context. Given the viewpoint we espouse, in which therapist, client, and treatment setting is each a part of the unit of treatment, the distinction among these parts can become blurred. Although this viewpoint is perhaps esthetically pleasing, we recognize that some therapists may find it pragmatically immobilizing and even irresponsible. However, such a conclusion does not necessarily follow. Rather, as Hoffman and Long (1969) discussed over a decade ago, the implication is that a "new type of helper" is needed who has the conceptual, relational, and tactical wherewithal to work with the various interlocking systems of which the family and the therapist are a part.

This "new type of helper" points to another difficult issue: What identity can therapists claim for themselves? Therapists who work only with families have an easy answer to this question: They are family therapists. At present there is no clear professional identity for therapists who work in the way we are describing—that is, as *systems therapists* rather than therapists whose identity is associated with any particular unit of treatment. This is an especially severe problem for students who cannot fall back on degrees or other professional labels, such as nurse, counselor, social worker, psychologist, or psychiatrist, to define themselves and who therefore cling to the unit they primarily treat as a source of their professional identity. In the projects we direct, we have had the interesting experience of having students follow us around asking questions like "When are you going to do therapy?" as if therapy occurred only within a particular setting and with a particular client unit, as if other things we were doing were not therapeutic. Peggy Papp has noted that systemic therapists often do not receive Christmas cards or other tokens of gratitude from their clients. In this kind of therapy, clients as well as trainees may not even recognize that therapy is taking place. Many useful things that therapists do while acting in a broker role do not look like therapy in its traditional sense but still need to be done—for example, helping a parent to find a job, preventing a school from placing a youngster in a special class without following procedures specified in Public Law 94-142, or filing a child abuse report with protective services.

An important part of the supervisor's job, then, may be to encourage trainees to question tying their professional identity to treating a particular unit or to operating in a particular modality. From our perspective, an alternative is for trainees to define themselves in terms of their ability to solve problems in systematically sound and sensitive ways. This self-definition allows for a professional role in which the therapist might provide or arrange for a variety of interventions traditionally associated with different levels (individual, dyadic, family, community) and approaches (compare Clark, Zalis, and Saccho, 1982). Decisions about the type, intensity, frequency, purpose, and framing of a particular intervention, along with how to coordinate it with other interventions, are informed by systems principles. For example, a traditional procedure such as psychological testing might be used not only to obtain information about a suspected learning disability in an underachieving adolescent (individual level) but also, depending on the results, to reframe the problem in family therapy in such a way as to change dysfunctional family interaction patterns (family level) and to implement new educational strategies at school (community level). Thus systems therapy cannot be defined in terms of particular interventions and procedures, as any intervention may have a perturbative effect on one or more levels of a family system (Montalvo and Haley, 1973). As numerous theorists remind us (see Hoffman, 1981), systems therapy offers a qualitatively different way of conceptualizing problems and their solutions rather than merely a set of technical maneuvers or interventions. That the authors of the chapters in this volume have been able to creatively implement systems therapy in contexts that on the surface appear ill suited for such work testifies to the flexibility as well as practicality of this superordinate view.

It is clear from the family therapy training literature (see, for example, Liddle and Halpin, 1978) that trainers currently do not know which methods are best suited for teaching particular aspects of systems therapy. We do not know either. Our goal in this section has been to identify a set of concerns that supervisors and trainers should consider if they wish to train students to do therapy in context. Our early experiences leading supervision groups alerted us to the importance of these issues. We discovered, for example, that when we did not pay explicit and detailed attention to the work settings in which our trainees were applying their newly learned skills and knowledge, many quickly got into trouble in all the ways described in this book. Some left their jobs; others abandoned the idea that systemic therapy was possible in their setting. These results not only were detrimental to the trainees but represented poor training on our part. We share this experience so that other trainees and trainers will not repeat it.

Implications for Social Policy

Auerswald (1983) recently described his work with the Gouverneur Health Services Program on the Lower East Side of New Yok City from 1964 to 1969, an innovative, ecologically oriented project that provided community-based health care for the poor. On the basis of his involvement and subsequent reflection on the program, he concluded: "I believe the major lesson to be learned from these events is that there is a gap in the socioeconomic ladder in our country. There are rungs missing between the poor at the bottom and those in the middle and at the top. And, there is a *qualitative* difference between the segments below and above that gap.

"This means that whenever people from the top segment design programs which are the same for both segments, such programs *will not fit* the bottom segment. The Gouverneur program was designed with only the bottom segment in mind, in cooperation with people from that segment. It *did* fit" (p. 22). Auerswald's comments echo those of nearly all the contributors to this book—namely, we need to look closely at the fit between the procedures of helping systems and the needs of families. When the fit is good, family needs are met, treatment is effective, and social service agencies are not iatrogenic. When the fit is poor, contact with the agency itself can increase the problems of families, and the agency itself, then, needs to change.

A change recommended by many of the authors involves placing greater emphasis on early intervention, especially before a family member receives a problem label (patient, delinquent, severely emotionally disturbed, and so forth). Once an individual is processed through official channels and labeled, the individual's family and social network, along with the helping system, tend to reorganize around his or her new status, making change more difficult.

A related issue is that each service system has its own unique way of defining and, in turn, treating problems. As the work of the various authors suggests, perhaps helping agents in different settings should pay greater attention to the helpseeker's definition of the problem even though it may not fit easily into their particular programmatic approach (Berger and Foster, 1976; Haley, 1976; Rosenheim, 1976). The literature on families with a handicapped child provides a striking example of the discrepancy between the ways clients and professionals view the needs of clients. Repeatedly, surveys of parents' needs have shown that what parents want is services to help handle day-to-day needs such as respite care, competent babysitters, and household appliances. Professionals respond by offering them therapy (Wolfensberger, 1967; Moroney, 1983; Wyngarden-Krauss, 1983). It would be intriguing, as part of an initial interview, to ask family members what they needed in order to get along and to see whether therapists could help them get what they needed. Such a change in orientation could very well make many time-consuming and expensive diagnostic procedures unnecessary and lead to more immediate and effective intervention.

It is also apparent in this book that the various helping agencies are much more interconnected (and even redundant in some cases) than would appear on the surface. Different agencies serve similar, if not the same, clients. Clients are routed from one agency to the next as problems arise which are outside the purview of a given agency or which do not respond to the change procedures of that agency (Carl and Jurkovic, 1983). Even referral patterns reflect the interrelated nature of the social service system. For example, according to the White House Conference on Children (1970, p. 374), "More children are committed to some reform schools and mental hospitals during the school year than during vacation periods, with highs at testing times." These interconnections deserve greater recognition so that agencies can develop a more coordinated approach.

Early intervention, client-centered problem definition, and interagency coordination are certainly consistent with a systemic orientation to treatment. Changes along these lines, however, will require broader-based reforms than even a systemic therapy can effect. Such factors as funding patterns and political power crucially affect the lives of families and the conduct of treatment settings but are generally neither considered nor easily influenced by therapists (Goldenberg, 1973; Sarason, 1972). It is presumptuous for therapists to think that they can practice unaffected by those factors, although we have stressed repeatedly that *in the short run* there is usually enough variability within the existing system to solve the problems of a particular client (Haley, 1976).

In the long run, however, for large numbers of families it may be necessary to change the treatment system radically. In addition to calling attention to family groups for whom the current helping systems do not work, therapists can facilitate such change by empirically demonstrating the specific effects of systemically based models of service delivery (see Auerswald, 1983). These efforts will necessitate that therapists cooperate with individuals and groups more directly concerned with institutional policy, such as public officeholders, economists, state and federal funding agents, media persons, citizen advisory councils, businesspersons, boards of education, and agency administrators. Such cooperation, of course, runs the risk that therapists will be coopted and become mere agents of the status quo, but it also provides them with the opportunity to influence social policies whose effects pervade the lives of families.

REFERENCES

Anderson, C. M., and Stewart, S. *Mastering Resistance: A Practical Guide to Family Therapy*. New York: Guilford Press, 1983.

Aponte, H. J. "The Family-School Interview: An Eco-Structural Approach." *Family Process*, 1976a, *15*, 303-311.

Aponte, H. J. "Underorganization in the Poor Family." In P. Guerin (Ed.), *Family Therapy: Theory and Practice*. New York: Gardner Press, 1976b.

Aponte, H. J. "Family Therapy and the Community." In M. Gibbs, J. K. Lachemeyer, and J. Sigel (Eds.), *Community Psychology: Theoretical and Empirical Approaches*. New York: Gardner Press, 1980.

Aries, P. *Centuries of Childhood*. New York: Vintage, 1960.

Asuni, T. "Aro Hospital in Perspective." *American Journal of Psychiatry*, 1976, *124*(6), 71-78.

Auerswald, E. "Interdisciplinary Versus Ecological Approach." *Family Process*, 1968, *7*, 202-215.

Auerswald, E. "The Gouverneur Health Services Program: An Experiment in Ecosystemic Community Health Care Delivery." *Family Systems Medicine*, 1983, *1*, 5-24.

Bane, M. J. *Here to Stay: American Families in the 20th Century.* New York: Basic Books, 1976.

Bell, J. E. *Family Therapy.* New York: Jason Aronson, 1975.

Berger, M. "Social Network Interventions with Families with a Handicapped Child." In E. I. Coopersmith (Ed.), *Families with Handicapped Children.* Rockville, Md.: Aspen Publications, in press.

Berger, M., and Dammann, C. "Live Supervision as Context, Treatment, and Training." *Family Process,* 1982, *21,* 332-334.

Berger, M., and Foster, M. "Family-Oriented Interventions for Retarded Children: A Multivariate Approach to Issues and Strategies." *Multivariate Experimental Clinical Research,* 1976, *2,* 1-21.

Berger, M., and Fowlkes, M. "The Family Intervention Project: A Family Network Approach to Early Intervention." *Young Children,* 1980, *35,* 22-32.

Bergman, J. S. "Paradoxical Interventions with People Who Insist on Acting Crazy." *American Journal of Psychotherapy,* 1982, *36*(2), 214-222.

Beroza, R., and Friedman, R. "John Hinckley's 'Leaving Home.' " *Family Therapy Networker,* 1982, *6,* 13-16.

Bowen, M. *Family Theory and Clinical Practice: The Collected Papers of Murray Bowen, M.D.* New York: Jason Aronson, 1978.

Bowen, M. "Foreword." In E. A. Carter and M. McGoldride (Eds.), *The Family Life Cycle.* New York: Gardner Press, 1980.

Bower, E. M., Shellhamer, T. A., and Dailey, J. M. "School Characteristics of Male Adolescents Who Later Become Schizophrenic." *American Journal of Orthopsychiatry,* 1960, *30,* 712-729.

Bradt, J. O. *The Family Diagram: Method, Technique, and Use in Family Therapy.* Washington, D.C.: Groome Child Guidance Center, 1980.

Bradt, J. O., and Moynihan, C. J. "Opening the Safe." In J. O. Bradt and C. J. Moynihan (Eds.), *Systems Therapy.* Washington, D.C.: Groome Child Guidance Center, 1971.

Brendler, J. "Crisis Induction with Hospitalized Families." Paper presented at New Directions in Family Therapy symposium, Downstate Medical Center, Brooklyn, N.Y., May 13, 1983.

Carl, D., and Jurkovic, G. J. "Agency Triangles: Problems in Agency-Family Relationships." *Family Process,* 1983, *22,* 441-452.

Chambers, J. M. "Cultural Sensitivity and Family Rights." *Legal Response: Child Advocacy and Protection,* 1980, *2,* 8-9.

Clark, T., Zalis, T., and Saccho, F. *Outreach Family Therapy.* New York: Jason Aronson, 1982.

Colón, F. "The Family Life Cycle of the Multiproblem Poor Family." In E. A. Carter and M. McGoldrick (Eds.), *The Family Life Cycle: A Framework for Family Therapy.* New York: Gardner Press, 1980.

Coopersmith, E. I. "The Place of Family Therapy in the Hierarchy of Larger Systems." In L. Aronson and B. Wolberg (Eds.), *Group and Family Therapy: 1982, an Overview.* New York: Brunner/Mazel, 1982.

Cowen, E. L., and others. "Long-Term Follow-Up of Early Detected Vulnerable Children." *Journal of Consulting and Clinical Psychology,* 1973, *41,* 438-446.

Cox, S. M., and Conrad, J. J. *Juvenile Justice: A Guide to Practice and Theory.* Dubuque, Iowa: William C. Brown, 1978.

Dammann, C., and Berger, M. "Household and Family: Creating a Workable Treatment Use." *Journal of Systemic and Strategic Therapy,* 1983, *2,* 67-73.

Dell, P., and Goolishian, H. Personal communication, March 17-18, 1979.

de Shazer, S. *Patterns of Brief Family Therapy.* New York: Guilford Press, 1982.

DiCocco, B. E., and Lott, E. B. "Family/School Strategies in Dealing with the Troubled Child." *International Journal of Family Therapy,* 1982, *4,* 98-106.

Emerson, R. M. *Judging Delinquents: Context and Process in Juvenile Court.* Chicago: Aldine, 1969.

Erikson, E. H. *Childhood and Society.* New York: Norton, 1950.

Fagin, C. "Concepts for the Future: Competition and Substitution." *Journal of Psychosocial and Mental Health Services,* 1983, *21*(3), 36-40.

Feigelman, W., and Silverman, A. R. "Preferential Adoption: A New Mode of Family Formation." *Social Casework,* 1979, *60*(5), 296-305.

Fisch, R., Weakland, J. H., and Segal, L. *The Tactics of Change: Doing Therapy Briefly.* San Francisco: Jossey-Bass, 1982.

Foley, V. "Family Therapy with Black Disadvantaged Families: Some Observations on Roles, Communications, and Technique." *Journal of Marriage and Family Counseling,* 1975, *1,* 29-38.

Foster, M., and Berger, M. "Structural Family Therapy: Applications in Programs for Preschool Handicapped Children." *Journal of the Division of Early Childhood,* 1979, *1,* 52-58.

Foster, M., Berger, M., and McLean, M. "Rethinking a Good Idea: A Reassessment of Parent Involvement." *Topics in Early Childhood Special Education,* 1981, *1,* 55-65.

Framo, J. L. "Chronicle of a Struggle to Establish a Family Unit Within a Community Mental Health Center." In P. J. Guerin (Ed.), *Family Therapy: Theory and Practice.* New York: Gardner Press, 1976.

Friedman, E. H. "The Nature of the Marital Bond." In J. Lorio and D. McClenathan (Eds.), *Selected Papers, Georgetown Family Symposia.* Vol. 2. Washington, D.C.: Georgetown Family Center, 1977.

Friedman, E. H. "Systems and Ceremonies." In E. Carter and M. McGoldrick (Eds.), *The Family Life Cycle.* New York: Gardner Press, 1980.

Friedman, E. H. "Bar Mitzvah when the Parents Are No Longer Partners." *Journal of Reform Judaism,* Spring 1981, pp. 53-66.

Friedman, E. H. "The Myth of the Shiksa." In M. McGoldrick, J. Giordane, and J. Pearce (Eds.), *Ethnicity and Family Therapy.* New York: Guilford Press, 1983.

Friedman, E. H. *Interlocking Triangles: Our Families, Our Congregations, and Ourselves.* New York: Guilford Press, 1984.

Garfield, S. R. "The Delivery of Medical Care." *Scientific American,* 1970, *222,* 15-23.

Gil, D. G. "A Sociocultural Perspective on Physical Child Abuse." *Child Welfare,* 1971, *50*(7), 389-395.

Goffman, E. *Asylums.* Garden City, New York: Anchor Books, 1961.

Goffman, E. *Stigma: Notes on the Management of Spoiled Identity.* Englewood Cliffs, N.J.: Prentice-Hall, 1963.

Goldenberg, I. (Ed.). *The Helping Professions and the World of Action.* Lexington, Mass.: Heath, 1973.

Goodman, P. *Growing Up Absurd.* New York: Random House, 1960.

Gorham, K., and others. "Effect on Parents." In N. Hobbs (Ed.), *Issues in the Classification of Children: A Sourcebook on Categories, Labels, and Their Consequences.* Vol. 2. San Francisco: Jossey-Bass, 1975.

Green, K., and Fine, M. J. "Family Therapy: A Case for Training School Psychologists." *Psychology in the Schools,* 1980, *17*(2), 241-248.

Gurman, A., and Kniskern, D. "Research on Marital and Family Therapy: Progress, Perspective, and Prospect." In S. Garfield and A. Bergin (Eds.), *Handbook of Psychotherapy and Behavior Change.* New York: Wiley, 1978.

Gurman, A., and Kniskern, D. (Eds.). *Handbook of Family Therapy.* New York: Brunner/Mazel, 1981.

Haley, J. *Uncommon Therapy: The Psychiatric Techniques of Milton H. Erickson, M.D.* New York: Norton, 1973.

Haley, J. "Why a Mental Health Center Should Avoid Family Therapy." *Journal of Marriage and Family Counseling,* 1975, *1,* 3-13.

Haley, J. *Problem-Solving Therapy: New Strategies for Effective Family Therapy.* San Francisco: Jossey-Bass, 1976.

Haley, J. *Leaving Home: Therapy with Disturbed Young People.* New York: McGraw-Hill, 1980.

Haley, J. *Reflections on Therapy.* Chevy Chase, Md.: Family Therapy Institute of Washington, D.C., 1981.

Hazard, G. C., Jr. "The Jurisprudence of Juvenile Deviance." In M. K. Rosenheim (Ed.), *Pursuing Justice for the Child.* Chicago: University of Chicago Press, 1976.

Helfer, R. E., and Kempe, C. H. *The Battered Child.* Chicago: University of Chicago Press, 1968.

Henry, J. *Culture Against Man.* New York: Pantheon, 1963.

Henry, J. "The Social and Behavioral Adjustment of the Child in Placement and an Assessment of the Effects of Separation Trauma." Unpublished research paper, Department of Behavioral Science, Shaw University, 1976.

Hines, P. M., and Boyd-Franklin, N. "Black Families." In M. McGoldrick, J. K. Pearce, and J. Giordano (Eds.), *Ethnicity and Family Therapy.* New York: Guilford Press, 1982.

Hobbs, N. *The Troubled and Troubling Child: Reeducation in Mental Health, Education, and Human Services Programs for Children and Youth.* San Francisco: Jossey-Bass, 1982.

Hoffman, L. "Deviation Amplifying Processes in Natural Groups." In J. Haley (Ed.), *Changing Families.* New York: Grune & Stratton, 1971.

Hoffman, L. "Discontinuous Change." In Z. Carter and M. McGoldrick (Eds.), *The Family Life Cycle.* New York: Gardner Press, 1980.

Hoffman, L. *Foundation of Family Therapy.* New York: Basic Books, 1981.

Hoffman, L., and Long, L. "A Systems Dilemma." *Family Process,* 1969, *8,* 211-234.

Hollingshead, A. B., and Redlich, F. C. *Social Class and Mental Illness: A Community Study.* New York: Wiley, 1958.

Illich, I. *Medical Nemesis.* New York: Random House, 1976.

Janeksela, G. M. "Mandatory Parental Involvement in the Treatment of 'Delinquent' Youth." *Juvenile and Family Court Journal,* 1979, *30,* 47-54.

Jegede, R. O. "Aro Village System in Perspective." In O. A. Erinosho and N. W. Bell (Eds.), *Mental Health in Africa.* Ibadan, Nigeria: Ibadan University Press, 1982.

Johnson, T. F. "Hooking the Involuntary Family into Treatment: Family Therapy in a Juvenile Court Setting." *Family Therapy,* 1974, *1,* 79-82.

Johnston, J. C., and Fields, P. A. "School Consultation with the Classroom Family." *School Counselor,* 1981, *29,* 140-146.

Justice, B., and Justice, R. *The Broken Taboo: Sex in the Family.* New York: Human Sciences Press, 1979.

Justice, R., and Justice, B. *The Abusing Family.* New York: Human Sciences Press, 1976.

Katkin, D., Hyman, D., and Kramer, J. *Juvenile Delinquency and the Juvenile Justice System*. North Scituate, Mass.: Duxbury Press, 1976.

Katz, L. "Older Child Adoptive Placement: A Time of Family Crisis." *Child Welfare*, 1977, *56*(3), 165-171.

Keeney, B. "Ecosystemic Epistemology: An Alternative Paradigm for Diagnosis." *Family Process*, 1979, *18*(2), 117-128.

Keeney, B. "What Is an Epistemology of Family Therapy?" *Family Process*, 1982, *21*, 153-168.

Ketcham, O. "The Unfulfilled Promise of the American Juvenile Court." In M. Rosenheim (Ed.), *Justice for the Child*. New York: Free Press, 1962.

Kirk, H. D. *Adoptive Kinship: A Modern Institution in Need of Reform*. Toronto: Butterworths, 1981.

Kopp, S. *If You Meet the Buddha on the Road, Kill Him!* New York: Bantam Books, 1976.

Langsley, D., and others. "Family Crisis Therapy—Results and Implications." *Family Process*, 1968, 7(2), 145-158.

Lemert, E. M. *Social Action and Legal Change: Revolution Within the Juvenile Court*. Chicago: Aldine, 1970.

Lewis, D. O., and others. "Introducing a Child Psychiatric Service to a Juvenile Justice Setting." *Child Psychiatry and Human Development*, 1973, *4*, 98-114.

Liddle, H. A. "The Emotional and Political Hazards of Teaching and Learning Family Therapy." *Family Therapy*, 1977, *5*, 1-12.

Liddle, H. A., and Halpin, R. J. "Family Therapy Training and Supervision Literature: A Comparative Review." *Journal of Marriage and Family Counseling*, 1978, *4*, 77-98.

Light, D. *The Making of Psychiatrists*. New York: Norton, 1980.

Lightfoot, S. L. *Worlds Apart: Relationships Between Families and Schools*. New York: Basic Books, 1978.

Lusterman, D. D. "School and Family as Ecosystems." Workshop presentation at annual conference of the American Association for Marriage and Family Therapy, Dallas, Oct. 28-31, 1982.

Madanes, C. *Strategic Family Therapy*. San Francisco: Jossey-Bass, 1981.

Meezan, W., Katz, S., and Russo, E. M. *Adoptions Without Agencies: A Study of Independent Adoptions.* New York: Child Welfare League of America, 1978.

Meiselman, K. C. *Incest: A Psychological Study of Causes and Effects with Treatment Recommendations.* San Francisco: Jossey-Bass, 1978.

Meyer, P. H. "Principles for Personal Definition in a Work System." In R. R. Sugar and K. K. Wiseman (Eds.), *Understanding Organizations: Applications of Family Systems Theory.* Washington, D.C.: Georgetown University Family Center, 1982.

Milan, M., and others. "The Implementation of Advocacy Training for Parents in Early Childhood Programs: A Model and a Rationale." *Young Children,* 1982, *37*(2), 41-46.

Minuchin, P., and others. *The Psychological Impact of the School Experience.* New York: Basic Books, 1969.

Minuchin, S. "The Use of an Ecological Framework in the Treatment of a Child." In E. J. Anthony and C. Koupernick (Eds.), *The Child in His Family.* Vol. 1. New York: Wiley, 1970.

Minuchin, S. *Families and Family Therapy.* Cambridge, Mass.: Harvard University Press, 1974.

Minuchin, S., Rosman, B. L., and Baker, L. *Psychosomatic Families: Anorexia Nervosa in Context.* Cambridge, Mass.: Harvard University Press, 1978.

Minuchin, S., and others. *Families of the Slums.* New York: Basic Books, 1967.

Monahan, J. (Ed.). *Who Is the Client? The Ethics of Psychological Intervention in the Criminal Justice System.* Washington, D.C.: American Psychological Association, 1980.

Montalvo, B. "Aspects of Live Supervision." *Family Process,* 1973, *12,* 343-359.

Montalvo, B., and Haley, J. "In Defense of Child Therapy." *Family Process,* 1973, *12,* 227-244.

Moroney, R. "Social Policy Implications of Research on Families with a Regarded Member." Paper presented at NICHD Conference on Families with a Retarded Member, Rougemont, N.C., Sept. 11-14, 1983.

Muir, K., and others. "Advocacy Training for Parents of Handicapped Children: A Staff Responsibility." *Young Children,* 1982, *36,* 41-46.

Mumford, E., Schlesinger, H., and Glass, G. "The Effects of Psychological Intervention on Recovery from Surgery and Heart Attacks: An Analysis of the Literature." *American Journal of Public Health,* 1982, *72,* 141-151.

Napier, A., and Whitaker, C. *The Family Crucible.* New York: Harper & Row, 1978.

Office of Technology Assessment. *The Efficacy and Cost Effectiveness of Psychotherapy.* Washington, D.C.: U.S. Government Printing Office, 1980.

Pabon, E. "Mental Health Services in the Juvenile Court: An Overview." *Juvenile and Family Court Journal,* 1980, *31,* 23-24.

Palazzoli, M., and others. "The Problem of the Referring Person." *Journal of Marriage and Family Therapy,* 1980, *6*(1), 3-10.

Paolino, T. T. J., and McGrady, B. "Joint Admission as a Treatment Modality for Problem Drinkers: A Case Report." *American Journal of Psychiatry,* 1976, *133,* 272.

Perosa, L. M., and Perosa, S. L. "The School Counselor's Use of Structural Family Therapy with Learning Disabled Students." *School Counselor,* 1981, *29,* 152-155.

Pinderhughes, E. "Afro-American Families and the Victim System." In M. McGoldrick, J. K. Pearce, and J. Giordano (Eds.), *Ethnicity and Family Therapy.* New York: Guilford Press, 1982.

Prentice, N. M., and Kelly, F. J. "The Clinician in the Juvenile Correctional Institution: Frictions in an Emerging Collaboration." *Crime and Delinquency,* 1966, *12,* 49-54.

Research Center, Child Welfare League of America. *The Sealed Adoption Record Controversy: Report of a Survey of Agency Policy, Practice, and Opinion.* New York: Research Center, Child Welfare League of America, 1976.

Robins, L. N. *Deviant Children Grow Up.* Baltimore: Williams & Wilkins, 1969.

Rosenheim, M. K. (Ed.). *Pursuing Justice for the Child.* Chicago: University of Chicago Press, 1976.

Rosman, B. "Developmental Perspectives in Family Therapy

with Children." Paper presented at annual meeting of the
American Psychological Association, New York, Sept. 1979.

Sarason, S. B. *The Culture of School and the Problem of Change.*
Boston: Allyn & Bacon, 1971.

Sarason, S. B. *The Creation of Settings and the Future Societies.* San Francisco: Jossey-Bass, 1972.

Sarason, S. B., and Doris, J. *Educational Handicap, Public Policy, and Social History.* New York: Free Press, 1979.

Scheflen, A. E. *Levels of Schizophrenia.* New York: Brunner/
Mazel, 1980.

Schein, E. H. *Organizational Psychology.* (3rd ed.) Englewood
Cliffs, N.J.: Prentice-Hall, 1980.

Schur, E. M. *Radical Nonintervention: Rethinking the Delinquency Problem.* Englewood Cliffs, N.J.: Prentice-Hall,
1973.

Schwartz, C. "Strategies and Tactics of Mothers of Mentally Re-
tarded Children for Dealing with the Medical Care System."
In N. Bernstein (Ed.), *Diminished People.* Boston: Little,
Brown, 1970.

Sgroi, S. M. *Handbook of Clinical Intervention in Child Sexual
Abuse.* Lexington, Mass.: Lexington Books, 1982.

Silverman, A., and Feigelman, W. "Some Factors Affecting the
Adoption of Minority Children." *Social Caseworker,* 1977,
58(9), 554-561.

Smith, A. H. "Encountering the Family System in School-Related Behavior Problems." *Psychology in the Schools,* 1978,
15(3), 379-386.

Sobel, B. "Applications of Bowen Family Systems Theory to
Organizational Systems." In R. R. Sugar and K. K. Wiseman
(Eds.), *Understanding Organizations: Applications of Family
Systems Theory.* Washington, D.C.: Georgetown University
Family Center, 1982.

Spiegel, J. *Transactions.* New York: Science House, 1971.

Stanton, A. H., and Schwartz, M. *The Mental Hospital.* New
York: Basic Books, 1954.

Stanton, M. D., and Todd, T. C. "Engaging 'Resistant' Families
in Treatment: II." *Family Process,* 1981a, *20,* 261-280.

Stanton, M. D., and Todd, T. C. "Engaging 'Resistant' Families
in Treatment: III." *Family Process,* 1981b, *20,* 280-293.

Stanton, M. D., Todd, T. C., and Associates. *The Family Therapy of Drug Abuse and Addiction.* New York: Guilford Press, 1982.

Stapleton, W. V., and Teitelbaum, L. E. *In Defense of Youth: A Study of the Role of Counsel in American Juvenile Courts.* New York: Russell Sage Foundation, 1972.

Steele, B. G., and Pollock, C. B. "A Psychiatric Study of Parents Who Abuse Infants and Small Children." In R. E. Helfer and C. H. Kenya (Eds.), *The Battered Child.* Chicago: University of Chicago Press, 1974.

Steinglass, P., Davis, D., and Berenson, D. "Observation of Conjointly Hospitalized 'Alcoholic Couples' During Sobriety and Intoxication: Implications for Theory and Therapy." *Family Process,* 1977, *16,* 1-16.

Stern, S., and others. "Anorexia Nervosa: The Hospital's Role in Family Treatment." *Family Process,* 1981, *20,* 395-408.

Task Force Report on Juvenile Justice and Delinquency Prevention. Washington, D.C.: U.S. Government Printing Office, 1976.

Tonry, M. H. "Juvenile Justice and the National Crime Commissions." In M. K. Rosenheim (Ed.), *Pursuing Justice for the Child.* Chicago: University of Chicago Press, 1976.

U.S. Senate. *Hearings Before the Subcommittee on Children and Youth of the Committee on Labor and Public Welfare, U.S. Senate, 93rd Congress, 1st Session, on S. 1191* (Child Abuse Prevention Act). Washington, D.C.: U.S. Government Printing Office, 1973.

Van Deusen, J. M., and others. "Engaging 'Resistant' Families in Treatment: I. Getting the Addict to Recruit His Family Members." *International Journal of the Addictions,* 1980, *15,* 1069-1089.

Viaro, M. "Case Report: Smuggling Family Therapy Through." *Family Process,* 1980, *19,* 35-44.

Wald, P. "Pretrial Detention for Juveniles." In M. K. Rosenheim (Ed.), *Pursuing Justice for the Child.* Chicago: University of Chicago Press, 1976.

Watzlawick, P., Weakland, J. H., and Fisch, R. *Change: Principles of Problem Formation and Problem Resolution.* New York: Norton, 1974.

Weakland, J. H., and others. "Brief Therapy: Focused Problem Resolution." *Family Process,* 1974, *13,* 141-168.

White House Conference on Children. *Report to the President.* Washington, D.C.: U.S. Government Printing Office, 1970.

Williams, H. "Village System in Nigeria: An Approach to the Rehabilitation of the Mentally Ill." Final Report, World Rehabilitation Fund, 1983.

Wolfensberger, W. "Counseling Parents of the Retarded." In A. Baumeister (Ed.), *Mental Retardation: Appraisal, Education, Rehabilitation.* Chicago: Aldine, 1967.

Woody, G. E., and others. "Program Flexibility and Support." In M. D. Stanton, T. C. Todd, and Associates, *The Family Therapy of Drug Abuse and Addiction.* New York: Guilford Press, 1982.

Worden, M. "Classroom Behavior as a Function of the Family System." *School Counselor,* 1981, *28,* 178-188.

Wyngarden-Krauss, M. "Families and Service Systems: Macro and Micro Analyses." Paper presented at NICHD Conference on Families with a Retarded Member, Rougemont, N.C., Sept. 11-14, 1983.

York, P., and York, D. *Toughlove.* Sellersville, Pa.: Community Service Foundation, 1980.

INDEX

A

Administration: and advocacy of family therapy, 324-325; analysis of, 301-331; and bureaucratic needs, 328-329; and case management and responsibility, 314-315; conceptual underpinnings for, 308-309; and coordination, 315-316; and diagnosis, treatment planning, and philosophy, 313-314; and diagnostic emphasis, 327-328; and family involvement, 320-322; in inpatient settings, 322-324; and intake policies, 311-312; literature on, 301-308; and medical/psychiatric responsibility, 317-319; and other treatment modalities, 319; pitfalls for, 317-325; program contexts for, 309-311; and program design aspects, 311-317; recommendations on, 330-331; of recordkeeping, billing, and statistics, 326-327; and remedicalization, 328; and resistance in helping

systems, 307-308; results of, 329-330; and scheduling, 313; and staff selection and training, 316-317; structure for, 317; and system factors, 326-330
Adoption: and child welfare agencies, 207-210; independent, 209-210
Aid to Dependent Children, 186
Anderson, C. M., 307-308, 345
Anorexia/bulimia, private practice intervention for, 36-40
Anxiety: in hospitals and clinics, 250-251, 257-258, 260, 267; premises about, 254-255; by staff, 255-256, 261, 265
Aponte, H. J., 8, 12-13, 120, 121, 227, 315, 332, 345
Aries, P., 237, 345
Asuni, T., 323, 345
Atlanta Institute for Family Studies, xiv, 79
Attempted solutions, and psychiatric inpatient unit, 66
Auerswald, E., 332, 333, 341, 343, 345